Laurie Gottlieb has her eye on the future of health care and what is now required for new directions, new paradigms, new thinking, to re-pattern our current outdated medical, illness-focused, problem-directed orientation, if not fixation. Strengths-based nursing is refreshingly liberating; it is focused on what is needed to sustain health and life itself. It is the necessary shift needed to redirect treatment and caring models from disease to health. It brings to the foreground strengths and positive options, and what is right, for our own daily living and health, versus what is wrong. This revolutionary work offers a breath of life into dominant medically oriented care models and liberates the human spirit of both nurses and those we serve.

Jean Watson, PhD, RN, AHN-BC, FAAN, Distinguished Professor Emerita
and Dean Emerita, University of Colorado Denver, College of Nursing,
Founder/Director: Watson Caring Science Institute

I enthusiastically recommend this book for every introduction to nursing course, and equally for graduate nurses in Advanced Nursing Practice Master's programs and nurses currently engaged in practice.

Patricia Benner, RN, PhD, FAAN, Professor Emeritus

Strengths-Based Nursing Care is a phenomenal book! Dr. Gottlieb has developed an approach to nursing that I believe holds a key in revolutionizing not only the discipline of nursing, but all of health care. She draws on the best traditions of nursing—the strengths of nursing itself that have endured for ages. As Dr. Gottlieb explains, nursing's deepest values have been derailed with the emergence of the "technocratic era." In this era, a deficit model prevails that emphasizes problems. Dr. Gottlieb proposes that we can and must turn our focus on strengths, and bring together four elements of strengths-based nursing—person-centered care, health promotion, collaborative partnerships and empowerment. I highly recommend this book for all nurses, and encourage all nursing faculty everywhere to embrace this book as a basic text.

Peggy L. Chinn, RN, PhD, FAAN, Professor Emerita, University of Connecticut

In the hallowed tradition of Florence Nightingale, who argued that nursing's mandate was *"to put the patient in the best condition for nature to act upon him,"* Gottlieb has captured the best within the philosophical core of nursing theorizing and modernized it for today's nurse. In *Strengths-Based Nursing Care*, she deconstructs the fine details of everyday nursing thinking and action, guiding the development of a thoroughly moral, optimistic and practical clinical wisdom within the practitioner across the spectrum of health and illness. Capturing our attention with examples and exemplars, she takes us on an engaging and highly reflexive journey through how the health care world looks from a genuinely nursing angle of vision. In an era of renewed interest in authentic patient engagement, Gottlieb's text will be an outstanding toolkit with which to support and develop the profession.

Sally Thorne, RN, PhD, FAAN, FCAHS, Professor, University of British Columbia

Laurie Gottlieb is an exemplary scholar who has produced a unique volume, which blends the accumulated wisdom of several decades' immersion in nursing with expert clinical testimony into a new synthesis known as the Strengths-Based Model of Nursing. The book will appeal to students and seasoned clinicians keen to expand and deepen their knowledge in their quest to unravel the enigma of expertise.

Anne Marie Rafferty, CBE, BSc, MPhil, DPhil (Oxon), RGN, DN, FRCN,
FKC, FAAN, Professor, King's College London

Strengths-Based Nursing Care is a welcome addition to the nursing literature. The author captures much of what has been implicit in nursing by focusing on the positive. In its emphasis on persons' strengths, this model has significant practice implications and provides considerable opportunities to advance nursing science.

Joyce J. Fitzpatrick, PhD, MBA, RN, FAAN, Professor of Nursing, Frances Payne Bolton
School of Nursing at Case Western Reserve University

Laurie N. Gottlieb, RN, PhD, is a professor at the Ingram School of Nursing, McGill University, Montreal, Canada, where she holds the Flora Madeline Shaw Chair of Nursing and is Nurse-Scholar-in-Residence at the Jewish General Hospital, a McGill University teaching hospital. She was the Director of McGill School of Nursing from 1995–2001. She is Editor Emeritus of the *Canadian Journal of Nursing Research (CJNR)*, a position she held for 22 years. She is the recipient of prestigious awards, including the Centennial Award, the first and one-time-only award from the Canadian Nurses Association recognizing the 100 most influential nurses in Canada; the L'Insigne du Merite in 2009, the highest recognition accorded to a nurse from the Order of Nurses of the Province of Quebec; and the Prix du Conseil Interprofessionnel du Quebec (CIQ). Laurie Gottlieb further developed, researched, lectured, and published extensively on the McGill Model of Nursing. This initial model served as the basis for the Developmental/Health Framework. Thus, Strengths-Based Nursing Care, a value-driven approach to nursing, represents a culmination of over 40 years of research and thinking into nursing's unique role in health and healing. Her books include *A Perspective on Health, Family, Learning and Collaborative Partnership* (an edited book on the early writings of the McGill Model of Nursing), *A Collaborative Partnership Approach to Care* (with translations in French and Japanese), and *Dreams Have No Expiry Date: A Practical Way for Women to Take Charge of Their Futures* (with translations in Spanish, Dutch, Korean, and Portuguese). Dr. Gottlieb is currently collecting stories of nursing practice for a book called *Exquisite Nursing*.

Collaborator:
Bruce Gottlieb, PhD, is a geneticist and a project director at the Lady Davis Institute of the Jewish General Hospital in Montreal, Canada. He is an adjunct professor in McGill's Ingram School of Nursing and a member of McGill's Department of Human Genetics.

Strengths-Based Nursing Care

Health and Healing for Person and Family

Laurie N. Gottlieb, RN, PhD

In collaboration with Bruce Gottlieb, PhD

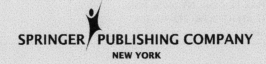

SPRINGER PUBLISHING COMPANY
NEW YORK

Springer Publishing Company, LLC
11 West 42nd Street
New York, NY 10036
www.springerpub.com

Acquisitions Editor: Allan Graubard
Production Editor: Michael O'Connor
Composition: Newgen Imaging

ISBN: 978-0-8261-9586-9
E-book ISBN: 978-0-8261-9587-6
Instructor's Manual ISBN: 978-0-8261-9597-5
Instructor's PowerPoints ISBN: 978-0-826-17249-5

14 15 16/ 8 7 6 5

Qualified instructors may request the Instructor's Materials by e-mailing textbook@springerpub.com

The author and the publisher of this Work have made every effort to use sources believed to be reliable to provide information that is accurate and compatible with the standards generally accepted at the time of publication. Because medical science is continually advancing, our knowledge base continues to expand. Therefore, as new information becomes available, changes in procedures become necessary. We recommend that the reader always consult current research, specific institutional policies, and current drug references before performing any clinical procedure or administering any drug. The author and publisher shall not be liable for any special, consequential, or exemplary damages resulting, in whole or in part, from the readers' use of, or reliance on, the information contained in this book. The publisher has no responsibility for the persistence or accuracy of URLs for external or third-party Internet Web sites referred to in this publication and does not guarantee that any content on such Web sites is, or will remain, accurate or appropriate.

Library of Congress Cataloging-in-Publication Data
Gottlieb, Laurie N.
 Strengths-based nursing care : health and healing for person and family / Laurie N. Gottlieb, in collaboration with Bruce Gottlieb.
   p. ; cm.
 Includes bibliographical references and index.
 ISBN 978-0-8261-9586-9 — ISBN 978-0-8261-9587-6 (e-book)
 I. Title.
 [DNLM: 1. Nursing Care. 2. Cooperative Behavior. 3. Nurse-Patient Relations. 4. Patient Care Planning.
5. Patient Compliance—psychology. 6. Professional-Family Relations. WY 100.1]

610.73--dc23   2012017008

Printed in the United States of America by Bradford and Bigelow

To my twin sister, Linda
"Born together, friends forever" (Author unknown)

And to my family, Bruce, Michah, Arielle, Ilana,
Gabriella, Jordanna, and Itai
"I sustain myself with the love of family" (Maya Angelou)

Contents

Our Expert Consultants

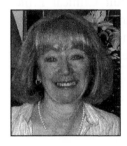

Sharyn Andrews, RN, BScN, is clinical nurse specialist, Reflective Practice in Nursing, McGill University Health Centre, Montreal, Quebec.

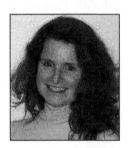

Cheryl Armistead, RN, MScN, is faculty lecturer and coordinator, undergraduate community health nursing program, McGill University School of Nursing. Cheryl interviewed the frontline nurses Maria Boggia and Charlotte Evans.

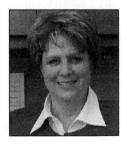

Sophie Baillargeon, RN, BScN, MScA, is nurse manager, Pediatric Intensive Care Unit and Hemodialysis Unit, Montreal Children's Hospital, McGill University Health Centre. Sophie interviewed the frontline nurse Monica Gallagher. *Current:* Sophie is assistant to the Director of Nursing, McGill University Health Centre.

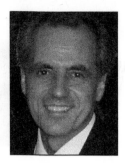

Franco Carnevale, RN, PhD, is chair, Pediatric Ethics Committee, and associate member, Pediatric Critical Care, McGill University Health Centre; clinical ethics consultant, Le Phare, Enfants et Familles (pediatric hospice and respite care); and associate professor as well as director of the master's program, School of Nursing, associate member, Department of Pediatrics, affiliate member, Biomedical Ethics Unit, and adjunct professor, Department of Psychology, McGill University. *Current:* Franco is professor and associate director as well as director of the master's program, McGill University School of Nursing.

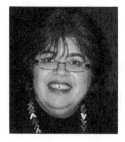

Jane Chambers-Evans, RN, MScA, MSc, is nursing practice consultant, clinical ethicist, and chair, Adult Clinical Ethics Committee, McGill University Health Centre; and assistant professor, McGill University School of Nursing. Jane interviewed the frontline nurses Maryse Godin and Gisèle Melanson.

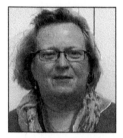

Luisa Ciofani, RN, MScA, IBCLC, is clinical nurse specialist in obstetrics, Royal Victoria Hospital, McGill University Health Centre; and faculty lecturer, McGill University School of Nursing.

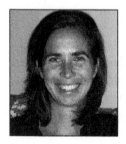

Christina Clausen, RN, BAH, MA, MScA, is nurse clinician in obstetrics and faculty lecturer, McGill University Health Centre. Christina interviewed the frontline nurses Lyne Charbonneau and Marie Grace Espinosa. *Current:* Christina is a doctoral student at the McGill University School of Nursing.

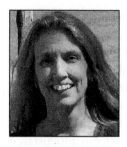

Joann Creager, RN, BA, MScA, is clinical nurse specialist in geriatrics and transition care, Montreal General Hospital, McGill University Health Centre; and lecturer in healthy aging, McGill University School of Nursing. Joann interviewed the frontline nurses Sharon Johnson and Line Pharand. *Current:* Joann is also nursing practice consultant for constant observation issues, Montreal General Hospital, McGill University Health Centre.

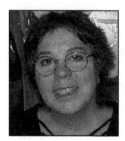

Cindy Dalton, RN, BScN, MScA, is community health nurse in psychogeriatrics, CSSS de la Montagne, Montreal; and faculty lecturer, McGill University School of Nursing. Cindy interviewed the frontline nurses Ora Alberton and Thi P. Hoang. *Current:* Cindy is nurse specialist in psychogeriatics and nurse consultant to frontline workers at CSSS de la Montagne.

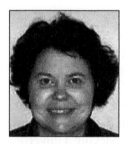

Lidia De Simone, RN, BA, MScA, is quality improvement coordinator, Kateri Memorial Hospital Centre, Kahnawake, Quebec.

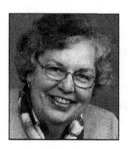

Margaret Eades, RN, MScA, is clinical nurse specialist in oncology, McGill University Health Centre; and assistant professor, McGill University School of Nursing. Margaret interviewed the frontline nurses Astride Bazile and Virginia Lee. *Current:* Margaret is retired but continues to teach in her role as assistant professor, McGill University School of Nursing.

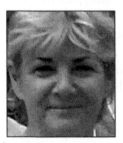

Lucia Fabijan, RN, BN, MScA, is nursing coordinator, Ambulatory Services, Neurosciences Mission, McGill University Health Centre; and assistant professor and clinical advisor for undergraduate and graduate students, McGill University School of Nursing. Lucia interviewed the frontline nurses Timothy Kavanagh and Sarah Shea. *Current:* Lucia is Associate Director of Nursing, Neurosciences Mission, McGill University Health Centre, and maintains a part-time private practice as a Registered Marriage and Family Therapist.

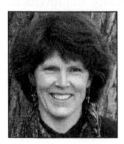

Catherine Gros, RN, MScA, is clinical nurse specialist, Douglas Mental Health University Institute; clinical consultant, Integrated Perinatal and Early Childhood Program, Cree Board of Health and Social Services of James Bay, Quebec; and faculty lecturer, McGill University School of Nursing. Catherine interviewed the frontline nurses Andrea Leimanis and Amy Nyland. *Current:* Catherine is assistant professor, McGill University School of Nursing.

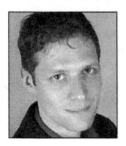

Heather Hart, RN, BEd, BScN, MScA, is faculty lecturer and clinical advisor for graduate students in family nursing, McGill University School of Nursing.

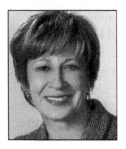

John William Kayser, RN, is a graduate student at the McGill University School of Nursing and motivational interviewing network trainer and master trainer, Freedom From Smoking program. John interviewed the frontline nurse Danielle Beaucage. *Current:* John is a doctoral student at Université de Montréal and a lecturer at McGill University School of Nursing.

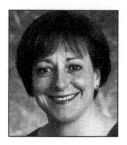

Diane Lowden, RN, MScA, is clinical nurse specialist, Multiple Sclerosis Program, McGill University Health Centre; and assistant professor, McGill University School of Nursing. Diane interviewed the frontline nurse Caroline Marchionni.

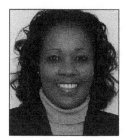

Althea McBean, RN, MScA, RN, MScA, is clinical nurse specialist in cardiology, Jewish General Hospital, McGill University Health Centre; and faculty lecturer, McGill University School of Nursing. Althea interviewed the frontline nurses Emilie Gauthier and Esther Laforest.

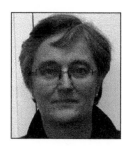

Catherine Oliver, RN, BA, MScA, is nursing practice consultant, Clinical Practice and Professional Development Service, Department of Nursing, McGill University Health Centre; and faculty lecturer, McGill University School of Nursing. Catherine interviewed the frontline nurses Siobhan Carney and Diane Lebeau.

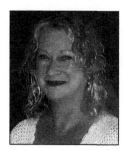

Christina Rosmus, RN, BScN, MScA, is clinical nurse specialist in pediatric pain management and multidisciplinary team member, Chronic Pain Service, Montreal Children's Hospital, McGill University Health Centre; and lecturer, McGill University School of Nursing. Christina interviewed the frontline nurses Sonia Castiglione and Devon Leguillette. *Current:* Christina is nursing consultant for advanced practice nursing, Montreal Children's Hospital.

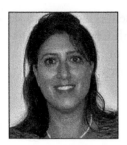

Rosalia (Lia) Sanzone, BScN, MScA, is former coordinator, Maternal-Child Family Program, CLSC community health centre, Montreal. *Current:* Rosalia is full-time faculty lecturer, McGill University School of Nursing.

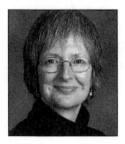

Gillian Taylor, RN, BSc, MScA, is clinical nurse specialist, Ambulatory Services (rheumatology clinic), Montreal Children's Hospital, McGill University Health Centre; and faculty lecturer, McGill University School of Nursing.

Our Frontline Nurses

Ora Alberton, RN, NScA, is staff nurse, Multidisciplinary Psychogeriatric Team, CSSS de la Montagne, Site Métro, Montreal, Quebec, Canada.

Astride Bazile, RN, BScN, MEdCON, is Nursing Practice Development Educator for Haematology/Oncology, McGill University Health Centre (MUHC), Montreal, Quebec, Canada.

Danielle Beaucage, RN, is Nurse Manager, Clinics, Montreal Chest Institute, MUHC.

Maria Boggia, RN, BScN, is Nursing Unit Coordinator, Neurology Program, Jewish Rehabilitation Hospital, Montreal, Quebec, Canada.

Siobhan Carney, RN, BScN, is Pivot Nurse, Cancer Nutrition Rehabilitation Program, MUHC.

Sonia Castiglione, RN, BSc, MScA, is, Advisor for Evidence-Informed Decision-Making, MUHC.

Lyne Charbonneau, RN, MN, is clinical nurse specialist, Neonatal Intensive Care Unit, Sir Mortimer B. Davis Jewish General Hospital, MUHC.

Marie Grace Espinosa, RN, BN, is Assistant Head Nurse, Postpartum Unit, Sir Mortimer B. Davis Jewish General Hospital, MUHC.

Charlotte Evans, RN, MScA, is senior staff nurse, West Island Palliative Care Residence, Kirkland, Quebec, Canada.

Monica Gallagher, RN, BScN, is staff nurse, Pediatric Intensive Care Unit, Montreal Children's Hospital, MUHC.

Emilie Gauthier, RN, BScN, is staff nurse, In-Patient Cardiology/Nurse Educator Cardiology, Sir Mortimer B. Davis Jewish General Hospital, MUHC.

Maryse Godin, RN, MScA, is clinical nurse specialist, Orthopedics/Emergency, Montreal General Hospital, MUHC.

Thi Phung Hoang, RN, BScN, is nurse clinician, Radio-Oncology Clinic, Sir Mortimer B. Davis Jewish General Hospital, MUHC.

Sharon Johnson, RN, is staff nurse, Acute Care Geriatrics, MUHC.

Timothy Kavanagh, RN, BScN, is staff nurse, Pediatric Intensive Care Unit, MUHC.

Esther Laforest, RN, BScN, is staff nurse, In-Patient Cardiology/Nurse Heart Function Clinic, Sir Mortimer B. Davis Jewish General Hospital, MUHC.

Diane Lebeau, RN, is Assistant Head Nurse, Palliative Care Unit, MUHC.

Virginia Lee, RN, PhD, is nurse researcher, MUHC, and Assistant Professor, McGill University, Montreal, Quebec, Canada.

Devon Leguillette, RN, BScN, is nurse clinician, Department of Ambulatory Services (Cardiology), Montreal Children's Hospital, MUHC.

Andra Leimanis, RN, is staff nurse/clinical nurse specialist in cardiology, Douglas Mental Health University Institute, MUHC.

Caroline Marchionni, BScN, MSc, MScA, is knowledge broker, Transition Support Office, and nurse clinician, Montreal Neurological Institute, MUHC.

Gisele Melanson, RN, is staff nurse, Intensive Care Unit, MUHC.

Amy Nyland, RN, MScA, is staff nurse in gynecology/oncology, Royal Victoria Hospital, MUHC.

Line Pharand, RN, BSc, is staff nurse in neurology/neurosurgery, MUHC.

Sarah Shea, RN, BScN, is staff nurse, Pediatric Intensive Care Unit, MUHC.

Foreword

I'm looking for the light; those little glimmers that make me think there's something there. I am looking for people's gifts of what they've got going for them.
—Nurse Heather Hart

Dr. Laurie N. Gottlieb has written a landmark book that should be required reading for all undergraduate and graduate nursing students and essential reading for all those involved in trying to redesign health care systems, reduce health care costs, and improve the health of people in any society. I cannot think of a better way to introduce student nurses, or others, to learning to think and act like a nurse than by referring them to this book. Dr. Gottlieb has articulated a commonly held stance and practice in nursing since Nightingale (*Notes on Nursing*, 1860). Nightingale was against a single factor: causal germ theory. Today, her more ecological stance of considering the person's own strengths, and the body's ability to repair itself when the environment is conducive to health, has much stronger evidence and validation than any single causal theory of disease. It turns out that Nightingale's more ecological model best fits the current social epidemiological scientific understanding of health and disease.

In the enlightening stories of wise nurses throughout this book, we learn about Strengths-Based Care (SBC), which seeks out the person's/family's strengths and helps people, families, and communities build on those strengths, marshalling them to cope with an illness or injury and recover so that they can resume their lives. This is truly a groundbreaking book! No one has written so clearly on the long-standing but underdescribed, poorly understood nursing goal and pervasive understanding of one's self and practice to work with patient/family strengths.

As Dr. Gottlieb points out, Nightingale did this work for her generation, but the forces for diagnosing deficits came to dominate health care discourse. The power to define and diagnose deficits became the received truth of the medical establishment's discourse. This book's narrative descriptions from nurses who practice SBC bring immediacy and clarity to SBC and to why it is an essential ingredient to health promotion and recovery. The nursing narratives demonstrate how nurses make transformative differences in patient care through noticing patient/family strengths and then encouraging and empowering those strengths. Students and nurses will read this work and find that it is almost impossible *not* to integrate its powerful message into their own work and life.

My own work in articulating knowledge embedded in nursing practice resonates with the pervasive nursing practice of looking for person's strengths, what matters to patients and families, and what works to support and encourage recovery and healing. Dr. Gottlieb clearly articulates what most nurses continue to claim in their practice, even when they lack good language to articulate and defend their approach, in the context of the dominance of a deficit-oriented, diagnosis-driven, and biomedical model in health care.

Nurses report in this book that they look for patient and family strengths and support those strengths in promoting well-being and assisting patients in their self-care and recovery. As Dr. Gottlieb states in Chapter 7: "Nurses who practice SBC are always responsive to the situation and never prescriptive."

This book is not doctrinaire, and Dr. Gottlieb makes it clear that she does not refer to, or intend to imply the "power of positive thinking" or ideologically static notion that "thinking makes it so" (variants of wishful thinking). SBC focuses on the patient, family, and community strengths in the moment and the context of the situation. SBC in nursing is about finding the *situated possibilities* of particular patients/clients/ families at particular points in time, in the midst of being confronted with particular challenges. Nowhere does Dr. Gottlieb imagine that patients, clients, or nurses have radical freedom to overcome any obstacle or challenge; instead, she carefully shows, in many clinical examples, patient-/client-/family-*situated* resources and possibilities. Dr. Gottlieb's goal is to enable student and clinical nurses to overcome the cultural and professional press to look only for deficits—that is, how far short the patient or family falls below normative expectations for performance or health. By accepting the inevitable vulnerabilities of being human and encountering injuries, illnesses, and situational and developmental challenges, Dr. Gottlieb guides the nurse to exercise the Nightingale tradition with new insights and skills. Throughout this book, she demonstrates how nurses look for strengths that currently exist in the person's and family's responses and then strengthen those resources through nursing skills of perception, relating, assessing, thinking, and action. This is thinking and acting like a nurse at its very best. In addition, one of the strengths of this book is in the detailed guides it offers, and its articulation of engagement, observation, and relational attunement skills.

I have no doubt that reading this book will spark the development of real skills and clinical imagination for the relational nature of nursing care. At the same time, Dr. Gottlieb has honed the guidance and message of this book over her entire research career; thus, it is a wise, seasoned, and unusually clearly written book.

SBC can only come from understanding the patient/client/family/community experience and a grasp of the situation...its meanings, challenges, threats, and felt resources and possibilities for meeting the challenges encountered. As Dr. Gottlieb writes in Chapter 4,

> A focus on strengths is not about ignoring weaknesses or downplaying a person's vulnerabilities. Moreover, it is not about reframing problems and weaknesses in terms of strengths. It is not about whether the glass is half-empty (i.e., weaknesses) or whether it is half-full (i.e., strengths); instead, it is about

understanding the whole. It is about finding strengths and recognizing that strengths coexist with weaknesses; about striking the vital balance between the two; and about understanding how strengths and weaknesses interact to promote health, recovery, and healing. A focus on strengths is about appreciating and discovering human strengths in the midst of problems and weaknesses and about how to work with strengths to mitigate vulnerability.

In the same chapter, one of the nurse clinicians backs up this message:

> Because I have seen in my practice that nurses can be a little overenthusiastic with our understanding of people's strengths and resources.... I think we have to remind ourselves that a strength two weeks ago in today's context might not be considered a strength anymore. That's where we try to figure out the balance.

Appropriate contextualizing caveats clarify the situated wisdom of SBC and its relational and contextual nature. For example, in Chapter 4, another nurse states: "When I talk about strengths, one of the caveats I have is, 'Be careful.' A person needs permission to say, 'Enough already! What worked in the past is just not sufficient now.'"

SBC is richly exemplified in nurses' first-person experience accounts of actual practice. This book is at once accessible and easy to read, but it requires much personal and professional reflection to put the rich wisdom and contextualized assessments and relational skills into practice. In this way, it is not a "one time only" read but what, in the heart of nursing practice, we understand what nursing practice is.

I enthusiastically recommend this book for every introduction to nursing course, and equally for graduate nurses in advanced nursing practice master's programs and nurses currently engaged in practice. This book is one of those rare treats that put into words what expert nurses come to know and experience over time in their best practice. By giving clarity, insight, and rigor to a central but poorly understood value and wisdom embedded in the best of nursing practice, Dr. Gottlieb has given nursing back a stronger, clearer self-understanding and social grasp of the best that nursing has to offer: SBC that can inform all diagnoses and health care design and implementation.

Patricia Benner, RN, PhD, FAAN
Professor Emeritus
University of California, San Francisco

Preface

Ideas, like everything else, find their moment to emerge and the right time to take hold. Focusing on and working with strengths rather than just on problems and deficits is an idea whose time has come. This idea has existed in some form for some time; however, in recent years this new way of thinking has moved from backstage, embraced by a few, to center stage, embraced by many. Focusing on person, family, and community strengths has always been an important value in nursing since the time of Florence Nightingale, but it has never been fully developed, that is, until now.

The strengths idea is gaining momentum. From such diverse fields as nursing, social work, psychology, education, community development, and the like, each field is developing its own understanding of why it is important to adopt a strengths-based perspective. The common thread that binds strengths-based work in different fields is that focusing on strengths brings hope because it engenders in people a sense of empowerment. People come to believe they have the power within to bring about change, exercise some control over their lives, and redefine the past to create a more desirable future.

Strengths-Based Care (SBC) represents a new way of thinking in nursing. It considers the positives, those things that are best, those that are working, and those areas that show potential. This does not mean that a strengths approach ignores problems, pretends that deficits do not exist, or turns a blind eye to weaknesses; instead, it is about finding the right balance between focusing on strengths while dealing with problems and deficits. It is about using strengths to minimize the deleterious effects caused by problems. It is about giving clients, patients, families, and communities the tools to improve their health. It is about knowing the individuals and their situation, placing their problems in context, and knowing their strengths in order to understand how to capitalize and mobilize them to support health, alleviate suffering, help in recovery, and restore wholeness through acts of healing. In other words, it is about working with strengths to tackle new as well as long-standing problems and then finding new ways to deal with them.

A strengths approach requires that new principles be articulated, a different set of structures and relationships be put in place, and a new language be developed to communicate this new orientation that is consistent with nursing values. A strengths approach, which on the surface appears to be a relatively simple idea, requires a profound shift in thinking about how we as humans relate to one another, whether it is in our own families, communities, and places of work, in different roles and capacities, or in our relationship with others on a global level.

A strengths approach reveals much about the nurse herself and how she chooses to express her humanity. As the famed late fashion designer Alexander McQueen said about himself, but could apply to anyone—"What you see in the work is the person himself."

STRENGTHS-BASED CARE IN HEALTH CARE AND NURSING

After many years of focusing on deficits and trying to fix problems, the results have been limited and, in many cases, disheartening. The deficit approach has yielded short-term solutions that often have proven to be nonsustainable in the long term. People have difficulty maintaining change when motivated by fear and when reminded of their weaknesses, what they are missing, and what is malfunctioning or dysfunctional. In fact, the opposite is the case: People often become depressed and demoralized by hearing repeatedly that something is wrong, missing, or lacking in their lives or health. In contrast, individuals, families, and communities are more likely to take charge of their lives and build a sustainable future for themselves and their children when they believe in themselves; focus on the positives in their situation; are treated with respect; and are given the help, support, and resources to come up with their own solutions to their problems. It is this philosophy about people that is transforming their everyday lives and bringing hope and renewal. Consider what happened when nurses working with high-risk teenage mothers during the first year of their infant's life focused on these young mothers' strengths. The turnaround was startling. These mothers, who were fortunate to receive such care, were able to get jobs, had fewer subsequent unplanned pregnancies, and their children had fewer behavioral problems. This early dose of nursing had a long-term sustaining effect on the mental health of both mothers and children (Olds et al., 1997).

In health care, the deficit model still remains the dominant model of care. This is hardly surprising given that health care professionals are trained to treat problems, correct weaknesses, and minimize deficits. Diagnosis is about interpreting and labeling the problem, whereas treatment is about removing the pathology, unblocking the obstruction, minimizing or eliminating the pathogen, and cutting away the diseased parts. But this is just one aspect of the healing process.

Health and healing are about wholeness. Health is about creating wholeness, whereas healing is about repairing and restoring wholeness. This is the work of nursing.

Wholeness is about the integration and coordination between and among every aspect of a person, including how he lives in and experiences his environments. It is in healing that the person discovers himself and, in the process, develops, evolves, grows, and is transformed. Health and healing require knowledge and skills that go far beyond the scope of what the deficit model can address. Both require knowledge of the human condition and human responses to a wide range of insults, including illnesses, injuries, and trauma, as well as anticipated threats to well-being. They draw their understanding from diverse bodies of knowledge from the humanities and from the physical, social, medical, and nursing sciences. It is only when nurses recognize the need for different types of knowledge that come from many sources that they are equipped to deal with patients' vulnerabilities and frailties and to work with them and their families to restore and recreate a new sense and level of wholeness. In fact, in the Institute of Medicine's report (2010) *Future of Nursing: Leading Change, Advancing Health*, considered the most significant report on nursing and the future of health care reform to be published in decades, one of the primary recommendations is that nurses "should practice to the full extent of their education and training." SBC allows them to do this because it requires a broad base of knowledge, education, and training.

Humans respond as whole people. When confronted by challenges and insults, all aspects of the person's being and many lifeworlds are affected. The only way to deal with the complexity in how humans respond to insults, challenges, and threats is to find ways to support innate health and healing systems. It is within these systems that specific strengths can be found. Thus, SBC capitalizes, mobilizes, and supports innate as well as learned mechanisms of health and healing.

All humans are vulnerable. All humans, at some point in their lives, will need to deal with expected and unexpected challenges, planned and unplanned changes, and ones that are manageable and ones that overwhelm. Yet it is when persons and families are at their most vulnerable and feel the most threatened that the human spirit is revealed. When humans feel, and are, threatened, they mobilize their resources to deal with these threats. Working with strengths is simply an extension of the natural way humans deal with threats by identifying, mobilizing, and capitalizing on existing strengths and developing new ones to help them ward off danger and threats and cope more effectively with their challenges. Nurses and health professionals are charged with the responsibility of helping individuals find their own strengths to deal with both everyday challenges as well as adversities that threaten their integrity, that is, their sense of wholeness as well as the intactness of their lives.

SBC shifts the focus from a narrow perspective on a problem or deficit to a wider perspective on the whole. The person, family, and community are situated in the context and history of their lives with their many facets, layers, and complexities.

SBC is better suited to the changes and challenges of today's complex and fragmented health care system. Individuals and families are expected to take charge of their health, assume greater responsibility for the health care of loved ones, and be an active partner in health care decisions. They are more likely to take charge when they are treated as partners in their own care, have a degree of self-confidence, and are helped to believe they can do it because they have the required strengths or will be helped to develop the necessary competencies. They are more likely to benefit from the support, teaching, and guidance of nurses when they have a fuller understanding of their own internal strengths and external resources.

This book is for nursing students who are developing their framework of nursing and for experienced nurses who are looking for a new way to practice that honors the uniqueness of each person, places the person and family as the focus and center of care, and understands that problems can best be understood if situated in context and understood within the person's personal history, culture, belief system, and values of what is important and what holds meaning for them. It is for nurses who want to create environments to support the person's innate mechanisms of healing. It is for nurses who believe that collaborative partnership is key to helping the patient, client, and family assume greater control over their health and health care decisions. It is for nurses who subscribe to the belief that focusing and working with strengths hold the key to helping the person and family learn how to become empowered.

HOW THIS BOOK CAME ABOUT

Although this book took five years to plan and write, its origins—working with strengths—began many years before. Having spent almost my entire career at the School of Nursing of McGill University in Canada—from an undergraduate and graduate student to researcher, professor, director, and professor once again—I have absorbed the school's values, only to rework and imbue them with new meaning in light of new understandings derived from empirical knowledge, personal experiences, an aesthetic approach to knowing, and an ethical and moral commitment to how nursing should be practiced. I have learned from my students and have benefitted from their experience and wisdom as practitioners. Many of the values in this book are rooted in the history and thinking of professors and graduates of the McGill University School of Nursing as found in Bertha Harmer's book (Harmer, 1922). Bertha was McGill School of Nursing's second director. For the most part these ideas were transmitted through an oral tradition from professor to professor, class to class, from one generation of students to the next. In the mid-1970s, Dr. Moyra Allen identified the six core features that distinguished the McGill approach to nursing, which she called Situation-Responsive Nursing or Complemental Nursing, that became the foundation for the McGill Model of Nursing (for a historical overview, see Gottlieb & Ezer, 2007). The beliefs and values underlying the McGill School of Nursing's approach include:

- The focus of care is on the person and family over many decades, not the system.
- Nursing is most effective when there is a genuine, deep abiding respect and valuing of the uniqueness of the person.
- Nurses care for patients with the disease and not the disease per se.
- Nurses are learners, and patients and families are the best teachers.
- Nursing requires a broad knowledge base about the human condition, and this knowledge derives from the integration of theory and practice and reflection on practice.
- Nursing is responsive to the needs of the person and family. It is not prescriptive and requires a way of being that is flexible, open, and nonjudgmental.
- People need to find their own solutions and take responsibility for their own health. Nurses create conditions by providing experiences to help this happen. They do so by working in partnership with patients and their strengths.

These values, which have guided the McGill School of Nursing for over 92 years, have also guided my own professional career, which now exceeds 40 years. One of the six core features that Dr. Allen identified was that nurses should work with strengths, not deficits, to plan care (Allen, 1977). However, the least developed and poorly understood feature was working with the person's and family's strengths. It was during my sabbatical in 1992 with Dr. Kathryn Barnard at the University of Washington that my attention shifted to strengths in a more deliberate way. Dr. Barnard underscored the importance of strengths when she called the McGill School of Nursing's approach to nursing as "that strengths model." Her comment caused me to ask myself: What did working with individual and family strengths look like in practice? How did strengths interface with deficits? What were its theoretical considerations? How did clients, patients, families, and communities benefit from a strengths approach? Her comment also set in motion a series of events and actions that culminated in my writing of this book, almost two decades later.

I have found that the best way to understand an idea is to teach about it. In 1997, I decided to choose "strengths" as the topic of that year's doctoral seminar in advanced nursing. The seminar proved to be a turning point. In teaching about strengths, I learned about strengths. The seminars were stimulating as ideas were discussed and debated, and important questions raised. As there was no book on this topic, the experience convinced me that a book on strengths was needed. I then invited expert nurses who had worked with me on a previous book to join me (Gottlieb & Feeley with Dalton, 2006). They enthusiastically embraced the idea of this project and agreed to join me in my latest adventure. To this original group of 10, 11 more expert nurses were invited to participate (see page ix for their photos and biographies). They agreed to first be interviewed by me about their own practice, and then to collect stories from frontline nurses whose nursing had impressed them. Their stories illustrated their understanding of what it means to work with strengths, and proved to be very moving. It was a privilege to hear about such exquisite and sensitive nursing. In fact, it is the stories about their practices and the insights gained from experience of working with strengths that give this book its "heart." These nurses provided me with the language and reinforced some of my own ideas about strengths that had already begun to take shape. It is their stories about practice that capture the essence of nursing and make these theoretical ideas accessible to nurses and other practitioners, alike.

ORGANIZATION OF THE BOOK

Henry Mintzberg (2009), the management guru and professor at McGill University, reminds us in his book called *Managing* that "We need to understand 'it' [in our, case SBC] for 'it' to be practiced better" (p. 2). This book sets forth to understand "it," that is, what it means to work with the person's and family's strengths to promote health and healing. It is a vision for nursing that blends art and science, formal knowledge acquired through education and practical knowledge gained in practice. It subscribes to the belief that when practice is informed by art, craft, and science, art gives rise to vision and creative insights, craft comes about through experience and practical learning, and science provides the best systematic evidence to guide clinical decision making (Mintzberg, 2009).

This book is organized into three sections: The chapters in Part I lay out the theoretical and conceptual foundations underlying SBC, how SBC is part of a web of other ideas that help the person and family empower themselves to promote their own health and embark on the road of self-healing. Part II examines the tools and strategies required to practice nursing. The chapters in Part III bring together two silos—theory and practice—and describe what working with strengths looks like in practice.

Part I, "Theoretical Foundations of Strengths-Based Nursing Care," consists of four chapters. Chapter 1, "Why a Strengths-Based Approach to Care?" places SBC in context. It examines the past and current health care systems, the shortcomings and limitations of the deficit approach, and why and how SBC can address many of these shortcomings. It demonstrates how the movements of person-focused care, empowerment, health promotion, and collaborative partnership are tied together by a common underlying substrate, namely, SBC. It provides evidence of how SBC improves quality care for patients and families and holds promise for transforming nursing practice and the health care system.

Chapter 2, "What Guides Practice?," asks students and nurses to consider this most basic question. The answer to this question reveals much about the values, beliefs, and attitudes that guide nurses' day-to-day decisions and nursing actions. SBC helps guide practice decisions, but it goes beyond that, to shape a nurse's professional identity. Chapter 3, "Values Underlying Strengths-Based Nursing Care," identifies and describes the eight core values specific to SBC. It reviews the different ways to conceptualize each value and then offers the way they are conceptualized in SBC. Taken together, they create a comprehensive and coherent orientation to practice. Chapter 4, "What Are Strengths? Characteristics of Strengths," sets out to define strengths and their characteristics. Consistent with a nonprescriptive approach to nursing, this chapter does not list specific strengths. It does provide examples of different classifications of strengths and why a discipline or profession has selected a specific set of strengths to achieve its goals. Most important, it describes nine key characteristics of a quality that makes it a strength. It draws examples from biological, psychological, and social strengths.

Part II, "The Essential Toolbox: Basic Skills Required to Practice Strengths-Based Nursing Care," comprises four chapters. In becoming a nurse, learners must acquire formal and practical knowledge and skills to meet that profession's focus, fulfill its role in the health care system, and meet its mandate to society. Nurses need to develop a broad repertoire of clinical and critical inquiry skills for clinical judgment and clinical decision making. All four chapters of Part II offer strategies and techniques that illustrate how one can develop the strengths and skills that transform the learner from a layperson providing care into a professional nurse. Chapter 5, "Essential Nurse Qualities Required for Strengths-Based Care," shifts the spotlight from the person to the nurse and the strengths that nurses must have, or need, to further develop in practicing SBC. It describes four categories of strengths with their specific subcategories (e.g., Category: Mindset Strengths, Subcategory: Open-mindedness). It describes each strength and why it is needed to practice SBC. It also offers suggestions on how to develop or acquire a particular quality to be used as a strength. Chapter 6, "Retraining the Eight Senses for Nursing Practice," examines eight senses, namely, the five traditional sensory systems (i.e., sight, hearing, smell, taste, touch) and three senses, required for practice, that monitor internal bodily sensations, thoughts, and feelings that are required for practice. This chapter examines what is involved in retraining the senses for practice and provides specific strategies, based on knowledge from the neurosciences, for how to retrain the senses. Chapter 7, "Nursing's Professional Gaze: Observations for Clinical Judgment and Decision Making," reviews why observation remains the cornerstone of practice and how observation is central to clinical grasp, a precursor of clinical judgment, clinical reasoning, clinical decision making, and nursing action. It provides readers with the knowledge underlying observation, the reflective and thinking processes involved, and the criteria for assessing quality observation, as well as specific strategies and techniques to improve observation. Chapter 8, "Reforming Skills of Social Involvement: Attunement, Authentic Presence, Attentive Listening, and Clinical Conversation," covers the skills involved in creating and maintaining the nurse–person/family relationship. It is during an encounter that the nurse develops a relationship, gets to know the person, works with her to promote health, and accompanies her on her journey from diagnosis and treatment through recovery and healing. This chapter focuses on adding to the nurse's toolbox by showing the importance of attunement, authentic presence, attentive listening, dialoguing, and questioning and provides the tools to develop these fundamental relationship skills.

Part III, "Strengths-Based Nursing Care in Practice," consists of two chapters that bring together all the threads that were set forth in the previous chapters. Chapter 9, "The Spiraling Process for Uncovering and Discovering Strengths," describes a four-phase process in the nurse–person relationship during which strengths are uncovered and discovered. Each phase of the process is described, along with specific approaches and techniques for nurses to use in uncovering and discovering strengths from getting to know the person and family to evaluating and reviewing care. Chapter 10, "Approaches for Working With Strengths," describes, in detail, approaches and techniques to create the conditions for SBC. It outlines how to work with existing strengths to deal with problems and concerns. It also details ways to develop new strengths by developing potentials into strengths, by transforming deficits into strengths, and by minimizing deficits.

FEATURES IN CHAPTERS OF THE BOOK

All chapters begin with Learning Objectives to help readers situate themselves in the content of the chapter and to guide them in what to attend to as they read through a chapter. At the end of each chapter are Key Summary Points, a quick synopsis of the major content covered in the chapter.

Every chapter contains tables and exhibits to help summarize and synthesize complex material to make it more accessible and understandable, and to facilitate recall, as well as figures to illustrate concepts and their interrelationships. Within the text, ideas are presented in list format to help capture, summarize, and communicate the material.

Each chapter has at least three other display items: an Empirical Study, a Personal Experience, and a Reflect and Connect exercise. These three represent approaches to how knowledge is learned and then constructed: use of the scientific literature (evidence-based practice), relating concepts to narratives or stories of actual patient experiences (narrative pedagogy), and reflecting on practice and connecting it to theoretical ideas or reflecting on a theoretical concept and then connecting it to practice or to a personal experience (reflective practice).

Concepts and ideas are brought to life with stories from the rich clinical experiences of our expert consultants and frontline nurses. These clinicians were asked to recall an experience with a patient/client and family that profoundly affected them and transformed their approach to practice. Years later, their experiences with these people remain vivid in their memories. Nurses could describe their patients and the experiences in minute detail because they touched something very deep within them.

In this book, the actual nurses' names are used. These are real nurses telling about real patients that they nursed. However, the first and last names of patients, clients, and family members have been changed to protect their confidentiality. Some details of their stories also have been altered for the same purposes.

The stories and direct quotes that appear in the book were interviews that were audio- or videotaped and then transcribed verbatim. They appear as told, with only some minor editing to put ideas into context and to make the transition from the spoken word to written form more readable.

INSTRUCTOR'S MANUAL

A companion to this book is the Instructor's Manual entitled Strengths-Based Teaching and Learning (SBTL). The manual has been developed as a resource for instructors/educators to assist them in transmitting the ideas and values of SBC to students, so that SBC becomes the students' theoretical orientation in practice. The manual provides instructors with a pedagogical approach to be used both in the classroom and clinical setting. It provides them with an orientation to teaching and learning that is consistent with the values of SBC. It also provides them with the skills to assist them to create a strengths-based learning environment for their students. It is my belief that when students experience a strengths-based approach in their education, they will understand its benefits at a deeper level and will adopt this way of being with patients, clients, and families. It is also hoped that when instructors teach from a strengths-based perspective they will experience firsthand its benefits. They will see how SBTL empowers students to become more engaged and self-directed in their own learning.

The Instructor's Manual contains two parts: Part I outlines the philosophy, values, and pedagogical principles underlying SBTL. It also contains the following sections: Instructors' Role in SBTL, Guidelines for Providing Feedback, and Instructor's Mirroring/Self-Reflection Activities. Part II of the Instructor's Manual includes specific activities designed to enhance teaching for a chapter. Each chapter begins with an overview of the contents and features contained within that chapter—*Chapter-at-A-Glance*. In addition, there are two enhancement activities that have been designed to engage students in selected content of that chapter's material. The Instructor's Manual is available to qualified instructors by contacting textbook@springerpub.com.

A NOTE ON TERMINOLOGY

In keeping with a nongendered approach, the terms *person* and *family* are used. *Person* refers to individuals, patients, clients, and consumers. The term *patient* is used to refer to an individual in the hospital, whereas *client* is used to refer to both the healthy and to the sick being cared for at home or in the community. I have tried to avoid using pronouns of *her/his, she/he*. When the sentence has required the singular, I have randomly used male or female.

The terms *clinician* and *practitioner* are used interchangeably. In general, I use *clinician* to refer to nurses practicing in hospitals and *practitioner* to refer to nurses practicing in the community.

A NOTE ON MY COLLABORATOR

Bruce Gottlieb reviewed drafts of this book, helped me sort out ideas, assisted in the research, wrote the boxes on the empirical studies, and worked with me on editing the book. As a biologist and geneticist, he provided many biological examples. He also wrote the feature Chapters-at-A-Glance for each chapter in the Instructor's Manual.

IN CONCLUSION

This book provides the knowledge and practical tools to practice nursing from a strengths perspective. SBC is not a prescriptive or a formulaic approach to care. It is not about creating standardized nursing care plans or care maps. "One size fits all" contradicts and violates the tenets of SBC. There is no magical formula or quick solutions or easy answers. People are complex, and they live complex lives. Nursing is about promoting health, helping to alleviate suffering, and caring for the sick. Nurses care for people throughout the life span. Nursing is also about caring for families. Health, wellness, and sickness are family events. Families need support to strengthen what they do in promoting the health of its members during all transitional life events; from conception to death and everything in between. They need help in caring for the sick, the injured, and disabled. Nursing is also about understanding communities. Families and health care systems are parts of communities. Communities either provide or lack resources that can make a difference.

Illness and tragedy are always unexpected and never welcomed; however, they do redefine people and reshape their lives. SBC is about understanding the whole person and understanding him in the context of his life. SBC is about understanding the profound effects that transitional events such as illness and tragedy have on people's lives. SBC is about bringing transformative change to lives that have become disrupted as people try to continue to live and find meaning and purpose in their lives while repairing that which has been broken. SBC is also about celebrations and triumphs that enable individuals and families to mature, grow, and develop. SBC is about honoring the human spirit.

SBC requires that nurses invest in individuals, families, and communities. To care for another person, especially a stranger, requires physical, mental, and emotional investments on the part of the nurse. Such investments yield indescribable dividends.

In today's health care climate, that which can be measured is most valued—this book bucks the trend. To care for others, be witness to their sufferings, find ways to help them maintain health, alleviate their suffering, and restore wholeness, often cannot be quantified. Such investments elude pricetags and dollar amounts. They may not translate into dollars, but they do translate into the knowledge that one stranger has touched and transformed the life of another. One person, one nurse, has the power to make a difference. The rewards are immeasurable.

SBC has the power to inspire, facilitate growth, and transform. This is true both for the nurse who is giving care and for the person and family who are receiving care. True power is distinguished by a concern for the powerless and the less powerful—the weak, the vulnerable, the ill and disabled, the dispossessed, the immigrant, and the stranger (Sacks, 2004). True power is the ability to hear the voice of the powerless and give them voice.

Everyone, at some time in their lives, undergoes change, is touched by disease, the ravages of illness, tragedy, and trauma, only to find themselves in positions of dependency and in need of the knowledge and skills of others. Yet this need not be the entire story. SBC helps people understand that although they did not choose to get sick or be touched by tragedy, they do have the power to choose how they will cope with what has happened to them.

Similarly, nurses have the power to choose how they will nurse. They have the power to choose how they will care for people by how they choose to be and what they choose to do. They have the power to choose how they will spend their time—whether they will spend time with their patients or spend time at the nursing station, whether they will monitor patients at their bedside or on a monitor and at a distance.

Nurses have the power to transform the current health care system, to be major players in bringing about health care reform given that they are by far the largest segment of the health care workforce (Institute of Medicine, 2010). They have the power to bring the human touch to a highly sophisticated, technological health care environment, and to touch the lives of many. They have the power to create a new culture, an ethos of caring rooted in values of compassion and knowledge that respects the human spirit and gives dignity to people. They have the power to restore the centrality of the nurse–patient relationship and the person as the focus of care. SBC gives nurses this power.

Laurie N. Gottlieb

Acknowledgments

This book has been a labor of love and has involved many people to whom I am deeply grateful. I begin my acknowledgments by thanking my editor, Allan Graubard, at Springer Publishing Company. From our very first correspondence, Allan recognized the potential of this book. He has been everything I could hope for in an editor: knowledgeable, insightful, understanding, supportive, fair, and wise. He has helped me through some very challenging times. His support in this project has been unwavering. I am also grateful to Margaret Zuccarini who, before joining Springer as their nursing publisher, suggested Allan's name. I have known Margaret for several years and hold her in the highest esteem.

The seed for a book on strengths, as explained in the Preface, was first planted by Kathryn Barnard of the University of Washington. I am grateful to my wise and insightful friend.

I began this book by approaching 10 expert nurse clinicians and inviting them to an initial brainstorming session. They enthusiastically endorsed the idea for this book, and all agreed to be interviewed by me and then to interview nurses who they knew practiced from a strengths-based perspective. I then invited another 11 individuals to become the expert consultants on this book. Dr. Judith Ritchie suggested some of the expert nurses to interview. To help these consultants prepare to become interviewers, I organized a training workshop. Franco Carnevale and Mary Ellen MacDonald graciously agreed to lead the workshop. Our training session took place in the then–newly opened Arnold and Blema Steinberg Medical Simulation Center at McGill University, as did all the interviews that I subsequently conducted with my expert consultants. I am grateful to Linda Crelinsten, Assistant Director of this center, who helped schedule the interviews, and to Robert Peuckert who videotaped them. I thank Sharyn Andrews, who invited me to attend one of her reflective nursing practice groups, and to Lidia De Simone, who allowed me to pilot my interview schedule. These first encounters met with such enthusiasm that they propelled me forward. The proposal for this book received institutional review board approval from McGill University ethics committee.

Over the course of writing this book, many individuals were involved. I thank Stephen Guy and Arielle Gottlieb for transcribing the video and audiotapes. Ulrika

Drevnick, Farrimnah Francis, Monica Parmar, and Melvin Yumang conducted some of the initial literature searches. Amanda Cervantes managed aspects of this project. I acknowledge the financial support of McGill Career Planning Service (CaPS), which matched funds to hire graduate students as research assistants.

Everyone needs a cheerleader, and Catherine Gros has been mine. I thank Madeleine Buck, Marcia Beaulieu, and Beverly Mendelson for their advice on the Instructor's Manual. Catherine Gros and David Wright made some invaluable suggestions and each co-wrote a section in the Instructor's Manual with me.

I thank my cousin Howard Richler, a logophile, who served as my consultant on the use and meaning of words and terminology. I also thank Franco Carnevale, Nancy Feeley, Ragnheidur Haralsdottir, Deanna Rosenswig, Linda Switkin, and Claire Thibault for their invaluable insights on different drafts of the book. Sean Clarke provided a summary of the research on the effects of downsizing found in Chapter 1. Claire Thibault has been a true partner in disseminating these ideas to the francophone nursing community in Quebec. Joanna Toti continues to impress me with her superb organizational skills and ability to get things done. I also thank Cait Beattie and Jane Broderick for help with the consultants' bios. I am particularly grateful to Deanna Rosenswig and Linda Switkin, who have encouraged, and guided me, and to my many friends for their support. I feel extremely fortunate to have such a cadre of devoted friends and talented colleagues.

I am also grateful to the Springer team, and in particular to Michael O'Connor and his team, in transforming my manuscript into a book.

I am indebted to Robert Vineberg for his sage professional and personal advice. He is a trusted friend—generous, compassionate, and extremely protective. I thank Adam Agensky for giving me a crash course in American intellectual property law and for his invaluable legal guidance.

I am grateful to Anne Marie Rafferty for inviting me to spend part of my sabbatical year at the Nightingale School of Nursing and Midwifery of King's College, University of London. Being close to where Florence Nightingale had lived and worked inspired me as I wrote.

I thank Helene Ezer, director of the McGill School of Nursing, for providing me with seed money to defray the initial costs of this book. She has been a wonderful friend and colleague. She has been generous in her praise and has been supportive in countless ways.

The soul of this book are the stories of nurses in practice, caring for patients, clients, and families when at their most vulnerable, yet focusing and seeing their strengths. As nurses shared with me their nursing experiences, I often found myself moved to tears. It was not just the poignancy of what people go through that revealed the human spirit, but the beauty of their nursing that touched me to my very core. These nurses are committed to those entrusted to their care and have a passion for their work. They recognize the importance of working with strengths, not only to empower patients and families but also to be empowered in their work as nurses to make a difference.

I am indebted to Patricia Benner, who wrote the Foreword for this book. When I invited Patricia to do so, I could never have anticipated her reaction to this book. Her understanding has been the best gift. I thank Judith Shamian for recognizing the importance of these ideas and for championing the book. I am honored that both Patricia and Judith have shared their insights and have situated this book in its broader context.

My final words of appreciation are reserved for my family. My husband, Bruce, has worked tirelessly with me on all aspects of the book. I am indebted to him for his unwavering belief in me and his commitment to the ideas in this book. His kindness, patience, and compassion know no bounds. His support and love have seen us through good times and bad. I dedicate this book to my twin sister, Linda, and my immediate family; Bruce; our children, Michah and Arielle; daughter-in-law, Ilana; and grandchildren, Gabriella, Jordanna, and Itai, from whom I draw my strength.

Laurie N. Gottlieb

Why a Strengths-Based Approach to Care?

1

After reading this chapter, you should be able to:

- Describe what Strengths-Based Care is.
- Identify the dominant approach to care in the health care system and its limitations.
- Identify four movements to address these limitations and their relationship to Strengths-Based Care.
- Compare Strengths-Based Care with Deficit-Based Care.
- Describe the evidence that indicates that Strengths-Based Care is effective.

Strengths-Based Care (SBC) is an approach that considers the whole person, focuses on what is working and functioning well, what the person does best, and what resources people have available to help them deal more effectively with their life, health, and health care challenges. It is about how nurses can best support what is working in order to help patients, clients, families, and communities cope, develop, grow, thrive, and transform. It represents a reconceptualization of what it means to care for another person. It returns nurses to their roots of caring for another human being by focusing on individuals' personhood and humanity and by asking them to see their faces, their uniqueness, and not just their diseases or problems. It asks nurses and health care professionals to gain a fuller appreciation of patients, clients, and their families by situating them and their issues in context, considering their situation and circumstances, getting to know their "story," and accompanying them on their health and illness journeys. It challenges nurses to work with patients, clients, and families in order to make health care decisions that are responsive to their needs and goals and to act in their best interests. Although SBC makes sense, it represents a radical shift in thinking and a new way of being and doing. It requires a new orientation on the part of most nurses, health care professionals, and the current health care system.

We live in a society in which deficit thinking is the norm. We tend to focus on the negative rather than on the positive, on what is wrong rather than what is right, on what needs fixing rather than what is working, and on the pains and sorrows of life rather than on its joys and celebrations. In short, we look for deficits, and thus we often miss the strengths and the many possibilities and opportunities for improving the quality of patients' lives.

Current health care systems exist to look for deficits at all levels, from cells to citizens to communities. Instructors in the health care professions train their practitioners to look for pathology to identify and treat problems. For example, microbiologists look for pathology at the cellular and tissue level. Doctors look for disease in organs and bodily systems. Nurses look for problems in individuals', families', and communities' responses to health and illness concerns. This is what they are trained to do, and this is what they should do, but this is not sufficient. By focusing on what is missing or deficient, they miss out on other aspects of the person that are functioning well and that are compensating for what is not working or is working below an optimal level. They often fail to see the person because they are blinded by the pathology, the diseased organ, or the dysfunctional family. They strip and reduce patients to their parts, ignoring their situations and circumstances, rather than seeing them for the unique individuals they are.

Nurses and other health professionals are all part of what is commonly referred to as the *helping professions*. The term *helping* implies the desire and willingness to assist, fix, and repair something that is lacking, missing, malfunctioning, or broken. There are, however, many ways of helping. A nurse can help people by focusing on the problem and trying to fix it, or a nurse can work *with* people and their strengths to help them deal with their concerns, find solutions to their problems, and choose how to live with them. The latter approach to helping is SBC, and it requires that a nurse knows, values, and respects the person and family who strive to live life and to find new meaning and purpose as they cope with the challenges of illness or other tragedies and work to achieve a higher level of health.

Nurse Gillian Taylor told the story of Sarah, who suffered from a severe, debilitating form of juvenile arthritis, previously misdiagnosed, that left her unable to walk; of her 20-year old single mother, Janice; and of Janice's parents, with whom they live. Gillian first met Sarah and her family when Sarah was 2½ years old: *"If I drew just a genogram* [a visual depiction of the structure of the family] *and wrote some facts about this mother and daughter on paper, any person would say, 'What a disaster and what misery'—and I would say: 'What resilience and what gutsiness!'"* Not only had Sarah not received the proper treatment after she stopped walking, having previously walked for a short time, but her mother also was told that Sarah's refusal to walk was because she wanted attention. As Gillian reported, *"Fortunately, the mom rejected this explanation."* During Gillian's first home visit, a number of things impressed her about Sarah and her mother.

"The first thing that struck me was Sarah's drive; her wish to do things on her own was fierce. She scooted around on her bum, asked for help when she needed it, and then pushed everybody away if they tried to do anything vaguely resembling help. She would say, 'Don't touch me! I'll do it myself! I'll do it myself!' And I watched how this mom responded. The mom put out a hand and gave her daughter a little help and then pulled away, so that her daughter could indeed say, 'I'm doing it myself'; and the mom could say, 'Yes you are! Yes

you are!' This was just phenomenal, because this child was very disabled and in a lot of pain. I remember thinking that this mom allowed this toddler her voice and control given a situation that was totally heartbreaking. Frankly, I just wanted to pick her up and take over because it all looked really difficult."

Another thing that Gillian observed was that, even though the grandmother was upset by the misdiagnosis and kept saying, "We should have gotten a second opinion earlier," Janice refused to feel guilty and disagreed with her mother by telling her that they had seen a second doctor. Gillian was impressed by Janice's attitude: *"I remember thinking she's struggling to have a version of this story that will allow her, like her daughter, to keep herself feeling OK."* What also impressed Gillian was that this young mother was able to develop a relationship with her and the doctor despite her negative experience with her previous physician and the health care system.

Sarah is now 8 years old. Gillian described the rollercoaster that Sarah and her family have been on together: *"From a medical point of view, this has been one of the toughest cases. Sarah has failed to respond to three different treatments. This means that at times her disease is under control and then it flares up and is out of control. She's tried experimental treatments and Janice has had to give her consent, which involves trust in the team that many families would find challenging."*

After all these years, Gillian continues to be impressed by this family. She described an incident that captures the spirit of this family and the way they work together: *"The other day, I was going over how to inject the new medication and the need to rotate the injection site. As I talked about rotating sites, Sarah said: 'No; I only get injections in my arms because once my mother gave me something in my belly it hurt, so no.' As the mom was listening to my explanation of why rotating sites would probably be necessary, the mom very quickly said: 'Well, for today we'll just do it in the arm and we'll let you know if we need to rotate.' Sarah quickly settled and I gave the injection in her arm. And that was the end of that. A couple of days later, Janice called because she just wanted to go over what had happened at our last visit. She said, 'I am trying to find a balance now that Sarah is old enough to understand some things. I want her to hear why it is important to rotate sites but she still needs to have some control and it is important that I give her as much as I can. And I've learned that she will change her mind about something when she has to.'"*

Gillian continued with her story: *"About two weeks later, they came in for an appointment and Sarah said to me, 'Now I like my needles best in my belly.' And so we looked at how that had come about. Sarah very generously said: 'You were right.' And that's a real strength, to be able to make a shift, to look back and say, 'Well, you know, that was OK.' And we talked about how it was a challenge to try new things. Janice, knowing her child's temperament and respecting Sarah in a way that acknowledges her drive and her gutsiness, also recognizes that Sarah is a child who will change when she needs to—when the timing is right. The mom is able to be both advocate and protector."*

Most clinicians would focus on Sarah's arthritis, her deformed joints, the pain, and the fact that her disability has prevented her from walking. They would fail to see Sarah the spunky toddler, who just happens to have juvenile arthritis. What are the things about Sarah and her family that impress Gillian?

Gillian sees a little girl with tremendous drive and an intense desire to do things by herself despite the pain and disability. She sees Sarah's mother not as a single teenage mother but as a mother who knows her daughter and what is best for her. Janice has a parenting style that meets her child's needs for autonomy and control, is able to advocate and protect her child, and can trust and work in partnership with the health care team to ensure that her child gets the very best care. Gillian, fully aware of Sarah's medical condition, sees a family who lives every day with the effects of juvenile arthritis and creates the conditions that enable them to cope and get the most out of life. She practices nursing from a strengths perspective.

The resiliency of the human body and spirit speaks to the human condition and its ability to rally from trauma, illness, and hardship; overcome vulnerabilities; cope and deal with problems; meet life's challenges, and find meaning in living. It is this recognition and appreciation of the human spirit that are at the heart of working with strengths. Consider how Sarah's inner spirit shines through despite incredible pain and deformity. Most nurses and health care practitioners, however, because they practice from a deficit perspective, are often blind to the human spirit and how that spirit informs and feeds a person's strengths. Why is this the case, and how did this come about?

> The resiliency of the human body and spirit speaks to the human condition and its ability to rally. Working with strengths begins by recognizing and appreciating the human spirit.

To address these two questions requires an understanding of how the deficit perspective became the dominant approach that most practitioners use to guide their practice.

BRIEF HISTORICAL OVERVIEW OF THE EMERGENCE OF THE DEFICIT PERSPECTIVE

What often determines the nature of a profession's practice is what society expects of it, how the members of that profession meets these expectations, and the rewards society bestows on that profession for meeting these expectations (Sullivan, 2005). Medicine is responsible for diagnosing and treating disease, whereas nursing is responsible for promoting health, caring for the sick, and alleviating suffering. The ways a profession fulfills its roles and societal obligations are affected in part by the social, political, and economic pressures of that period in time. Although nursing is primarily responsible for caring for the sick, the way nursing fulfills its mandate looks very different today than it did 10, 20, 50, and even 100 years ago, as outlined in Table 1.1 (Hallett, 2007; D'Antonio & Lewenson, 2010).

During the 19th and first half of the 20th centuries, health care delivery was radically different from what it is today. Each family had its own family physician who was intimately involved with and knew them well (Howell, 2001). Family doctors and public health nurses were part of the family's community and accompanied the family through all major life events, from pregnancy, births, illnesses, accidents, and traumas, to death and its aftermath. Doctors and nurses knew their families from cradle to grave. They saw them at schools and visited them in their

TABLE 1.1

A "gallop" through nursing history

Period	Major Feature	Values and Qualities
15th to 19th centuries	Caritas Era	Nursing emerges in an era that subscribes to an ethos of caring and self-sacrifice. It is a time of: • Charity • Strong resonance of spiritual love, self-sacrifice • Precursor to modern caring
1850s to 1950s	Heroic Era	Nursing roles are forged during wartime (Crimean War, the Boer War, World Wars I & II): • Calculated risk taking • Courageous • "Angels" • Compassionate care
1950s to 1980s	Professionalizing Era	Nursing begins to forge its knowledge base with a focus on logico-scienctific systems but has difficulty finding acceptance.
1980s to the present	Technocratic Era	Nursing embraces medical technology with its link to status and power and loses its identity and purpose.

Source: Based on Hallett (2007).

homes, and when a family member had to be sent to the hospital it was for a specific medical treatment. They knew each family member's strengths, weaknesses, vulnerabilities, and frailties. They knew which families had the emotional and financial resources to cope and which ones did not. They knew which family member could provide accurate information and which ones could not. They knew who would comply with treatment and who would not. They knew who was at risk for disease and who was not.

The primary responsibility for health maintenance, prevention of disease, and the care of the sick and dying rested with the family, extended family members, friends, and their community. Nurses visited families in their homes and worked alongside family caregivers in partnership with doctors and other health care workers when patients succumbed to illness (Reverby, 1987). They were the primary health care workers who cared for the population during life-threatening epidemics, such as the Yellow Fever epidemic in the U.S. Deep South (Sabin, 2010) or the major influenza epidemic of 1918 (Keeling, 2010). Health care providers were an important part of the family's social network. They were called on at the appropriate time when their expertise was needed.

With industrialization and the move to cities, along with the growth of scientific knowledge, the development of new technologies to diagnose, and changes in medical therapeutics, care shifted from family caregivers in the home to professional caregivers in hospitals. Beginning with the first world war, and increasingly so during the second world war, hospitals supplanted care in the home, and nurses became primary caregivers (Howell, 2001; Lynaugh & Fagin, 1988; Reverby, 1987).

The division of labor between nurses, physicians, and other health care providers was clear. Physicians were responsible for overseeing the patient's care, whereas nurses were responsible for carrying out doctors' orders and reporting to them about any change in the patient's condition (Barnes, 1961). Nurses came to know their patients by ministering to their physical needs, providing physical care, and listening to their stories (Sandelowski, 2000). Hospitals took care away from families and transformed the illness experience. In the new modern hospitals, family visitation was neither desirable nor acceptable, and families were seen as more of a nuisance than as a help (Barnes, 1961; Markel, 2008). Hospitals made little provision for family members. Often, they did not provide a place even to hang up a hat or coat or a chair on which to sit (Barnes, 1961). Family members were relegated to a visiting role and had limited access to their loved ones. The premise was that this would be "best" for the patient, who would be protected from infection and could direct his energy to healing. Families were tolerated at best, viewed as interfering with treatment at worst, and certainly not treated as partners in care.

A study in the late 1950s of patients' experiences in hospitals found that they were expected to be passive and submissive (Barnes, 1961). Now that doctors had at their disposal new treatments, surgeries, and drugs brought about by advancements in the biological and physical sciences, they, as well as the general public, saw the medical profession as responsible for curing whatever ails people. Physicians, particularly surgeons, were elevated to the status of gods and considered omnipotent. In exchange for being cured, patients were expected to ask few questions; cooperate with treatment; and submit body, mind, and soul. Often, patients and families were left in the dark, knowing little, and were also expected to ask little (Barnes, 1961).

Patient hospital stays were lengthy, and patients were discharged only when all symptoms had abated and when minimal home care was needed. During the 1950s and 1960s, the average length of hospital stay for commonplace procedures, such as a tonsillectomy, cholecystectomy, or cataract removal, was five to fourteen days. Today, these procedures are routinely conducted in day surgery. Because patients were in the hospital for a relatively lengthy period of time, they were often assigned to the same nurse. Nurses were responsible for caring for three to five patients, of whom only one or two were acutely ill, with the remainder in various stages of recovery. Patients and nurses got to know one another. Direct patient care was only part of a nurse's responsibility. Although they were the record-keepers, message carriers, caretakers, organizers, and housekeepers of the ward, nurses were expected to give bodycare (bathing, backrubs, and the like) and find time to listen to their patients as well (Barnes, 1961).

In addition to hospital care, community care nursing focused on home visiting, public health education, prenatal and postnatal care, immunization programs, lifestyle counseling, school nursing, occupational health, and the like. Public health nurses visited patients at home to give treatments, educate, and support families in the care of their ill member.

THE GROWTH OF THE DEFICIT MODEL AND ITS INFLUENCE ON HEALTH CARE PRACTICE

At the present time, the deficit model dominates thinking in the health care system. In part, this is due to the prevalence of the *biomedical model*, which was developed over the course of many generations to help doctors understand their patients' medical problems, arrive at an accurate diagnosis, and find the best treatment. Thus, the biomedical model is a method for, or an approach to, systematically collecting, organizing, and categorizing clinical data (D'Antonio & Fairman, 2004). Physicians are attuned to what is wrong and are focused on understanding the cause of the symptom; the underlying pathology; the malfunctioning organ or system; and how to cure, correct, or minimize the problem. There is a downside here: The biomedical model has become a reductionist approach in which patients are reduced to, and thought of, in terms of their body parts: the diseased heart, the malfunctioning lung, the pain in the stomach. Their personhood is ignored, and their strengths go unnoticed.

There are a number of reasons why the biomedical model has come to dominate the health care system and is used by so many other health care practitioners as their orientation to practice. First, patients often seek out medical care because something is bothering them. The medical model has been shown to be a highly effective and systematic approach to address such concerns. Second, the current health care system is primarily a medical one that is devoted to the treatment and cure of disease, not one that primarily promotes health and helps patients heal. Third, the biomedical model provides a common language within the health care system for health care professionals to communicate with each other. However, the unintended consequence of the dominance of the biomedical model is that the culture it fosters in the health care system roots it in deficit-type thinking. Most health care professionals are preoccupied with what is not working and ignore what is working. Finally, medicine has been and continues to be the dominant member of the health team, which garners the most attention in the system. Nurses and others believe that, by identifying with and adopting the medical model they will, by association, elevate their status within the organization they practice in. This observation, which was made in hospitals over 50 years ago (Barnes, 1961), is just as real today.

The power of the powerful to shape others' thoughts and action should not be underestimated. Harris (1998), through her groundbreaking insights into how children turn out the way they do, alerted readers to the power of the group in socializing an individual to a particular role, a specific way of behaving. At a very early age, children select a group with which to affiliate because there is something in that group that they want or that resonates with them, so they then adopt the ways of thinking and behaving of a group that is perceived to be more powerful. This pattern of socialization continues throughout an individual's life span. One of the first things a person does when he enters a new environment is scan the environment for the *attention structure* that is in place; that is, he appraises the different social groups; categorizes the groups in terms of power, status, attention, interests, values and the like; and then decides on the group he would like to join. Shortly thereafter, he quickly learns to behave like the other members of that group (Harris, 1998). In hospitals and the health care system, there is an attention structure as well: the group that gets the attention, the profession to which everyone looks when they are unsure about what to do. Those individuals who are high on the attention structure often get privileges and rewards that those low on the structure could never dream of having, let alone hope for (Harris, 1998). Medicine has enjoyed being on the highest echelons of the attention structure. This has been going on for a very long time. In fact, a study of the inner workings of hospitals conducted during the 1950s found that nurses derived much of their satisfaction from doctors' approval of what they did, and things that doctors did not consider important, useful, or proper were not considered important (Barnes, 1961). Although today's nurses derive their job satisfaction from being given the autonomy to carry out responsibilities that are commensurate with their knowledge and experience, job satisfaction is still related to a positive relationship and clear communication with physicians (Wanzer, Wojtaszczyk, & Kelly, 2009). Attention structure theory may explain in part why nurses and others have muffled their voices and diminished their own roles by adopting medical language and the deficit discourse.

CAVEAT

The medical model need not be a deficit model. The two are not mutually exclusive. Physicians can diagnose and treat problems and also have a strengths perspective and practice whole-person care.

WHAT EFFECT HAS DEFICIT THINKING HAD ON PRACTICE?

The first effect of deficit thinking is that many nurses and health care practitioners view their patients through a negative lens. As a result, behaviors that seem unfamiliar or unusual are interpreted in clinical terms, such as *abnormal, deviant, pathological,* or *dysfunctional.* Because clinicians focus on problems, there is a tendency to frame a patient's behavior negatively. Even healthy responses can be labeled pathological. Consider the story of Mrs. Coreen Kennedy, who was diagnosed with advanced rectal cancer when she was in her first trimester of pregnancy. The doctors advised Mr. and Mrs. Kennedy to abort the pregnancy, so that Coreen could start treatment immediately. This couple agonized over what to do and, after much discussion with their minister, family members, and health care professionals, decided to continue with the pregnancy until the earliest date at which time Coreen could safely give birth to a viable baby. She would then have surgery to remove the malignant tumor and begin chemotherapy and radiation therapy. Once the couple had made their decision, Coreen became calmer. The doctors were disturbed by her calmness and interpreted Coreen's calmness negatively. Christina Clausen, Coreen's primary nurse, described the medical team's response: *"There were questions among physicians of whether Coreen was coping appropriately because she was so strong. And they're thinking—'She must be in denial, someone this positive and this able to manage; well, that just can't be!'"* Yet Christina knew this mother was not in denial. She knew what this couple had gone through in arriving at their decision. Christina saw that her role was to support the Kennedys' decision and advocate for them. She believed that the decision the Kennedys had made was right for them. Both Coreen and her infant daughter survived.

A second effect of the widespread adoption of the biomedical model, with its associated deficit thinking, has been to deconstruct and depersonalize the individual who is seeking care. Part of diagnosing the problem is to identify, locate, and understand symptoms. What becomes problematic is when the process of diagnosing becomes generalized to the person; that is, when the person is reduced to her symptoms, as if symptoms can exist separate from the person, instead of the patient being viewed as a person who is experiencing a symptom or illness. In other words, patients may be referred to and treated as Mrs. Wallis—"the amputee," or Mr. Roberts—"the stomach ulcer."

> Diagnosis involves understanding the nature and meaning of signs and symptoms. Just focusing on the diagnosis, however, has its risks: the person will be known by their symptoms and not their personhood.

Another reason for this state of affairs lies in the nature of the work. Many medical treatments cause pain. Think of the effects of surgery or invasive procedures, such as taking blood, inserting lines, and catheters and tubing in different orifices (e.g., feeding tubes). Nurses often have to inflict suffering in order to alleviate suffering. Most procedures and treatments cause bodily pain. It is easier to cause pain if the nurse or physician or any health professional is detached from the patient. It is easier on the doctor or nurse to inflict pain on a body part or target a specific symptom, rather than cause pain to a person (Barnes, 1961). Thus, depersonalizing a patient and reducing him to a symptom or bodily part has become a defense learned early in a person's professional career.

A third effect of the dominant medical model is that nurses who practice deficit thinking have relinquished many of their traditional roles of caregiving in favor of taking on more medical tasks and functions. Traditional caregiving roles gave nurses their distinct role in the health care system. Many of the relinquished tasks (e.g., bed baths, backrubs, patient positioning) involved caring for the person by caring for the person's body and attending to her bodily needs. It was in the act of doing these tasks that nurses came to know their patients as individuals and could assess at close hand their health and healing status (Wolf, 2009).

Finally, the focus on disease and problems has stimulated the invention of ever-more-sophisticated technologies to help practitioners diagnose and treat medical conditions. In short, health care systems tend to be problem centered rather than person centered, yet they can be both. The focus needs to be on understanding the disease, its cause, and how to cure it, or at least manage it. The approach to healing patients needs to focus on the persons and use their strengths and capabilities to manage their problems. These two approaches can be compatible, as I describe in more detail in Chapter 3, Exhibit 3.6.

EMERGENCE OF THE TECHNOLOGICAL ERA

Beginning in the 1960s, with the advent of new technologies for diagnosis and treatment (e.g., imaging scans) and advances in pharmaceutical technology and therapies, the health care system underwent radical changes. Intensive care units were created to deal with the most seriously ill patients. Health care became more specialized; services became more technologically driven; and traditional health care professions, such as medicine and nursing, had to rethink their roles as new groups of health care technicians and therapists were trained.

New technologies have ushered in a new era of treating diseases, extending life and, for many, improving the quality of their life. Such advances, among them noninvasive surgeries, have minimized the trauma of major surgery, have reduced complications, and enabled individuals to resume their normal activities within a relatively short period of time following treatment. A case in point is cholescystectomy surgery. Until the early 1990s, the removal of a gall bladder required a five- to ten-day hospital stay because the surgery was invasive, requiring a large incision in the abdominal wall. The development of laparoscopic surgical equipment offered general surgeons the ability to complete cholecystectomy surgeries and send patients home the very same day. Patients often resume their normal routines within the week.

> While the introduction of new technologies has vastly improved our abilities to restore the person to health, nurses who rely too heavily on technology can lose sight of the person.

Nurses have identified both positive and negative effects of technology on their practice (Zuzelo, Gettis, Hansel, & Thomas, 2008). On the positive side, nurses have reported that technology has increased their efficiency and saved them time, as well as helped them keep their patients safe by detecting subtle changes in their patients' condition so that they could intervene early to prevent deterioration, injury, complications, and infection. Technology also contributed to shortened hospital stays by promoting healing and helping nurses prepare patients for discharge. In addition, the new technologies better prevented nurses from injuring themselves while providing care. However, there are negatives associated with the new technologies, such as the challenges associated with broken equipment, how to operate/use complicated equipment, and how to keep up to date with changing technologies. Another downside of technology is that it can be addictive. Professionals and the public have come to believe that technology can solve all problems.

We live in a culture fascinated with new technology, almost to the point at which there is overconfidence in what technology can achieve and an overreliance on its use. Many people believe that technology can address and correct what is wrong, repair what is broken, and cure what ails us. Health care professionals are increasingly reliant on these technologies as their primary source of information. At times, technology has diverted nurses' attention away from the patient as a person (Barnard, 2009). In other words, nurses often find themselves watching a machine instead of observing, interacting with, and developing a relationship with the person who is attached to the machine. Direct care of the patient has been replaced by care of the patient via a machine! When nurses view patients in this way, what patients and their families have to say can be more easily ignored or discounted.

Doctors, nurses, and other health care professionals have come to believe that they alone are responsible for curing the patient and that the patient plays a minor role in their own recovery. This assumption is clearly erroneous. As Florence Nightingale, the founder of modern secular nursing, observed in the first book ever written on nursing, *Notes on Nursing,* back in 1860,

> It is often thought that medicine is the curative process. It is no such thing; medicine is the surgery of functions, as surgery proper is that of limbs and organs. Neither can do anything but remove obstructions; neither can cure; nature alone cures. Surgery removes the bullet out of the limb, which is an obstruction to the cure, but nature heals the wound. So it is with medicine; the function of an organ becomes obstructed; medicine, so far as we know, assists nature to remove the obstruction; but does nothing more. And what nursing has to do in either case is to put the patient in the best condition for nature to act upon him. (p. 133)

Nightingale's observation is no less true today than it was in 1860. Ultimately, the ability to rally and recover from disease and trauma resides in the person, and the role of the nurse (as well as that of other health care professionals) is to create the conditions that encourage and support the person's health and natural healing processes. Creating the conditions for health and healing can best take place when nurses develop a relationship with their patients. SBC is about "putting the patient in the best condition" by capitalizing on the person's strengths and supporting those areas that are functioning to allow the body and mind to heal.

THE CURRENT HEALTH CARE SYSTEM: A SYSTEM IN CRISIS

The past 20 years have been a period of major upheaval in health care systems worldwide. With escalating medical costs primarily brought on by the high demand for costly technologies and an increase in chronic care services due to an aging population, health care costs are spiraling out of control (Rachlis, 2004). Regardless of whether health care is publically funded, as in Canada, the United Kingdom and France, or partially government funded (e.g., Medicaid, Medicare), as in the United States, the challenge for all governments and health care systems has been how best to contain costs while meeting increasing expectations and demands on the part of their citizens for the latest medical technologies and providing quality health care.

Many hospital administrators have even turned to business models to find solutions to control and contain escalating costs. During the 1990s, hospitals merged to reduce duplication, eliminate waste, and consolidate services. Because nursing accounted for the largest portion of hospital budgets, nursing management and front-line nursing positions were slashed as hospitals downsized and merged and many services were transferred from tertiary hospitals (a hospital with a full complement of services) to community facilities or to home care (Rachlis, 2004). The effects were devastating on both patients and the nursing workforce. The loss of nursing expertise put patients' safety at risk, as reported in a landmark nursing study conducted by Linda Aiken and her colleagues at the University of Pennsylvania (Aiken, Clarke, Sloane, Sochalski, & Silber, 2002). They surveyed 10,000 staff nurses and 232,000 surgical patients. When the nurse:patient ratio went above four (i.e., when a nurse was assigned to care for more than four patients), for each additional patient cared for there was a 7% increase in the odds of a patient dying within 30 days. Moreover, nurses were more likely to experience burnout and job dissatisfaction. Six years after this study was published, Aiken and her group reported more specific features of the care environment on which the quality of patient care depends (Aiken, Clarke, Sloane, Lake, & Cheney, 2008). This study is described in Exhibit 1.1.

Patients and families became numbers and statistics. Health care services and professional values shifted from a focus on patients to a focus on the bottom line, the financial cost of care (Weiss, Malone, Merighi, & Benner, 2001).

Another measure taken to contain costs was to shorten hospital stays and send patients home early. Hospital stays are expensive when the costs of salaries, housekeeping, equipment, and food are all factored in. Administrators reasoned that

---

EXHIBIT 1.1

Empirical study *Downsizing and mergers of hospitals: Effects on nurses and patients*

The Problem
Does the environment in which a nurse practices make a difference to nurse and patient outcomes?

The Issues
It is known that the environment in which nurses practice can have a profound effect on both them and their patients. In particular, do management skills and their effects on staff relationships make a difference?

The Study
Aiken et al. (2008) collected data from more than 10,000 nurses and more than 230,000 surgical patients in 168 Pennsylvania hospitals. The care environments were classified according to the following two criteria: (a) quality of staff development and management and (b) interpersonal relationships. They then measured and analyzed outcomes that included nurse job satisfaction, burnout, intent to leave, and reports of quality of care, as well as mortality and failure to rescue in patients.

The Findings
Nurses reported more positive job experiences and fewer concerns with care quality in better practice environments. In these environments, there were significantly lower risks of death and failure to rescue. The care environment elements that had a positive effect on nurses and their nursing included staff development and the quality of management, nurse manager abilities, support given by management to nurses, and the collegial quality of the nurse–physician relationship.

The Bottom Line
The quality of patient care depends on the care environment in which nurses practice. In particular, the leadership and management of the nursing staff as well as their interactions with physicians can have a profound effect.

Source: Adapted from Aiken, Clarke, Sloane, Lake, & Cheney, (2008).

hospitals could save significant amounts of money by discharging patients home early or sending them to less expensive facilities, such as rehabilitation or convalescent institutions.

For the most part, people do recover faster and without complications in the comfort of their own surroundings, particularly when they and their families have access to professional support and advice. However, this is not always the case. When patients are sent home to be cared for by family members who feel ill prepared or have inadequate support, family caregivers often feel stressed and burdened themselves (Bull, 1990; Scherbring, 2002).

These are some of the changes that people have been dealing with as the health care system transforms itself. Although many of these changes have brought about improvements, they have also resulted in citizens experiencing high levels of dissatisfaction and frustration with the health care system and health care professionals.

Indicators That Something Is Amiss

There are many indicators that something is amiss within the current health care system. These indicators range from job dissatisfaction and nurse burnout, concern for patient safety, difficulties in patient–professional communication, increase in litigation suits, and an overall deterioration in quality care. A sample of studies illustrating that something is amiss is summarized in Table 1.2.

What do these responses have in common?

Many of these responses are primarily the result of health care professionals' failure to establish a connection with their patients and families and to work with them in ways that are meaningful to them. For professionals who care about patients and want to get to know them, the failure to develop a relationship with patients and advocate on their behalf have given rise to a new condition health professionals suffer. *Moral distress*, as it is called, surfaces when doctors and nurses feel trapped by the competing demands of the health care system and are unable to do what they believe to be right for their patients (Chen, 2009). In other words, the health care system puts system needs first and patient needs further down the priority list, causing health professionals to experience a sense of helplessness because they are unable to do what they believe is right for their patients.

By depersonalizing people, and treating them more as symptoms or numbers than as human beings, the health care system has unduly put people at risk rather than safeguarding and protecting them (Kohn et al., 2000).

HOW HAVE PEOPLE RESPONDED TO THE EFFECTS OF A DEFICIT-DOMINATED HEALTH CARE SYSTEM?

In response to the growing dissatisfaction with and mistrust of health care providers and the deterioration in the quality of health care services, citizens, professionals, organizations, and governments have organized to lobby for a different type of health care system based on a different set of values. Although many proposals have been

TABLE 1.2

Evidence that something is amiss in the health care system

Indicator	Study	Sample	Findings
Nurses' job satisfaction	Aiken et al. (2001)	43,000 nurses in 500 hospitals, five countries	Widespread dissatisfaction among nurses. High demands on nurse workforce, with reports of nurses having insufficient time to teach and counsel patients and families.
Patient safety	Kohn et al. (2000) Baker et al. (2004)	Meta-analysis of U.S. studies; Washington, DC The Canadian Adverse Events Study: the incidence of adverse events among hospital patients in Canada	Between 44,000 to 98,000 people die each year as a result of preventable medication errors, compared with fewer than 50,000 people who die of Alzheimer's disease. About seventy thousand (7.5%) of hospitalized patients experience preventable adverse events (estimated 9,000–24,000 preventable deaths in Canada annually due to error).
Patient–practitioner communication	Levinson et al. (1999) McGlynn et al. (2003)	Focus group of the frustrations among patients and physicians with managed care organizations American patients in hospitals	Disagreements between physicians and patients involved three areas: (a) allocation of resources, (b) access to care, and (c) financial arrangements. Patients expect a level of quality care that physicians cannot provide. Patients and physicians are not communicating, leading to patient and physician frustration. Fifty-five percent of patients are not getting treatment for which a sound evidence base exists, and approximately 10% are getting inappropriate treatments linked to problems in system design and provider–patient communication.
Quality of patient care	Jha et al. (2008)	Patients in U.S. hospitals, perceptions of care	Patients expressed need for improvement in nursing care, communication about medications, pain control, and provision of clear discharge instructions.

advanced to address these problems, the four key approaches to reorient health care service delivery are as follows:

1. Patient/person/family/relationship-centered care
2. The patient/person empowerment movement
3. Health promotion, illness prevention, and self-care
4. Collaborative partnership care

CAVEAT

Although each approach is discussed separately, it is important to keep in mind that they are interrelated (see Figure 1.1). They are derived from many of the same beliefs and core values about the person, a person's role in the health care system, and a person's relationships with health care providers.

Patient/Person/Family/Relationship-Centered Care

Person-centered, patient-centered, family-centered, and *relationship-centered care* are buzzwords being touted by health care institutions and practitioners to signify a "new" approach to care that is sensitive and responsive to patient needs. Person-centered care is about practitioners and the health care institution holding the patient's "personhood" central in clinical decision making (McCormack, 2003). Personhood is the right of people to have their values and beliefs respected. Each profession has its own concept of what person-centered care means.

Patient-Centered Medicine. In medicine, patient-centered care was proposed as a model to redress the public's dissatisfaction with the care they received from physicians, a dissatisfaction that arose because of physicians' education and training in the

FIGURE 1.1

Interrelationships among the four approaches.

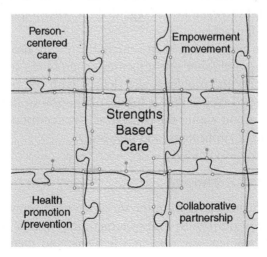

biomedical model, which focuses almost exclusively on the disease or problems rather than on the person who is dealing with the disease or problem (Stewart et al., 2003). The patient-centered model of medicine was developed to transform physicians' clinical method of practice and to incorporate ways to improve how they communicate with their patients. Patient-centered medicine, as conceptualized by Stewart and her colleagues, incorporates six interactive processes into medical clinical practice:

1. Exploring disease as well as the illness experience
2. Understanding the person at the personal level (i.e., life history), proximal level of influence (i.e., family, social support) and distal level (i.e., culture, community)
3. Finding common ground.
4. Enumerating problems, priorities, goals of treatment and/or management of the disease
5. Incorporating prevention and health promotion
6. Enhancing the patient–doctor relationship
7. Being realistic

Person/Family/Relationship-centered care in nursing. In nursing, person-centered care is not a new idea. The term has been around for over 50 years. It was coined in the 1960s by early nurse theorists, such as Faye Abdellah and Ernestine Wiedenbach, to shift the focus of nursing away from tasks and techniques to the patient or family as the center of the nurse's attention and their care (Abdellah, 1960; Wiedenbach, 1964). Dr. Myra Levine, another early nurse theorist, used the term *patient-centered nursing care* to refer to individualized nursing or care that was tailored to the unique needs and concerns of each patient (Levine, 1973). Patient-centered or individualized care required that nurses know their patients as unique human beings in order to be able to promote their recovery and help them return to a better state of health (Dunphy, 2009). In fact, hospital life during this period was fraught with some tension on the wards between the head nurse and her nursing battalion and the doctor-in-chief and his physician battalion. As Barnes (1961) summed up, the tension between these two factions was due to a difference in orientation: "Patient-centered nursing techniques and interest in human needs versus disease-centered medical techniques and interest in pathology" (p. 50). Moreover, nurses regarded the patient and human problems as their special domain of practice.

It is important to note that person-centered care can also be practiced from a deficit lens when the practitioner solely focuses on problems or weaknesses without considering or balancing the problems and deficits with the person's strengths. The appeal of person-centered care is that it brings the person to the forefront. The person's problem is understood within the context of his circumstances, past experiences, relationships, different environments, and lifeworlds.

Patient/Person Empowerment Movement

The idea of empowerment derives from the social action movements of the 1960s and the self-help ideology of the 1980s. Empowerment movements such as those seeking equal civil rights for women, gay men and lesbians, and members of racial/ethnic minority groups were borne out of frustration; a lack of control; and feelings of powerlessness, helplessness, hopelessness, and oppression. These groups felt marginalized and silenced at many levels of society.

The patient empowerment movement traces its roots to the rise of the consumer movement of the 1960s. Ralph Nader, an American lawyer and early consumer activist, was the David who took on Goliath, the giant automobile industry, to advocate for safer cars. His actions resulted in legislation that mandated the use of many safety devices in cars that we now take for granted, such as seat belts. Nader showed that one man could change a system to make it more responsive and accountable to the needs of its citizens. The idea that citizens could empower themselves to create change spread to other sectors of society, including the health care system (Sullivan, 1998).

Empowerment movements are grassroots or "bottom-up" movements whereby individuals and communities come together, find their voice, and organize themselves to change the status quo. Citizen empowerment movements advocate for better care in dealing with specific diseases, for the right of individuals to be treated with respect and dignity, to choose treatments, and to participate in decisions affecting their own health. Consider one of the earliest patient empowerment movements, the breast cancer movement, which showed how citizens could empower themselves to advocate for changes in their own health care as well as change in the health care system itself (see Exhibit 1.2).

What is meant by personal "empowerment"?

Empowerment is "a social process of recognizing, promoting, and enhancing people's abilities to meet their own needs, solve their own problems, and mobilize the necessary resources in order to feel in control of their own lives" (Gibson, 1991, p. 359). Thus, empowerment is the process of helping people help themselves to assert control over the things that matter to them and affect their health. Empowerment requires a number of qualities in order to be effective (Chamberlin, 1997), including

- access to information to help people make decisions,
- having a range of options from which to choose,
- assertiveness to express ideas and to stand up for oneself,
- the belief that one can make a difference, and
- learning to think critically.

Empowerment is premised on the belief that every person, family, and community has the capabilities, capacities, skills, competencies, and potential to assume responsibility for their own health as well as to gain some mastery over their own lives. It encompasses the belief that people, not health care professionals, empower themselves. Health care practitioners create the conditions that enable people to acquire the skills to foster their own empowerment (Gibson, 1991). Again, this approach requires an emphasis on the inherent and acquired strengths residing in individuals, families, and communities.

Health Promotion, Illness Prevention, Self-Care Culture

The current health care system is a misnomer. It is not a health care system but rather a disease care system. The majority of health care dollars are spent on diagnosing and treating disease; the sum is vast compared with the amount of money spent on

EXHIBIT 1.2

History The rise of the breast cancer movement

The breast cancer movement that arose in the 1970s in the United States is an excellent example of patients seizing the initiative for their own care. Up until then, it was virtually unheard of for a patient to challenge the opinion of a physician, because it was always assumed both by patient and doctor that all the relevant diagnostic and treatment data were solely in the possession of the physician.

This changed in 1975 when a young journalist named Rose Kushner questioned why she had to undergo a radical mastectomy procedure known as a Halstead, when data showed a modified procedure that involved only a partial mastectomy had been proven to be just as effective. Following her own diagnosis with breast cancer, she had to go to nineteen different surgeons before she found one who would consider this procedure. She then conducted extensive research that culminated in her publishing *Why Me? What Every Woman Should Know About Breast Cancer to Save Her Life*. This book proved to be the impetus that launched a patient-based movement that totally changed the dynamics of the patient–doctor relationship.

Within a short period of time, Kushner helped found the Breast Cancer Advisory Coalition (now known as the National Breast Cancer Coalition), which became not only a powerful advocate for breast cancer patients but also a key player in determining research funding and policy in the United States. This coalition included breast cancer patients as well as politicians, physicians, nurses, members of Congress, and media personalities. Together, they raised the public profile of breast cancer.

Ironically, when Rose Kushner first addressed a meeting of oncologists in 1976 she was booed off the platform. When she died in 1990, the American Medical Association gave her fulsome praise as a fighter against the war on breast cancer. Her activism provided a model for other patients suffering from high-profile diseases, such as heart disease, and stigmatized diseases, such as AIDS.

Source: Adapted from Casamayou (2001).

promoting health or preventing illness. Health promotion and disease prevention programs, such as parenting programs, school health, and safety and injury prevention, receive a relatively small proportion of the total health care budget. In the United States, for example, less than 5% of health care expenditures are dedicated to health promotion and illness prevention (Jacobs & Rapport, 2004).

A new culture of health promotion is starting to take hold. The cost of preventing a disease is significantly lower than the cost of treating the disease once it has occurred. Advocates of health promotion use the arguments that are captured in the phrase "PAY A SMALL AMOUNT NOW OR PAY A LOT MORE LATER." In other words, invest now in health education and the determinants of health that affect people's lifestyle choices with respect to diet, physical activity, sexual behavior, substance abuse, coping with stress, and the like in order to save money and lives later (McGinnis, Williams-Russo, & Knickman, 2002).

Take, for example, the diseases associated with smoking, such as lung cancer and heart disease. Consider what the costs of treating lung cancer and heart disease are. Now compare these costs with the costs of educating young people about the dangers of smoking; supporting smoking cessation programs; or getting at some of the root causes of smoking, such as stress, poverty, low self esteem, and peer pressure. Also, consider the cost of treating car injuries caused by a failure to use seat belts. What is the cost of intensive care and rehabilitation for a person involved in a car crash versus the cost of educating people in the proper use of car seats and safety belts?

Self-Care

Self-care is an important aspect of health promotion that is concerned with issues of autonomy, self-determination, and independence. In the 1970s, knowledge about self-care reached a broader public because of the wellness and self-help movements. It stressed that people "should gain confidence as health care consumers and that there were many options on the road to health and within medical treatment" (Kickbusch, 1989, p. 125).

In Canada, self-care was proposed as one of three key mechanisms in a health promotion framework aimed at achieving health for all Canadians, commonly referred to as the *Epp Report* (1986). This report defined health promotion, using the World Health Organization definition, as "the process of enabling people to increase control over, and to improve, their health". In addition to self-care, mutual aid, and the creation of healthy environments were the mechanisms advanced to promote health. In this context, *self-care* referred to "the decisions and actions individuals take in the interest of their own health". The Canadian self-care framework involves supporting the person, sharing knowledge, facilitating learning and personal development, helping the person build support networks, and providing a supportive environment (see Table 1.3; Health Canada, 1997).

A culture of health promotion, illness prevention, and self-care is premised on the belief that people can change their health behaviors and that they possess within themselves the power to change. It requires that people make better lifestyle choices for themselves. It also requires a different mindset on the part of individuals, families, communities, and government. People at each level need to rethink how to build and make better use of their strengths and assets. It also requires communities to provide environments that support health. For example, consider the recommendation that a healthy diet includes daily portions of fruits and vegetables. Fulfilling this requirement may be difficult for low-income families if they live in neighborhoods where there are few stores that sell fresh fruits and vegetables (Kawachi & Berkman, 2003). Although the change toward health promotion is primarily economically motivated to relieve the burden on the health care system by keeping people healthy, the culture of health promotion also requires a change in attitude on the part of many including communities, policy makers, and local and federal governments. However, most important it requires a change in attitude on the part of both the person and the health care professional. It requires that people want to assume greater responsibility for their health and make better lifestyle choices. It also asks nurses and health care professionals to make health promotion an integral part of their practice.

TABLE 1.3

Self-care framework

1. Supporting the person	• Conveying acceptance • Creating a climate of trust • Listening • Focusing on the person's strengths • Helping the person build self-confidence • Being accessible • Developing a relationship over time
2. Sharing knowledge	• Recognizing the experiential knowledge of the person • Providing information • Teaching skills • Suggesting resources
3. Facilitating learning and personal development	• Helping the person understand and name problems • Helping the person set goals • Going at the person's pace • Dividing learning into small steps • Encouraging the person to try things out • Modeling ways of approaching health problems • Focusing on strategic moments and key transitions
4. Helping the person build support networks	• Helping the person identify sources of support • Facilitating roles of natural caregivers and family members • Suggesting programs that provide support, e.g. support groups and self-help groups
5. Providing a supportive environment	• Providing an environment that is supportive in terms of its psychological, organizational and physical aspects

Source: Health Canada (1997).

Collaborative Partnership

Changes in the health care system have necessitated that roles and relationships between the person and health care provider be redefined. With the shift in care from hospital to home, individuals and families have had to assume greater responsibility for their own health care decisions and the management of their own care.

A collaborative partnership signifies a different relationship between the person and nurse and redefines the boundaries between them. Rather than the person being a passive recipient of care, she becomes a partner in her own care. This new relationship replaces the traditional hierarchical (paternalistic) relationship in which the health care provider is the expert, knows what's best for the person, and expects the person to comply with the prescribed treatment regimens. In contrast, the collaborative partnership approach to care requires, among other things, a willingness on the part of the nurse to share power with the person and to work together on mutually agreed upon goals (Gottlieb & Feeley, 2006). This approach recognizes and respects the experiences and expertise of both partners. It does not mean that the nurse relinquishes responsibility to the person. It does mean that the nurse listens to the person, recognizes the person's expertise, and together they work out a plan of care that is tailored to the person and famiy's goals, needs, lifestyle preferences, and circumstances.

This relationship encourages individuals to become more involved and to take greater responsibility for their care. People feel empowered when they are encouraged to express themselves and to believe that they have the capacity to find solutions to their own problems. Collaborative partnerships also encourage people because it enables them to get the help that best suits them.

Dr. Mary Grossman (2011) narrated the story of Eleanor Johnson, who was diagnosed with a very aggressive, Stage IV form of breast cancer. When Eleanor was given the diagnosis, she believed she would surely die. Eleanor was lucky to find an oncologist who saw her as a person with an illness and not just a case of breast cancer that needed to be treated. In Exhibit 1.3, Eleanor tells how her doctor entered into a collaborative partnership with her and how this partnership made all the difference in how she coped with the diagnosis. Eleanor's doctor made a difference in how Eleanor faced the long journey that awaited her: Fear and anxiety were replaced with feelings of calm and being in control.

WHAT DO THESE FOUR APPROACHES HAVE IN COMMON?

SBC brings these four approaches together under one umbrella. At the heart of person-centered care, the empowerment movement, the culture of health promotion, and collaborative partnership is the belief and valuing of the person and their strengths (see Figure 1.1). These approaches aim to create a more humane health care system that puts people first and is responsive to their needs. Although these four approaches may differ in focus, they share many common elements:

- A shift from illness, problems, and disease to health, coping, and development
- A shift from a disease model to a process model of a person living with an illness or condition
- A shift in focus from the practitioner and organization to the person and his personhood
- A rebalance in the power between practitioners and persons
- Recognition that the person, not the practitioner, is ultimately responsible for his own health.
- Recognition that a person is a unique human being who has the right to be treated with respect and dignity.
- Recognition that within every person, family, and community reside actual and potential strengths.

WHAT IS STRENGTHS-BASED CARE?

SBC is an orientation to guide practice:

- SBC places patients at the center of their own care (person-centered care).
- SBC empowers persons to achieve their own goals and find new meaning in their lives (empowerment movement).

- SBC is a prerequisite for change, a requirement for self-care that encourages a person to take charge of and be responsible for her own health, recovery, and healing (health promotion and illness prevention, self-care).
- SBC requires a collaborative relationship between the person and health care provider (collaborative partnership).
- SBC works with biological, intra- and interpersonal, and social strengths (resources, assets) to help the individual deal with challenges, meet goals, and function as integrated, whole person.
- SBC is a commitment to the person's development.

EXHIBIT 1.3

Personal experience *The story of Eleanor Johnson: The visible woman*

Eleanor Johnson had never been sick a day in her 45 years. So when her arm accidentally brushed against a solid lump lying along the outer aspect of her left breast, during her exercises that evening, she was momentarily incredulous but also knew instinctively that she was in trouble. When the doctor removed the aspiration needle from the center of the huge lump the next morning, she did not need to be told the significance of the empty syringe. A swell of anxiety and fear overcame her normally collected composure. She was going to die. "You know what this means," the doctor said, oblivious to the fact that she was struggling to concentrate on what he was saying. "You have cancer. You need a biopsy. You'll need to be booked for surgery and then chemotherapy. Come back in a couple of weeks for the biopsy results." And that was that.

Eleanor took control over her own health care by deciding the type of oncologist she wanted and seeking out one that would fit her way of doing things. When Eleanor received the biopsy report, she learned that the news was extremely grim, stage 4 of an extremely aggressive tumor that had a poor prognosis. She made the decision to find an oncologist with a team approach. "Yes, it is aggressive but there are things we can do. Remember that a prognosis is about the natural trajectory of the illness before the medical intervention. Statistics say nothing about how you personally will respond to treatment." With that, the load of fear and anxiety started to lift. "Don't forget," the oncologist added, "there is a whole team behind you. We have an idea of what we want to do- but we also are consulting with colleagues at several leading cancer centers." For the first time, Eleanor began to feel safe. But there was still something else she needed to understand. "But I don't fit a protocol? Her anxiety soared again. "True, but we have something else- your cancer to help direct us to the best combination of treatments. We think the surgery should be delayed until we try to make the tumor smaller- and then we can monitor its response to the chemotherapy." "Ok" she persisted. "But I have a hard time just doing nothing." "Who says you have nothing to do? Your work is to eat healthy food, stay calm, and walk everyday. My job will be to take care of your treatment." He could see she was hesitating, not

(continued)

EXHIBIT 1.3 (*Continued*)

totally convinced. "I know you have a PhD in physiology—are you interested in me sending you a key article before our next meeting so we can review the pros and cons of the options I'm considering?"' And then Eleanor knew that she was fortunate. This was not for every patient, but it was perfect for her.

Source: Story told in Grossman, (2011).

The SBC approach varies from discipline to discipline. For example, the positive psychology movement uses the word *positives* to refer to qualities that work best (i.e., strengths). Its focus includes the mental processes involved in happiness, well-being, quality of life, self-actualization, flow and personal growth, and it looks to those positives within the person so that the person can better enhance them (Snyder & Lopez, 2002).

The field of social work uses a strengths perspective to develop strengths and resilience to help persons, families, and communities overcome adversity (Saleebey, 1996; Saleebey, 2008; Walsh, 2006).

Counseling psychology professionals and early childhood special educators have as their overriding goal the facilitation of growth by focusing on individuals' innate strengths and the promotion of social change (Smith, 2006). They often use strength-based interventions to support families in which children are at risk for psychopathology and delinquency. These programs target families who may be experiencing pervasive poverty, a history of family and community violence, inadequate health care, substance abuse, and the like (Powell, Batsche, Ferro, Fox, & Dunlap, 1997). Counseling psychology and early childhood education professionals focus on strengthening families to create health-promoting environments for its members, particularly young children.

Medicine uses a strengths perspective when subscribing to whole-person care. Physicians who practice whole-person care continue to diagnose and treat patients through a biomedical lens; however, their focus is on treating the whole person and that person's medical condition in the context of her life. They consider the impact of the medical condition on the person and are sensitive to patients' suffering and their personhood and how these relate to their health care (Hutchison, 2011; Mount, 1993).

For nursing, working with the person's and family's strengths allows patients to maximize and support their responses, in order to deal with everyday events and difficult life challenges (including illness, injury, disability and trauma) and to meet their goals (Allen, 1977; Feeley & Gottlieb, 2000). This approach has also been used in health promotion, to enhance wellness and well-being (Leddy, 2006). Strengths can be biological, intra- and interpersonal, and social. Biological strengths are related to the biochemical, genetic, hormonal, and physical qualities within each individual. Intrapersonal and interpersonal strengths reside in the person and define his personhood and are considered a part of a person's inner resources. Social strengths, commonly known as *resources* or *assets*, reside in the person's environment and are available to him.

Working with strengths enables a person to get the most out of living in order to cope, recover, heal, and discover new purpose and meaning in living. SBC is an approach to care in which the nurse identifies and develops the person's and family's strengths. The nurse, in collaborative partnership with the patient and family, then works with their strengths to help them deal with their problems to achieve their health goals. As Nurse Andra Leimanis explained: "*Working with strengths is the major part of what I do. You want to build on those strengths, to work through those problems areas, to work through that dark cloud. As a nurse, you need to ask yourself 'What's going to be the driving force? What's going to support you (during these dark periods)?' It's fundamental to gain awareness of those positives and work with them because it is the person's strengths that will help them to face their dark clouds.*"

SBC does not ignore or negate problems; neither does it turn a blind eye to weaknesses or deficits. Instead, it uses strengths to balance or overcome them. SBC, at its core, is about looking for what is working and capitalizing and mobilizing those areas within the person, and in the person's life, that are working. In SBC, the conversation shifts from "What is wrong?" to "What is right?" and "What has happened or is happening?" to "What is working?" This change in thinking places the problem within the context of what else is happening in a person's life that may directly or indirectly affect how the patient and family are responding to and coping with their challenges.

> SBC is not about ignoring or negating problems rather it is about using strengths to counterbalance, contain, or minimize weaknesses to allow what is working to function effectively.

Practitioners who subscribe to SBC begin with an appreciation of the complexity of the human being and the innate strengths of the human spirit. They have the knowledge, judgment, and skills to recognize, support, and develop the person's strengths—which can be biological, psychological, and/or social in nature—to achieve better health outcomes.

Nurse Sophie Baillargeon summarized what SBC is: "*Every person has some kind of strength within them. It is there for the nurse to find. It is how the nurse can help them work within their situation to deal with their concerns. Some issues are difficult. Some situations may not be going well, but it is how the person goes through the situation and the way they cope with it that is important. That's the strength. As nurses, we are here to help them see that they can cope. We help them build on what they have and give them other ways to get through difficult situations.*" Sophie continued: "*. . . Strengths are the person's tools to help them work around their more problematic issues. If you only work at problematic issues, you deplete the person's energy. By bringing strengths, people come to believe in themselves. And then as a nurse you can help them figure out other ways to work through their more difficult issues.*"

How Does Deficit-Based Care Compare to Strengths-Based Care?

The major features of SBC are summarized and compared with deficit-based care (DBC; Table 1.4) and are briefly described below.

The *primary focus* of DBC is to understand what is not working (deficits) and how to correct or "fix" it. In contrast, the primary focus of SBC is to understand what is working and to use what is working, what the person is capable of doing, as a means to minimize symptoms and find solutions to help the person develop—and, in the case of

TABLE 1.4

Comparison of the deficit-based care and strengths-based care

Distinguishing Features	Deficit-Based Care	Strengths-Based Care
Primary aim	A focus on problems, what is missing (deficits), not working, malfunctioning and dysfunctional. Labels behaviors by giving a diagnosis or slotting the person into a category. Requires patient compliance with treatment decisions. Looks to "fix" problems.	A focus on what is working, what capabilities the person has while dealing with concerns and problems. A focus on how the person copes or deals with adversity and rallies from insults. Avoids labels and instead focuses on the person and her personhood. Uses strengths to build confidence to deal with concerns. The person is responsible for finding his own solutions; the nurse supports, creates conditions, scaffolds, compensates, and encourages. Supports and facilitates innate mechanisms of health, recovery, and healing.
Context	Context-stripped: Problem is viewed in isolation with little or no consideration of the person's situation, past experience, or current circumstances.	Context is critical to understanding the person's concerns and goals. All issues are "situated." Health and illness are understood in light of the person's situation, past and current experiences, culture, relationships, and the social/economic/political environment.
Language	Negative language: *disease, dysfunction, deficiency.* Language of fear.	Positive language: *strength, energy, challenges, opportunities, possibilities.* Language of hope.
Relationship	Traditional hierarchical relationship; "practitioner-knows-best" model. The person is expected to assume a passive role, as a recipient of care.	Collaborative partnership in which the nurse, the team, with the person and family jointly make decisions, create the plan, and work together to find solutions.
Primary source of information	Values objective data over subjective data. Focuses on the medical and health status. Nurses use multiple sources of information but rely heavily on technological equipment and machines for information, such as laboratory tests, biopsies, X-rays.	Values subjective information: what the person feels, thinks, and experiences. Focuses on the person's health and life. The person and family are primary sources of information. Importance is placed on the person's story, narratives, reflections, experiences as gained during clinical conversations. Values multiple sources of information, including objective data from laboratory tests, biopsies, and X-rays. Values, appreciates, and requires different ways of knowing, including empirical data, personal experience, moral/ethical comportment, and aesthetics to understand the whole.

(continued)

TABLE 1.4

Comparison of the deficit-based care and strengths-based care   (*Continued*)

Distinguishing Features	Deficit-Based Care	Strengths-Based Care
		Knowledge is derived from formal education and practical experience and is created through experience and reflection.
Basis for decision-making: Plan of care	Differential diagnosis, diagnostic reasoning, and problem-based approaches to diagnosis are the tools for decision making. Plan of care is based on what needs "fixing." Prescriptive: One size fits all. Nurses carry out doctors' orders when plan is medical. In decisions governing nursing action, nurses diagnose the problem and use a standardized care plan to fix or correct the problem.	Knowledge is derived from a complex process of clinical reasoning and clinical judgment. Plan of care is built on the person's strengths. Situation responsive; one size fits no one. The nurse works in partnership with the team and the patient/client/family to plan and manage care. The plan is customized to the uniqueness of the person and family and their situation.
Outcomes	Measured in terms of how well the practitioner was able to "fix" the problem. A dead end. If the problem is not satisfactorily resolved, the nurse and team may feel they have run out of options.	Person and family determine outcomes: what is important to them including subjective well-being and their quality of life. Focus is on strengths, possibilities, empowerment, engagement, and energizing the person. Effects can motivate; energize; increase self-awareness; promote self-discovery; improve rallying, rebounding, and recovery; create hope; empower; and promote development through growth and transformation.

Source: Based on a synthesis of ideas from Allen (1977); Benner, Sutphen, Leonard, and Day (2010); Carper (1978); Gottlieb and Feeley (2006); Gottlieb and Gottlieb (2007); Maddux (2002a); McAllister (2003); Saleebey (2008); and Sullivan (2003).

a patient, to recover and heal. For example, in treating pain, a nurse who uses DBC may give a medication without exploring other ways to treat the pain. On the other hand, a nurse who uses SBC may know her patient and has learned that this patient enjoys music. The nurse knows that the patient's hearing is intact (a capability or strength) and may suggest that the patient listens to music as a way of distracting her when the pain is most acute and before the medication has had time to reach its peak effect.

Nurses who practice from a DBC perspective believe that the problem can be understood in its own right without placing the problem in *context;* that is, without reference to or knowledge of the person's situation, history, or circumstance. For example, a nurse may find that a patient is rude and withdrawn. She may interpret the patient's behavior as negative and label the patient as antisocial, disturbed, or difficult. In contrast, SBC nurses believe that the patient's behavior can best be understood by knowing that person, her situation, and the circumstances affecting her. The nurse looks for patterns of response. Is this patient's behavior unusual? In taking the time to talk with the patient, the nurse comes to learn that the patient has recently lost her grandson in an automobile accident and that today is the 6-month anniversary of his untimely death.

These two approaches also differ in the *language* they use. In DBC, clinicians often use a lot of "D" words as part of their vocabulary, such as *disaster, deficit, detrimental, dysfunction,* and so on. It is language that is associated with criticism and blame. This language sets a tone for confrontation that often leads to fear and despair (another D word!). For example, when a patient does not improve, the patient may be "blamed" for not following the medical regimen or for not taking the medication as prescribed. On the other hand, SBC language is more positive in tone and uses language that communicates hope. The nurse looks to encourage and reinforce what the person does well, what is working. He seeks to understand the patient's capabilities and capacities. SBC language uses words that communicate growth, energy, transformation, possibilities, and opportunities.

In DBC, the practitioner tends to view the person as a "case" or "disease," not as a person who has experience, knowledge, and capabilities and who is competent to make decisions. DBC practitioners believe they have to do *for* the person rather than *with* the person. In SBC, the *relationship* is collaborative. The person and nurse respect each other's expertise and trust each other's judgment. Nurses see themselves both as learners as well as educators. They knows that patients are their best teachers and that they have much to learn from them. They also see themselves as educators and teachers, guiding patients in making decisions in matters of health and health care.

DBC and SBC both rely on multiple *sources of information*, including the results of objective testing (e.g., laboratory reports, X-rays), visual images, empirical research, and the like to understand the problem. In addition to objective, technical information, SBC nurses place high value on the person's subjective understanding of how they view themselves and what is happening to them by talking, listening, and piecing together their narratives.

In DBC, creating the person's treatment plan and making decisions is primarily the responsibility of the practitioner, whereas in SBC the nurse and person, where appropriate, devise a customized plan that capitalizes on the person's strengths and capabilities. Together, they fashion a plan that is responsive to the person's situation because such a situation-responsive plan is believed to have the best chance to succeed. When patients have a say, they devise plans that take into account their realities and that which they realistically can follow. In contrast, DBC practitioners give patients plans that are prescriptive. In other words, every patient with that condition is prescribed the same, one-size-fits-all treatment that in reality

> When nurses capitalize on the person's strengths, they are creating conditions that support and encourage the person's innate health and natural healing processes.

fits no one. It does not take into account the possibility that the person' has a unique way of responding physiologically, psychologically, and behaviorally.

The *effects* of focusing on deficits can be demoralizing and lead to a sense of frustration for both the nurse and the person. This sense of frustration results when clinicians play on patients' fears, intentionally or unintentionally, to convince them to comply with what they believe to be is in the patients' best interest. Often one hears a well-intentioned nurse warn patients of the dangers of their actions, thereby playing to their fears: "If you don't lose weight, you will have a heart attack." They can often reach a dead end when all options to resolve a situation have been exhausted. In contrast, working with strengths may require more effort, yet it also opens up more possibilities. Together, the nurse and the person can explore different treatment options. Looking for different solutions often generates hope, and hope is in and of itself often empowering.

Nurse Danielle Beaucage clearly identified the effects of SBC on both the nurse and patient: *"[SBC] works because if somebody focuses on your strengths you tend to trust that person more. There are strengths in every individual. It makes nursing more relevant and more fun. Working with a person's strength helps to establish a collaborative partnership. It also helps the patient and nurse to have more realistic goals because you're building on something together. Even to acknowledge strengths is in and of itself an extremely valuable nursing intervention."*

Danielle describes caring for a patient with whom other nurses had difficulty dealing: *"Once I reframed his stubbornness as a strength, as a positive side of his personality, I saw him differently. I often thought, 'If he did not have this personality he would be dead.' It really helped me to take care of him."*

Now reread the story told earlier in this chapter by Nurse Gillian Taylor, who cared for Sarah and her family. Reflect on the features of SBC and then connect them to Gillian's care of Sarah and her family. Take a few minutes to complete the exercise in Table 1.5.

THE EVIDENCE THAT STRENGTHS-BASED CARE BENEFITS PERSONS AND FAMILIES

Focusing on strengths has been found to be effective with different populations (e.g., adolescents, parents, elderly individuals), in dealing with a wide range of problems and conditions (e.g., acute and chronic illness, mental health, health promotion), and in different settings (hospital, ICU, community, workplace; for relevant review articles and book chapters, see Hodges & Clifton, 2004; Powell et al., 1997; Snyder & Lopez, 2002). Studies have found that persons cared for by practitioners who focus on positives and strengths have shown improvements in their health and quality of life (Bluvol & Ford-Gilboe, 2004), better subjective well-being (King, 2008), improved resiliency (Walsh, 2006), greater personal growth, more positive relationships (Fredrickson, 2008), and increased control and self-efficacy (a can-do attitude; Maddux, 2002b). Moreover, health care professionals who subscribe to a strengths-based philosophy have developed therapies that cultivate specific strengths, such as hope (Worthington et al., 1997), optimism (Carver & Scheier, 2002; Seligman, 2006), subjective well-being (King, 2008), positive emotions (Fredrickson, 2008), better mental health outcomes (Klausner, Snyder, & Cheavens, 2000), and improved couple relationships (Worthington et al., 1997). Consider the strength of hope. Klausner et al. (2000) found that a hope-focused group intervention conducted with depressed elderly individuals

TABLE 1.5

Reflect and connect: Strengths-Based Care in practice

Distinguishing Features	Strengths-Based Care	Nurse Gillian Taylor and Sarah and Her Family
Primary aim of care	Focuses on what is working, what is best, while dealing with concerns, problems, illness, and disability. Focus is on how the person copes or deals with adversity and rallies from insults. Avoids labels and categories and focuses on the person and her personhood. Uses strengths to build confidence to deal with concerns. Looks for solutions instead of dwelling on problems. Supports and facilitates coping, healing, and development.	
Context	Context is critical to understanding the person's concerns and goals. Health and illness are understood in light of the person's situation, past and current experiences, culture, relationships, and the social/economic/political environment.	
Language	Language is positive, associated with words such as *strength, energy, challenges, opportunities, possibilities.* Language of hope.	
Relationship	Collaborative partnership in which practitioner and person jointly make decisions, create the plan, and work together to achieve the person's health goals.	
Primary source of information	The nurse's primary source of information is the person and family. Values subjective information: what the person feels, thinks, and experiences. Importance is placed on the person's story, narratives, reflections, and experiences as gained during clinical conversations. Values multiple sources of information, including objective data from laboratory tests, biopsies, and X-rays. Values, appreciates, and requires different ways of knowing, including empirical data, personal experience, moral/ethical comportment, and aesthetics to understand the whole person. Knowledge is derived from formal education and practical experience and created through experience and reflection.	

(continued)

TABLE 1.5

Reflect and connect: Strengths-Based Care in practice   *(Continued)*

Distinguishing Features	Strengths-Based Care	Nurse Gillian Taylor and Sarah and Her Family
Basis for decision making: Plan of care	Knowledge is derived from a complex process of clinical reasoning and clinical judgment. Plan of care is built on the person's strengths. Situation responsive; one size fits no one. The nurse works in partnership with the team and the patient to plan and manage care. The plan is customized to the uniqueness of the person and his situation.	
Outcomes	Focuses on strengths and possibilities that empower, engage, energize, motivate, energize, increase self-awareness, promote self-discovery, improve rallying and recovery, create hope, and promote development through the person's growth and transformation.	

Reflect and Connect Instructions:

1. Reread Gillian Taylor's nursing of Sarah and her family.
2. Reflect on the features of SBC and then connect them to Gillian's care of Sarah and her family.
3. Identify the behaviors that illustrate these features.

reduced mild depression and anxiety and promoted adjustment. When used with couples, hope-focused therapy enhanced the couples' relationships by improving relationship satisfaction and quality-of-couple skills (Worthington et al., 1997). Moreover, when practitioners direct therapy to cultivating positive emotions, the effects of this therapy not only counteract negative emotions but also build on personal resources that enable people to cope with and optimize their own feelings of health and well-being (Fredrickson, 2000).

One of the only nursing intervention studies to use a strengths-approach was a randomized controlled trial that examined whether children with chronic physical disorders had better psychosocial adjustments if they and their family received care by nurses whose nursing was guided by the McGill Model of Nursing (Pless, Feeley, Gottlieb, Rowat, Dougherty, & Williard, 1994). (The McGill Model of Nursing focuses on understanding the person, family issues, and working with strengths within a collaborative partnership; Gottlieb & Rowat, 1987.) The results of this study are summarized in Exhibit 1.4.

As part of the study described in Exhibit 1.4, some of the parents were randomly selected from families who had received the specialized care (i.e., SBC) for an in-depth interview about their experiences (Ezer, Bray, & Gros, 1997). Parents assigned to the intervention group were asked to describe what they thought about the nursing they had received. Parents reported positive child- and family-related changes following the intervention. Almost 89% of families reported that their children took more responsibility

EXHIBIT 1.4

Empirical study *The effects of specialized nursing (strengths based/collaborative partnership) on children with chronic physical disorders*

The Problem
Could specialized nursing care (strengths-based care) help prevent or reduce psychosocial problems among children with chronic physical disorders?

The Issues
Children with chronic physical disorders often suffer from psychosocial problems. Does specialized nursing care help prevent or reduce psychosocial problems?

The Study
Pless et al. (1994) investigated whether a strengths-based form of nursing care could help prevent or reduce psychosocial problems among children, aged four to sixteen years, with chronic physical disorders. A randomized clinical trial was conducted in which 332 children and their families were randomly assigned either to receive this specialized nursing for a one-year period or to remain in the control condition. Three measures of psychosocial functioning administered before and after the intervention were the basis for assessing its efficacy.

The Findings
Statistically significant positive differences were found in those families who received the nursing intervention: The children were reported by their parents to be less anxious and/or depressed after the intervention, and their scholastic competence and behavior improved, as did their global self-worth.

The Bottom Line
Specialized nursing intervention (Strengths-Based Care) can help children with chronic disorders deal with their medical conditions by preventing or reducing any psychosocial problems they may have.

Source: Adapted from Pless et al. (1994).

for their health. Moreover, parents noted improvements in almost all aspects of their child's life, as reflected in the following themes from the interviews: "doing better at school," "having greater self-confidence," and "spending more time as a family." Parents also reported that they liked the approach that nurses took with them. They felt that the nurses treated them as unique individuals and gave them "time to discuss all kinds of things," which made them feel that they were "more than just a number." Families explained that when nurses focused on strengths, it helped them to see themselves in a new light and proved to be an important first step in considering what to change. For many of these parents, who were not used to hearing what they were doing right, they said that it was good to "[hear] that we were doing something right."

Consistent with these findings, in another study that evaluated the effects of a family systems nursing intervention that included commendations (i.e., nurses noting what families were doing well) for families found that families reported that focusing on strengths was very therapeutic (Robinson & Wright, 1995). In a more recent, small qualitative study of adolescents who were at risk for suicide, patients were asked what nursing interventions they found to be most helpful (Gros, Jarvis, Mulvogue, & Renaud, 2011). Of the many things that these adolescents reported about the nursing they had received, what they found most helpful was when the nurse focused on their strengths. These adolescents commented or advised the following: *"Focus on the positive," "Notice the parents care…that will help so much, cuz…if you're going to therapy, you're saying your problems. It's negative, negative, negative."* Another patient linked nursing action to patient outcome and in so doing sent a powerful message: *"Pointing out the things you're good at makes you want to live. It really does. It makes you think that you're not completely worthless."*

Our consultants and front-line nurses provided further validation of the effectiveness of SBC from the feedback they have received from their patients and clients. Many felt that focusing on the person and family strengths played an important role in helping patients find new directions and helping them take greater responsibility for their own health. Some of their patients credited their nurses with helping to improve their self-confidence and to feel more empowered.

The following insights are a selection of statements from some of the expert consultants' interviews of why they value and have adopted SBC as their nursing orientation and approach.

Nurse Lidia De Simone explained her rationale for using a strengths approach: *"It is important not to lose sight of a person's strengths because if you lose sight of their strengths, their unique qualities, the person's confidence goes down and they won't have the energy to deal with whatever it is that they are dealing with."*

Nurse John Kayser told of the feedback he has received from the patients he works with on addiction issues: *"My patients tell me: 'You believed in me when I didn't believe in myself and your belief in me raised doubts in my own mind that if you think I can, well maybe I can,' and that moves them forward."*

Nurse Catherine Gros summarized why this is an important approach for the person: *"Not listening, not tuning in to that person can be very damaging. I have never had a case in which understanding and working with someone's strengths has had a bad outcome. Even when the person is dying and may not survive, there is a good outcome in terms of the relationship I am able to develop with them."*

The Benefits of Strengths-Based Care for Nurses

Clinicians who choose to practice from a strengths perspective reveal something about themselves, their values, and what they feel committed to and passionate about, what they oppose and what they are willing to advocate for. As Charles Taylor (1991), the renowned philosopher observed that we become what we are by virtue of how we decide to look at others as well as ourselves. Nurse Sharyn Andrews, one of our consultants, affirmed Taylor's observation. She reported that nurses who practice from SBC have told her, *"I feel good about myself when I work with families in this way."* In working with strengths, nurses reveal and find expression of their own humanity.

Nurses who see the person rather than the disease or condition learn about the human spirit. They come to appreciate that people find courage even when tragedy strikes. It is working with people during periods of vulnerability that nurses find themselves admiring and being inspired by their patients. This type of respect at times borders on awe. It brings nurses great satisfaction and fosters a special connection between them and their patients. Nurses have used phrases such as "amazing people" and "I feel honored and privileged to care for them" to describe their patients.

Nurse Charlotte Evans cared for Diane, a woman suffering from the debilitating neuromuscular condition, amyotrophic lateral sclerosis, during the final weeks of an eight-year battle. Charlotte summarized her feelings of admiration for Diane, who handled herself with great dignity, continued to protect her husband despite her own rapid deterioration, and remained involved in all the decisions concerning her care up until death. Nurse Evans: *"I know this sounds cheesy, but she was very strong. She was an amazing woman, really an amazing woman. I think I was so privileged to have known her and cared for her."*

Nurse Margaret Eades believes that SBC is the key that fosters the nurse–patient relationship and facilitates the health work that they do together: *"Using a strengths approach helps me get right to the heart of where I can begin to work because whatever I do is of no consequence unless the person is interested in what I have to offer. And I have to find that kernel (key) to build the relationship. Focusing on the person's strengths is that kernel."*

Nurse Caroline Marchionni summed up what focusing on strengths "buys" her that a deficit approach just doesn't: *"I use strengths because what else are you going to focus on, the negative? 'You didn't get out of bed today?' or 'We don't have your pain under control.' Then why bother?... Positivity breeds positivity in the same way that negativity breeds negativity. When you're around somebody who's in a bad mood, then you often find yourself in a bad mood. Positivity is contagious, too."*

Nurse Lidia De Simone described how SBC has added value to the way she nurses: *"I learned that focusing on people's strengths was really going to help them use what tools they have. I remember saying 'I can do more with this interaction, but I didn't know what to do or how to do it..' Working with strengths was the key. I could continue the conversation with people. I didn't focus on deficits and I didn't say to them everything that was wrong or what they couldn't do. Working with their strengths either gave them some 'gas' because they felt good about themselves and they would say to me, 'Oh yeah, you know, that's true; maybe I could do that if I approached it in this way.'"*

Nurses are in a privileged position because they often are privy to the inner world of the person who is suffering. If they are able to connect with their patients and create a relationship of trust, patients will share their most intimate thoughts and feelings of vulnerability as well as their dreams and goals for the future.

Health care practitioners have generally measured the effectiveness of their work in terms of morbidity and mortality outcomes. There is some recognition that these outcomes do not capture the things that are important to patients. If the aim of patient-centered care is the patient's health, helping the person recover and heal, and to find new meaning and purpose in living, then different outcomes must be considered in addition to morbidity and mortality. There is a need to shift from solely measuring health status via the body to those outcomes that concern the patient's quality of life and whatever is important to them (Sullivan, 2003). As Sullivan (2003) astutely observed,

> Each step in this direction (towards measuring outcomes in terms of health or patient's life rather than in terms of outcomes of the body) brings medicine

(medicine being used here in its generic sense to encompass all health care practices) closer to pursuing "what really matters to patients" and also brings greater scientific, ethical, and social complexity. Subjective health is more meaningful to patients than objective health measures such as coronary artery stenosis or joint space narrowing. But it introduces many complex factors into the core of medicine beyond tissue diagnosis or organ impairment. Now medicine must concern itself with the perceiver of ill health as well as the ill body. (p. 1602)

SBC is an approach to care that enables nurses to broaden their scope of practice and sphere of influence by improving the lives of the person and family with whom they are called to care for, regardless of whether it is during normative life transitions or during unexpected, unplanned and often unwelcomed and undesirable life events.

Key Summary Points

- SBC is an approach to care that focuses on and works with a person's and family's strengths to promote health, recovery, and healing.
- The medical model is a systematic approach to diagnosis and treatment of disease that, when used to reduce the person to a diseased body part rather than to understand the person as a whole, has contributed to DBC.
- Although the growth of technology has improved medical diagnoses and treatment, it has also contributed to a distancing between the nurse and the patient.
- Patient/person-centered care, the empowerment movement, health promotion/self-care, and collaborative partnership have been proposed to address the shortcomings of the current health care system. The underlying foundation of these four movements is a focus on a person and family's strengths.
- SBC restores the person to the center of care and helps empower patients to take greater control over their lives and their health care decisions.
- SBC places illness care in the context of knowing and appreciating the whole person situated within their own context and lifeworlds.
- SBC works with what is working and what is functioning best. Strengths can be biological, intra- and interpersonal, and social (resources and assets) that enable people to deal with challenges and function as integrated whole human beings.
- SBC differs from DBC in terms of its purpose, consideration of context, use of language, nature of the nurse–patient relationship, source of information, how decisions are made, and types of outcomes considered important.
- Nurses and health care practitioners who practice SBC look to discover potentials, possibilities, and opportunities to help people manage their illness and deal with life events.
- SBC is a rewarding approach for both the person who seeks help and for the nurse who gives care.
- SBC helps to define nurses' professional identity by how they care for others, how they see themselves, and how others see them.

What Guides Practice?

2

LEARNING OBJECTIVES

After reading this chapter, you should be able to:

- Define three significant forces that guide nursing practice
- Describe how values, beliefs, and attitudes develop
- Describe why it is important for nurses to identify the values underpinning their practice
- Describe what a theoretical perspective is
- Describe what happens in the absence of a theoretical perspective
- Explain how a theoretical orientation can affect a nurse's work environment

One of the most important questions that nurses can ask themselves is "What guides my practice?" (Cody, 2006). The reason this is such an important question is because the way the nurse answers it can provide insights into what influences those automatic, almost intuitive practice responses, or those deliberate day-to-day decisions of care. Nurses may be able to describe what a good nurse is, or what constitutes good nursing care; however, when they examine their actual nursing there may or may not be a disconnect between what they think they do and how they actually practice.

Most nurses are unaware of why they do what they do, but when they stop to reflect on what they do and the reasons why they do what they do, they discover that their practice is rooted in tradition, knowledge, and experience, as well as the culture and practice norms of their work environments. It is also very much rooted in the nurse's social imaginings, that is, how he imagines things to be, how he sees himself, and his ways of

> When nurses become aware of their values, they are more likely to practice in ways that inspire them to nurse in a manner that reflects who they are, what is important to them, and what they believe to be morally right.

behaving (Taylor, 2004). What may be less obvious to many nurses is the powerful role that values, attitudes, and beliefs play in shaping their practice decisions. When nurses become aware of their values, attitudes, and beliefs they are in a better position to control their own practice so that they can perform their professional duties that is consistent with what is important to them. Such an awareness puts them in a better position to practice in ways that reflect who they are and what they believe to be the right way to nurse.

When Nurse Sophie Baillargeon began as a head nurse on a neurological intensive care unit, children under age 18 were not allowed to visit their gravely ill parents. Sophie, who had previously worked at a children's hospital, believed that children should be encouraged to visit their ill parents to help them understand what is happening and that this was critical in how they eventually would deal with their parent's illness—or, in some cases, how they would come to terms with their parent's death. Sophie noted that many of the very ill patients on her unit were in their 40s and 50s and were parents of young children. She believed that the current hospital visiting policies did not meet the needs of these families, and so she began the process of revising the visiting policy on her unit to allow young children to visit their critically ill or dying parent.

The first step to changing the visiting policy was to prepare the staff by talking about families, what family members needed, and how best to work with them and their children. Sophie described the process she undertook: *"My assistant head nurse and myself tried to bring the children to see their parents in the [intensive care unit], especially when the parent was dying. When we did this there were a lot of emotions and opinions on the part of the staff nurses. Nurses were saying: 'That could be my child. I would never bring my child here to see me with all those drains, tubes, and all that is going on.' I invited the nurses to join us in working with these children and families. Together, we read the literature on child development—how children think, how they talk, and how we can talk with them. The assistant head nurse gave some children teddy bears when they visited their critically ill parent. It was interesting to see what the children did with those teddy bears. Children used the teddy bears very differently. Some hugged them. Some cried in them. Some left them with their parent, and some brought the teddy bear home."*

In this chapter, I return to Sophie's story to examine how her imaginings, values, beliefs, and attitudes guided her nursing and the decisions she made.

WHAT ARE SOME OF THE FORCES AND FACTORS THAT GUIDE PRACTICE?

Many forces and factors influence practice, such as the nurse's knowledge, life and work experiences, the policies and attitudes of the workplace and so forth. The most significant forces, however, are the nurse's own personal and professional values, beliefs, and attitudes.

Values, Beliefs, and Attitudes

Values are powerful determinants that guide human actions. Values are those things that really matter to a person. Because they really matter, values hold great sway in influencing how a person thinks, feels, and behaves, and the choices she makes.

What does Nurse Baillargeon value? Sophie values family relationships, including children and their development. She also values collaborative partnerships with colleagues, that is, working through issues together.

Different sets of values govern different aspects of a person's life. For example, values encompass personal–cultural, ethical–moral, political–religious, social, and aesthetic domains (see Table 2.1).

Beliefs are the lens through which a person views the world. Beliefs are convictions that a person thinks is true. Beliefs are a person's explanations of how they understand themselves, their world, and what has happened to them. Beliefs help a person make sense of what is happening to them (Wright & Bell, 2009; Wright, Watson, & Bell, 1996). Beliefs underpin and guide behavior and actions.

People can hold beliefs about another person (e.g., "I believe he is trying to gain control over the situation and that is why he is so difficult and hard to get along with") or an event (e.g., "I believe that I got sick because I drank a cold drink with hot food"). People hold beliefs about almost everything that affects their lives. What is important to know is that people's health and illness beliefs are at the heart of what they do and how they respond, either to promote their own health or in their reactions to sickness and suffering. These health/illness/suffering beliefs guide them in their everyday living.

Now let us return to the case of Nurse Sophie Baillargeon. What are Sophie's beliefs that guided her decision to allow children to visit their critically ill parents in the hospital? Sophie believes that children need to see their parents in hospital, no matter how ill the parent is, because she believes this will help them deal with their parent's illness or impending death. This belief is informed by her values; personal and clinical experiences; and knowledge of children and how children cope with serious illness, loss, and death.

Think of other beliefs that affect how clinicians behave. For example, if doctors and nurses believe that they are the primary source for transmitting infection from patient to patient, then they may be more careful to wash their hands between seeing patients. Consider the empirical study of hand-washing practices with hospital-based physicians and how their beliefs influenced their behavior as described in Exhibit 2.1 (Pittet et al., 2004).

TABLE 2.1

Sets of value systems

Sets of Values	Examples of Values
Personal/cultural	Always do the right thing. There are rewards in working hard.
Ethical/moral	People have a right to make choices related to their care. People have a right to be treated with respect and dignity.
Political/religious (doctrinal/ideological)	Health care is a right, and the state should provide and pay it. Health care is a privilege; people are responsible for taking care of themselves.
Social	Be compassionate to strangers.
Aesthetic	Pleasant physical surroundings is important for a person's healing.

EXHIBIT 2.1

Empirical study   *Performance, beliefs, and perceptions of hand hygiene in hospital-based physicians*

The Problem
Physicians' adherence to hand hygiene remains low in most hospitals.

The Purpose
To identify risk factors for nonadherence and assess physicians' beliefs and perceptions about hand hygiene.

The Study
Pittet et al. (2004) conducted a survey of 163 physicians in a large university hospital to determine their practices, beliefs, and attitudes toward hand hygiene. They observed physician hand hygiene during routine patient care. They followed up their observations with a self-report questionnaire to measure their beliefs and perceptions.

The Findings
Fifty-seven percent of physicians practiced correct hand hygiene. The factors influencing adherence were associated with their belief in being a role model to others, a positive attitude toward hand washing, and easy access to hand-rub solutions. The highest rate of nonadherence were physicians from the specialties of surgery, emergency medicine, and intensive care medicine. Although the rate of adherence was relatively low, this rate was hypothesized to be higher than what actually happens in part because physicians knew that they were being observed.

The Bottom Line
Physician adherence to hand hygiene is associated with work and system constraints, as well as knowledge and cognitive factors. At an individual level, strengthening a positive attitude toward hand hygiene and emphasizing the importance of individual behavior influencing group behavior may improve adherence among physicians. It was recommended that physicians who worked in technical specialties should also be targeted for improvement.

Source: Pittet et al., (2004).

Some beliefs are based on scientific evidence; others are learned from parents and transmitted by peers; others come from observing others and how they behave; others are learned from previous experiences; and still others are reflected in the prevailing views of a particular society, religious, or cultural group.

Consider the story of how beliefs are linked to health behavior as told by Nurse Catherine Gros, a clinical nurse consultant, of a young pregnant woman, Marie, who has been diagnosed with schizophrenia. Marie was hospitalized on an inpatient psychiatric unit. Marie continued to smoke despite the nurses' best efforts to help her to stop smoking. The nurses knew, on the basis of scientific evidence, that smoking can harm a developing fetus. No matter what they said to Marie, their efforts met with little success: Marie continued to smoke. Then, one day, Marie told Catherine that she believed that smoking was good for the baby. In exploring this belief further, Catherine learned that Marie had been pregnant the year before. In Marie's last trimester of her pregnancy, she was in a car accident and had lost the baby. This current pregnancy was planned. As Catherine related, *"When we started listening to her, she said, 'I've wanted a child all my life. All my life, I've wanted to be a mother and smoking is good for my baby because last time, with my last pregnancy, I quit smoking and my baby died. I could not handle another dead baby.'"* This statement came as a revelation to the nurses. They then began to understand the power of beliefs in directing Marie's behavior and why they had failed in their attempts to get Marie to stop smoking. It also helped them view Marie in a different light. As Catherine explained the nurses now saw Marie *"not as a bad mother who didn't care about her baby because she was smoking but rather as a good mother who really did care and who really wanted this child."* The nurses' beliefs were based on what they knew from the scientific literature, whereas Marie's beliefs were informed by her own personal experience of having lost her last baby after she had quit smoking. Marie was engaged in what is known as magical thinking, which is one of the hallmarks of schizophrenia. Knowing what Marie believed to be true required the nurses to rethink their strategies on how better to nurse her.

In the early 1980s, some people believed that HIV/AIDS was transmitted through human touch. This was a widely held view in society. People who believed this would not touch or come in contact with a person suffering from HIV/AIDS. When the late Princess Diana of Great Britain visited patients with HIV/AIDS and held their hands and hugged them, her actions did more to change societal beliefs than all the scientific information had done up until this point in time.

A nurse needs to consider not only her own beliefs to guide her actions but also those of the patient, family, and other nurses and colleagues as well as the prevailing societal beliefs. These beliefs must be considered in light of existing scientific evidence, personal knowledge, and ethical and moral considerations.

Now take a moment to reflect on your own health practices and how they have been influenced by your health beliefs by completing the exercise in Table 2.2.

Attitudes are the third major influence that guides practice. Attitudes are judgments that comprise three components: (a) **A**ffective (i.e., emotion), (b) **B**ehavioral, and (c) **C**ognitive (i.e., thinking), otherwise known as *ABC* (Solomon, 2009).

Consider the nurses' attitude on Sophie Baillargeon's unit. Many nurses felt that children should not visit hospitals, especially not the intensive care unit. These nurses feared that children would become distressed (affective, emotions) when they saw their parent with tubes, drains, and monitors (behavioral), and they thought that this experience would traumatize them (cognitive).

Values, beliefs, and attitudes are so highly interrelated that it is often difficult to separate them. In fact, some authors prefer to use only the term *values* and to define values in terms of both beliefs and attitudes (Uustal, 1978), whereas others prefer the term *beliefs* and define beliefs in terms of values (Wright et al., 1996). This is not surprising given that values are often aligned with a person's beliefs and are reflected in a person's attitude. Over time, values, beliefs, and attitudes become more integrated as they shape a nurse's personal and professional identity, which is then reflected in

TABLE 2.2

Reflect and connect: Health practices to health beliefs

Health behavior	Describe your health practice	What do you believe about this health practice?	Where did this belief come from?
Exercise			
Brushing your teeth			
Suntanning			
Washing your hands before eating			

Reflect and Connect Instructions:

1. For each health behavior, describe your own health practice.
2. What beliefs influenced your health practice?
3. Where did this belief come from?

her practice orientation. This integration is important to ensure that the way a nurse practices reflects what matters most to her.

The important point here is that nurses need to get in touch with their own values, beliefs, and attitudes so that they can understand how these forces serve as guiding principles that shape their clinical judgments, decisions, and actions. Consider a story told by Nurse Esther Laforest, who recalled that as a student nurse she held certain beliefs about what a "good" mother was and what a "bad" or inadequate mother was. During a home visit, she met Joyce, an adolescent mother, who was pregnant with her second child. Esther recalls that she was able to see only the bad in the situation, what Joyce was doing wrong, and was blinded to her many strengths. Although Esther had been taught in her nursing program about the importance of focusing on strengths, as a student she either did not understand what this meant or did not fully appreciate its importance. Thus, she says she gave lip service to having a strengths approach when in reality she was nursing from a deficit orientation. When she found herself in the practice setting with a real patient, her already-held beliefs about what a "good" mother and a "bad" mother were began to surface. All Esther could see in Joyce were the things Joyce was doing wrong, and as a nurse she thought her role was to "fix" things. It was only years later, after several years of practicing as a nurse clinician that Esther came to understand and then value the importance of practicing from a strengths perspective. She began to understand how her own values, beliefs, and attitudes directed her nursing action. She also understood that, with a different attitude, her nursing of Joyce would have been very different. Esther recounted her experience with Joyce and described what led to her new insights about that situation. Her story is told in Exhibit 2.2.

Where Do Values, Beliefs, and Attitudes Come From?

Beginning in infancy and continuing throughout a person's life, individuals develop, rework, and revise their values, beliefs, and attitudes as a result of changing circumstances, acquiring new information and knowledge, and personal and professional experiences. Values, beliefs, and attitudes are deeply embedded in the culture of a person's family, community, and society. They are transmitted through family, friends,

EXHIBIT 2.2

Personal experience *Through dark-colored glasses: Nurse Esther Leforest links beliefs to nursing responses*

In every nurse's career there are patients and families that she never forgets because of what she learns about herself as a nurse. These experiences become sentinel events in that they provide insights into how one's own values, beliefs, and attitudes guide one's assessment and subsequent actions.

Nurse Esther Leforest recalled a visit that she made as a student nurse during her community placement to an 18-year-old mother, Joyce, who was expecting her second child. Esther explained why she decided to share this story: "*The reason I am bringing up this case is because, as I look back, the potential for observing strengths was tremendous and only now I realize that I approached the whole situation from a deficits point of view.*" She went on to explain: "*Joyce was considered a high-risk patient from a psychosocial point of view because she had spent most of her adolescent years in and out of juvenile detention centers and halfway homes. She had been followed by a social worker very closely since the age of ten. At sixteen, she was discharged from the system to be basically on her own. She was on welfare and was with no consistent partner. She was having a healthy pregnancy. However, she smoked (cigarettes) and marijuana, which caused us a lot of concern…So right away, when we approached the situation, my preceptor and I, we had the idea that this was a family in desperate need of nursing follow-up because of all these issues in spite of the fact that Joyce took excellent care of her child.*"

Esther continued to identify the information that reinforced her belief that this was a mother who needed to be changed: "*On one of my visits, it was 10 in the morning and Joyce was feeding her child chocolates and cola. And right away the hair on the back of my neck stood up and I thought 'Oh my goodness, weaknesses, we have to do something, we have to do something.' And all I could think of was 'What am I going to do in this situation? How am I going to change this obviously troublesome situation so that there is a healthy baby and a healthy family—how am I going to fix this, because this is so wrong, there's so many wrong things: she smokes, she smokes marijuana, the nutrition is poor, the apartment is not necessarily as clean as it could be, she was a single mother on welfare, cash is an issue. There was this idea that we had to fix things—this was a high-risk situation and we had to fix it. I wanted to impress her. I wanted to fix things. I had the 'fix-things' mentality that was not the orientation of the McGill Model of Nursing that I was being taught—this is not what I believe in now. And in that tunnel vision of fixing, I completely ignored everything that was right and all of the innate strengths in the situation and in this mother.*"

Years later, something happened that caused Esther to reevaluate and reflect on her nursing and what she had missed.

"*Joyce was fiercely independent and had a strong internal locus of control. She had lived through drug abuse, through very difficult family relationships, [so] she did not open up during our time together. She had probably sustained a certain amount*

(continued)

EXHIBIT 2.2 (Continued)

of abuse herself from her various relationships. Yet, here was also a woman who was fiercely devoted to her children. Perhaps some small things, such as nutrition, were overlooked, however, in a general sense, these children were always well cared for. Joyce was a deeply resourceful woman who could always find what she needed. And despite whatever amount of welfare checks she was on, when the baby was born she found herself an apartment with more space to take care of the baby. She was a master in making contacts, in interacting with the people in her life to support her family. And it may not have been what a health care professional would have considered optimal to support her family but it was supportive of her family nonetheless.

Esther recognized how she was blinded to Joyce's many strengths: "*I completely ignored that, from her own perspective, she was right where she needed to be because she had made it. She had gotten past the halfway home and she had made a good life with what she had. So for her, she was just fine. And there was no need to fix anything at this time.*"

Esther recalled why she reevaluated her initial assessment: "*I ran into Joyce a few years later. Yes, she is still managing with her welfare, and her daughter, who was born while I was working with her, is healthy and well, and her son is healthy and well, and they are managing their day-to-day life very well. If I had approached her based on her strengths, viewing her as an individual who really had it together and who could always find what she needed and who stayed positive throughout really difficult situations, I think that I would probably have been able to work with her a lot better. There would probably have been a lot more trust rather than imposing myself and looking at only the deficits... Reflecting back on it makes me feel differently about her. I wish I could go back and deal with Joyce on that level, and I think we would have gotten a lot further than we got.*"

school, community, neighborhoods, religious groups, and class structure. They are learned by observing, reading, and interacting. They are shaped by the political, social, and economic context of the time as well as knowledge of history. Values are learned through formal and informal education. Finally, values are affected by experiences: planned and unplanned events that transform lives and set a person in different directions and on new paths of discovery.

In addition to having personal values, nurses need to develop a set of professional values. For some nurses, personal values may be inconsistent with professional values. This may cause a nurse distress and may be a source of inner conflict. It is desirable to have personal values and professional values that are congruent and consistent. A study of nurses that intended to determine the values that shaped their personal and professional identity revealed that human dignity and altruism were the most prominent moral values that contributed to the nurses' overall philosophy and shaped their nursing practices (Fagermoen, 1997). Often, personal values influence professional values, and professional values alter personal values. If the person believes that relationships with family and friends should be built on respect and trust, it is likely that these values will be reflected in how that person relates to patients, colleagues, family members, friends, and strangers.

Professional values are acquired through reading, discussing, trying out, observing, rehearsing, and reflecting. They are shaped by and reinforced by the type of feedback received from patients, teachers, colleagues, and team members. Recall that in the study of what influenced physicians to adhere to the principles of sound hand hygiene, one of the important factors shaping the physician's behavior was the need to serve as a good role model to others (see Exhibit 2.1).

It is important, first as a student and then as a nurse clinician, to take the time to reflect on what matters most to you and where your values come from, because it is these values that will shape and guide your practice.

Why Is It Important For Nurses to Identify the Values That Shape Their Practice?

When nurses are aware of the forces that guide their own practice, then values, beliefs, and attitudes become a more integral part of how they practice. By becoming aware of their values, nurses are capable of the following:

> When nurses feel pride in what they do and have a strong sense of themselves as a nurse, they are more likely to exercise control over the way they practice nursing.

- They are more likely to act in ways that are considered, reasoned, and deliberate rather than haphazard or automatic.
- They are in a better position to detect inconsistencies between their core values and their actual practices. When there is a discrepancy between values and actions, this often is the root of unexplained anxiety, concern, and guilt—that is, moral distress.
- They are better able to articulate, both to themselves and to other team members, the basis underlying their decisions. They are able to defend and rationalize practice choices and are in a more informed position to know what causes to embrace and which ones to oppose.
- They are able to resist pressures from others that could undermine their nursing or what they believe is the right thing to do.

Nurses can evaluate the extent to which their decisions and actions reflect what is important to them and practice in a way that is moral and ethical and that in turn makes them feel good about themselves and the way they nurse patients and families. Consider Nurse Sharon Johnson's experience of caring for Mr. Splane, a 72-year-old policeman who was in the terminal stages of pancreatic cancer. He had prided himself as being a man who took care of his family, a man who was in charge and always in control. His doctors had told him that his cancer had metastasized and that they could offer no further treatment other than to make him comfortable. He was in need of palliative care and would be transferred shortly to the palliative care unit.

Although Mr. Splane understood what was happening to him, he had decided not to share this information with his family. Sharon was disturbed by this; she worried about Mr. Splane and the effects that his decision would have on himself and on his wife and children. As Sharon recalled: *"I had been off for about four days, and during those four days the medical team had done the final workup on him, and it was decided that he was now palliative. They had consulted with the palliative care unit and were actually supposed to transfer him. And his wife came in and she was sitting there and they were still asking questions as if he was going to be having lots of treatments, and I thought to myself, 'Well, something is missing here because I am reading in his chart one thing and the family is working from a different perspective.' I took a couple of minutes and sat down with Mr. Splane and asked him what exactly did the family know, and had he spoken to his daughters about being transferred to the palliative care unit? He told me he hadn't talked to them because he didn't think they could handle it and he wanted to know what the unit was like. It was one of the first times that I decided that I was just going to put everything aside and just focus on him. I spent the next three hours sitting with him and going through his life, his history. I learned that here was a man who was proud and who was passionate about his work as a policeman. You could see he was always accustomed to being in control. He was the one who was still running his home from the hospital, still giving his daughters advice and stuff. Here he was facing this thing and was totally afraid that his family would see him in a different light if he let down his guard and told them that he was now going to palliative care and would just be treated for comfort measures.*

Sharon spent three hours with Mr. Splane, talking about palliative care. She even took him to visit the unit, spoke to some of the nurses, and talked about the treatment. Sharon recalled that conversation: "*We spoke about what it was like, if the family could come in, if there were psychologists that could work with them and everything.*" Sharon talked to him about telling his family, and they even improvised and rehearsed how he would tell them. When she left him that evening Mr. Splane said that he was going to think about whether to tell his family. As Sharon later recalled, he had decided to tell his family about the transfer, and when she offered to be there he told her that he preferred to do this alone. A few days later, he did tell his family. The other nurses told Sharon what had happened: "*There were lots of tears and lots of sadness, they were hearing everything but nothing was going in.*"

That afternoon, about an hour and a half after Mr. Splane shared this information, the palliative care unit called and he was transferred. The next day Mr. Splane's daughter asked to speak to Sharon. Sharon recounted what happened:

"*The daughter asked me 'Do you mind if we go sit?' and then she started to cry and said 'Thank you.' She said 'Do you know you made the difference by just taking the time to just sit there, showing him the palliative car unit, explaining to him exactly what it was, explaining to him why he needed to go there versus staying here and putting the time in.' And then she said something to me. She said 'My father has never been able to let go being the dominant male counterpart in this family.' She said it had been a battle. She said cancer was just not something that he was going to deal with, he was just going to ignore it. She said the man who is on the 10th floor (referring to the hospital unit her father was on) speaking to my family is not the man who was here a couple of days ago.*"

Sharon recalled that an unexpected and unpleasant encounter greeted her the next day. One of her colleagues angrily scolded her: "*'Do you know you forgot to chart yesterday?' And I said, 'Yeah.' And she said, 'Well, what the hell were you doing?' And I said, 'What do you mean, what was I doing? I took Mr. Splane down to the unit, spent the time with his family, and did a lot of patient teaching. I took the time to be with his family.' This nurse then turned to me, and she said, 'I just wish you would pay attention and do real nursing.' I responded, 'Thank you, but in my opinion I was doing real nursing.'*

And I think that is why it's so vivid for me because I remember walking in the next morning and her being so angry because I didn't sign off and I was thinking, 'I spent three and a half hours with this patient bringing everything into perspective, bringing somebody who was petrified, giving him the support, allowing him the time to go through everything at that time, to open up to his family, to share, to take him down to the palliative care unit, and here my colleague, in her opinion, didn't think I had done any nursing!'"

Sharon's nursing was guided by her beliefs and orientation of what "real" nursing was. She had a completely different orientation than her colleague. Sharon took her cues from her patient, and from her colleague, to evaluate the effectiveness of her nursing. She felt good about herself and the quality of the care she had given to Mr. Splane and his family. She knew her choice made a difference because she practiced family-centered, whole-person care. She understood Mr. Splane—who he was, what he valued, what was important to him—and worked with him collaboratively for his benefit and the benefit of his family. In contrast, her colleague placed more value on paperwork than on being with the patient. This is not to say that charting is not important. Both are important—being with the patient and then documenting one's nursing. However, the actions of these two nurses reveal what they believe is nursing and what they feel is important. Sharon values patients and families and sees her role as helping them work through painful issues. Sharon's colleague values paperwork. This is reflected in how they choose to spend their time.

When ideas and actions are driven by both the nurse's values and beliefs and those of her patients and are used to guide actions, values can transform practice, make a difference in people's lives, and ultimately have the power to change health care systems.

VALUES, BELIEFS, AND ATTITUDES GUIDING PRACTICE: A CASE ANALYSIS OF NURSE SOPHIE BAILLARGEON

Let's return to Sophie to examine her values, beliefs, and attitudes and the forces and factors that shaped her nursing actions with a young boy and his dying mother. As you read at the beginning of this chapter, Sophie values a family-centered approach to care and believes that it is in a child's best interest to be allowed to visit his dying parent. After working with the nursing staff to change their attitudes, Sophie was now ready to act on these values, as illustrated in the story of Peter and his mother.

Sophie described how she prepared six-year-old Peter to visit his dying mother, Mrs. Pinker. She was suffering from encephalitis and was on life support, and her condition was deteriorating rapidly. Mr. Pinker had told the nurses that he was concerned for his young son. He didn't know how to prepare him for what was happening to the boy's mother. He felt it best to protect Peter from pain by not discussing what was happening. Sophie described nursing this family: *"The assistant head nurse approached Mr. Pinker: 'Maybe we can help you with your son?' We can give you some ideas and we can work together."* They suggested bringing Peter to visit his mother.

Sophie continued, *"I shared with Mr. Pinker what I knew about children. I prepared some articles for him on children's grief and circled the key ideas to make it easier for him to read. We talked about how children grieve. We talked about his son being part of the story, the hospital story. It would be difficult for a child to understand what had happened to a parent—going from seeing his mom at home who was not too well and then seeing her in a coffin or never seeing her again. If Peter had never seen his mother in the hospital it would make it difficult for him to understand what had happened to her. Mr. Pinker decided to bring Peter the next day to visit his mother.*

Sophie recounted what happened next: *"We took Mr. Pinker and Peter to a quiet room and began to prepare Peter for seeing his mother. We talked to Peter about what was happening to his mom. We had asked Mr. Pinker to have Peter bring the things he liked to play with. Peter came with his cars and little soldiers. While Peter played with his cars and soldiers, I spoke to him. He never looked up at us but he was really listening. We took our time and explained things in very simple words. After awhile I said, 'I think you're ready now to go and see your mom.' We went slowly to the door and I explained that the tube in his mother's nose was like a big straw to help her breathe. We put his toys on the bed so that he could play with them if he wanted to. He took his cars out and the assistant head nurse saw there were ridges (lines) in the blanket and said to Peter, 'Oh, it's like a little street.' We wanted to go at his pace. Slowly Peter went closer to his mom's head. And we told him, 'Your mom can hear you. You can speak to her.' He then touched her and told her what had been happening at school. After a little while he said he had had enough. He was ready to go."*

Sophie took Peter and his father to a room and spoke with Peter: *""What did you see? Did you find something that you didn't like?' And Peter replied: 'Yeah.' And I said: 'What was it?' And he said: 'The tape on her nose.' He didn't talk about the tubes, the drains, and the monitors. And then he drew a picture of his mom and talked about sending the soldiers into his mother's blood to fight the really bad guys. They were the enemies in her brain. And at one point I said to him: 'I'm not sure that these great soldiers that you're sending are going to win the battle. I don't think they'll win the battle.' He never looked at us. When I told him about the little soldier that might not win, I think he understood."*

Sophie knew about Mr. Pinker prior to meeting him from listening to the nurses' reports. She also knew about children, having nursed children for many years, and had the confidence and skills to work with them (**factors:** knowledge, experience). She knew the scientific literature on how children grieve and the importance of having children visit a dying parent in understanding their parent's death and their subsequent long-term adjustment (**factor:** formal education). In her role as head nurse, Sophie valued families and the importance of working collaboratively with them (**values and beliefs:** her philosophy and theoretical perspective of nursing). She also had the confidence to know how to approach Peter and gauge his readiness, by communicating at his level through the play soldiers (**factors:** knowledge, experience, skilled know-how).

Sophie also knew that she needed to understand Mr. Pinker's values because it would be his values that would direct whether or not he would bring Peter to visit his mother (**factor:** took the time to establish a relationship by engaging, observing, attuning, listening attentively, and engaging in clinical conversations [see Chapters 7 & 8]). In order to decide whether to even suggest to Mr. Pinker that he bring Peter to see his mother, Sophie had to assess whether Mr. Pinker would be open to such a suggestion (**factor:** clinical judgment). In talking with Mr. Pinker, Sophie and the other nurses were impressed with his openness and concern for Peter (**value:** noticing and working with strengths). Mr. Pinker was a caring, loving father who was worried about 6-year-old Peter and wanted to protect him from pain but wasn't quite sure what to do (**value:** love for his son; **belief:** children need to be protected; **attitude:** open to professional opinions and doing what was in his son's best interest). Having observed and talked with Mr. Pinker, Sophie and the assistant head nurse felt that Mr. Pinker was open to their suggestion and that he was ready to consider bringing Peter to visit (**value:** importance of readiness).

In her position as head nurse, Sophie had the power to change the visiting policy to allow for liberal family visiting hours that also included young children. She had the support of the assistant head nurse and the other nurses to allow children to visit their dying parents because they shared her vision and values (**values:** collaborative partnership among team members, institutional support).

It was Sophie's belief that you nurse not just the patient, but the whole family, that led to her interest in how family members cope with the impending death of a loved one, including children. She determined that children should be allowed to visit their dying parents. These values and beliefs led Sophie to prepare the nurses on her unit to work with families. With the support of the assistant head nurse, they worked with the other nurses on the unit to overcome their own fears and deal with their emotions of witnessing children visiting their dying parents. Sophie modeled for the nurses certain ways of behaving, how to be responsive, attune to and attend to cues, and in the process provide exquisite nursing care.

WHAT IS MEANT BY A THEORETICAL PERSPECTIVE?

In the course of individual development, each person constructs a personal philosophy, social imaginings (i.e., how an individual imagines himself to be and to behave), and a set of theories about life. Together, these make up that person's theoretical orientation or perspective. All people use their theoretical perspective to better understand themselves and how their world and the universe work. These theoretical perspectives are continuously being updated, reworked, developed, and revised in light of new knowledge and new understandings. Individuals have several perspectives for different aspects of their lives: personal, professional, relationship-based, and the like.

A theoretical perspective becomes so integrated into a nurse's way of thinking that it becomes a way of being that affects how the nurse practices and conducts her personal life, as Nurse Caroline Marchionni explained when referring to Strengths-Based Care. *"It is a mindset that colors everything you do in your life. It colors your interactions with your peers. It colors your interactions with your own family and of course, it colors your interactions with your patients."*

A theoretical perspective serves to inspire and guide action. Nurse Andra Leimanis, in talking about working with strengths, explained, *"It's like a guiding philosophy. Nothing is black or white; there are always shades of grey, and within those shades of grey, there's always some kind of positive somewhere."*

The Role of Nursing Theory in Strengths-Based Care

The term *theory* refers to "a well articulated system of concepts and propositions rooted explicitly in a specific philosophy that serves to guide practice and research" (Cody,

1994, p. 144). A profession requires a theory to describe and explain the phenomena that define its practice. Nursing theories are rooted in the discipline's history and traditions and evolved meanings, and they develop over time in response to changing knowledge and societal expectations (Meleis, 1997).

The most important test of a good theory is how well it "fits" with the realities of practice and the degree to which nurses see that their nursing is able to achieve the desired outcomes. All nurses need to construct their own particular theoretical perspective. They do this by reworking their theoretical orientation in light of their own personal and professional experiences and knowledge, by reflecting on their own experiences with patients and families; acquiring new knowledge; and then adding to, modifying, and developing their personal orientation accordingly. Consider the McGill Model of Nursing, which begins with a set of values and assumptions that has been developed collaboratively with practicing nurses and in light of the latest scientific thinking. It is a model that continues to develop and evolve but is grounded in and derived from practice (Gottlieb & Rowat, 1987; Gottlieb & Ezer, 1997; Gottlieb et al., 2006; Gottlieb & Gottlieb, 2007).

Nurses, for the most part, are unaware of their own theoretical perspectives that underpin their practice because these perspectives tend to operate just below the surface and go undetected until something happens that causes a nurse to stop and reflect on the connections among her values, beliefs, attitudes, as they are reflected in her nursing practice. For example, a nurse may say that she believes that every person has strengths. She may tell the patient that each person is unique and that it is that person's strengths that define his or her uniqueness. Yet the nurse may fail to mention any strengths when she describes the person or family. In fact, the nurse may know very little about a specific patient, his biological responses to the disease, how his illness has affected his way of life, the impact that his illness has had on his family, or how that family has coped.

The best way to know whether nurses practice what they preach is to look at how they actually talk to, talk about, and interact with patients. Nurse Caroline Marchionni described an incident that called into question a practice that did not fit her nursing theoretical orientation, the McGill Model of Nursing, with its focus on person-centered care, collaborative partnership, and strengths-based care (SBC; Gottlieb & Rowat, 1987; Gottlieb & Gottlieb, 2007).

As Caroline explained, *"It's important to have direction in your practice and the McGill Model of Nursing gives that to me. It gives me the idea that the patient and family are the experts in their care. I will ask my patients: 'What do you usually do?' 'What do you usually take for pain?' 'What usually works for you?' And then I go about seeing if I can get whatever pain medication that works best for them. If it's just a case of having their meds changed I will go to the physician and say 'At home, they take this, at home they do it this way, and they say it works for them.' We are very lucky that when I advocate for the patient, the doctors are very receptive. I've even had a resident make fun of me once when I mistakenly referred to a patient by the room number because I couldn't pronounce the patient's name. I wanted the doctor to know exactly who I was talking about and he said 'What's this? You are referring to the patient by the room number. I thought you believe in empathy and all of that stuff— that's not very empathic—talking about a patient by a room number?' And when he told me this he was laughing at me and I thought 'Oh man, you're so right!'"*

Caroline could see a discrepancy between her theoretical perspective, what her colleagues knew she valued, and this one incident that was inconsistent with her values and did not reflect her usual way of talking about her patients.

It is important to keep in mind that the way a nurse practices and talks about his practice reveals much about how the nurse sees himself and expresses his own humanity.

What Happens When Nurses Practice Without a Nursing Theoretical Perspective?

Having a unique theoretical perspective gives a profession and its members an identity. It also provides them a framework and language with which to communicate to others. For nursing to survive and flourish in the health care system, it must contribute a unique service that no other health profession can provide (Gottlieb & Gottlieb, 1998). Nurses who understand, are in touch with, and can articulate their theoretical orientation are in a better position to defend their positions, exercise control over their own practice, and function more autonomously. They hold themselves in high esteem, derive satisfaction from their work, and function as an equal member of the team. They garner respect from their colleagues and most importantly, their patients, clients, and families. In short, they have clarity and direction. Together, these factors contribute to a sense of pride and lead to feelings that their work is meaningful and valued. What happens when nurses lack clarity and direction?

A Confusion of Identity and Roles: Nursing and Medicine

The field of nursing has had its own share of identity crises and has suffered from role confusion. Many factors have contributed to this state of affairs, such as nursing's relationship to medicine, women's role in society, nursing's status in society, the resources and rewards available in the health care system, and so forth (Carpenter, 1995; Gordon, 1996). For the purposes of this discussion, my focus is on nursing's relationship with medicine and their overlapping and interdependent functions.

Since the time of Florence Nightingale, nursing has found itself in a somewhat difficult—and at times, untenable—situation in regard to the field of medicine. Unlike most other health care professions, nursing has historically been closely tethered to medicine. Both are concerned with health, and both focus their attention on the condition of the human body, the care of the sick, and the alleviation of suffering. Nightingale recognized that there was an inherent and unavoidable tension that existed between nursing and medicine because of the overlap of their respective work. In 1869, she wrote the following:

> Nursing and medicine must never be mixed up. It spoils both. Keep medicine and nursing perfectly distinct. Do not let a nurse fancy herself a doctor. If you have medical women let them be as entirely distinct from nurses as medical men are...a smattering of nursing does a doctor good. A smattering of medicine does a nurse harm. (Rafferty, 1996, p. 44)

Some of these tensions continue to this day. Some nurses have difficulty describing what it is they do apart from medicine. More important, they often fail to recognize that what they do makes a difference to the person's health and recovery. They downplay or discount the relationship between themselves and their patient (Weinberg, Aranda, & Brown, 2006). Instead, they embrace the work of medicine with its emphasis on diagnosis, techniques, and reliance on medical therapeutics. This is an important part of nursing, but it is just one part of the nurse's role.

The complexity of nursing and the breadth and depth of knowledge and technical skills required to nurse, even at the most basic level, has been often underestimated by doctors and the public, but most seriously by nurses themselves (Nelson & Gordon, 2006).

Nursing is more than compassion and having a caring attitude; it is about understanding the human condition, in all its complexity, to help people deal with day-to-day life events and choices that affect their health, as well as recover from insults to the body. Skilled nursing requires depth of knowledge, skill in clinical reasoning and judgment, and a broad range of technical and thinking skills that have been honed through years of practice that blend both the art and science of caring and curing (Weinberg et al., 2006). Thus, nurses need a broad theoretical orientation to guide their work.

What Was Responsible for This State of Affairs?

Florence Nightingale created the structure to organize knowledge for nursing practice around health, person, environment, and nursing, which Fawcett (1984) labeled and then claimed as nursing's meta-paradigm. Nightingale, in setting down her thoughts about nursing, distinguished nursing from medicine and in the process created a separate profession. Hers was the first nursing theory to describe the nature of nursing; delineate the scope of nursing practice; the knowledge involved in skilled know-how; and the roles, obligations, duties, and responsibilities of nursing separate from medicine (Nightingale, 1860).

From the turn of the 20th century until today, hospitals became the center of the health care system and medicine emerged as the dominant profession (Reverby, 1987). The alliance of medicine with science and the development of medical education within the university system also helped medicine dominate the way health care and the health care system were funded and defined (Wuest, 1994).

The field of nursing worked alongside medicine but did not progress in parallel partly because of the way nurses were educated (Reverby, 1987). The majority of nurses were trained in a hospital to provide cheap manpower through an apprenticeship system whose focus was on acquiring practical skills, often learned on the job and through trial and error. With few university-educated nurses, there were few nurse–scientists to develop the discipline's theoretical and scientific base to guide nurses in their daily practice. In short, with the growth of hospitals as the cornerstone of the health care system, medicine emerged and nursing became submerged.

Nursing's Search for Its Own Voice

By the late 1950s, nurses began to return to universities in greater numbers. Armed with knowledge and theories in the natural and behavioral sciences, nursing scholars now had the foundational basis to formulate theories to guide practice. Nursing models and theories proliferated as nurse–scientists provided the theoretical orientations to guide practice.

By the early 1970s, many nurses wanted to expand their role to more accurately reflect what they knew, what they were doing, and what they knew they could do. Moyra F. Allen (1977) framed the debate, in effect, as follows: "Should nurses expand their role into medicine, taking on those functions that physicians were relinquishing due to the growth of medical specialization, or should nurses develop their own unique role in the health care system?" Allen envisioned a role that would complement medicine in which nursing would focus on family health work practiced from a strengths perspective rather than replacing physicians' role, practiced from the medical model perspective (Allen, 1977). Since the heady debates of the 1980s, what has emerged is a blending of roles (e.g., assistant-to-the physician, replacement, and complementary), but in different ratios depending on the nurse's values, the workplace values and rewards systems, and whether the nurse has a clear nursing theoretical perspective.

Can a Nurse Practice Without a Theoretical Perspective?

The answer to this question is a resounding "No!" As Cody (1994) reminded us, "History tells us plainly that nursing not guided by nursing theory becomes something else" (p. 145). In the absence of a well-articulated theory of nursing, nurses will construct their own theoretical perspective to guide their practice (Adam, 1991) or will adopt the dominant model in practice. This is just what nurses did when they opted for the medical model to guide nursing practice.

Consider a story told by Nurse Caroline Marchionni, who believes that at the heart of nursing is the nurse–patient relationship. It is by connecting and by being fully present with the person that she is able to understand a patient's distress and alleviate her anxiety. The belief in this type of nursing is not shared by all nurses, however. A colleague of Caroline's, who did not have a clear nursing orientation, told Caroline what guides her practice. As Caroline recounted, *"One of my colleagues said to me 'You don't need to have a relationship with your patient, you can just give them pills. Go and get some pills and give it to them and that's it—that's all you have to do.' "* Caroline responded, *"Wait a minute. You can't be a nurse without developing a relationship with your patient."*

Caroline then reflected on what this nurse had told her. *"I suppose you could just give the pills and not really care about your patient and just do what you're instructed to do on your shift—change the dressing or whatever and not actually ever talk to the patient. But what I enjoy most about my job is the connection I have with my patients. If I just handed out pills and wiped bums all day long, I'd be completely miserable. It really is the connection with the patient that is important and gives meaning to my work as a nurse."*

The Importance of Having a Nursing Theoretical Perspective to Guide Practice

In recent years, some nursing leaders have been alarmed at the growing medicalization of nursing as nurses relinquish their more traditional roles of caregiving (Fawcett, 2006; Keighley, 2006). There is evidence that people have suffered from the lack of skilled, professional nursing (see the section titled *Indicators That Something Is Amiss* in Chapter 1). A clarion call has been sounded to rediscover nursing practice rooted in nursing's traditional values of caring, wholeness, person-/family-centered care and to reclaim nursing's intimate care of the body to support and facilitate health and healing (Gottlieb & Gottlieb, 2007; Locsin & Purnell, 2009; Nelson & Gordon, 2006). These values appreciate that health and healing result from both those big and small acts of nursing, such as providing comfort, giving physical care, being with the person and dealing with body, mind, and spiritual issues through knowledgeable, compassionate, caring. These are some of the values that underlie the theoretical orientation of SBC and are described and elaborated on in Chapter 3.

A nursing theoretical orientation is the result of selecting and integrating different bodies of knowledge that accurately reflects nursing's value systems. This orientation becomes an integral part of the nurse's personal and professional identity (Fagermoen, 1997; Ohlen & Segesten, 1998). In short, a theoretical perspective becomes the nurse's internal compass to guide his practice. It allows the nurse to answer the following questions:

- What are the issues that require my expertise and skills?
- How do I conduct myself as a professional?
- How do I go about creating a meaningful connection with this person and family? What should the nature of the relationship be?
- What information do I need to gather to nurse this person and family? What should I be observing? Attending to? Listening for?
- What knowledge and skills do I need to have to nurse this person and family?
- How do I know when the actions and activities that I have taken are right or best for the person?
- How do I know what I know?
- What counts for me as evidence?

CREATING AN ORGANIZATIONAL CULTURE TO SUPPORT STRENGTHS-BASED CARE

Nurses practice within hospital units, medical institutions, and other organizations. Their work environments can play an important role in shaping their nursing orientation. When the nursing leadership adopts a strengths philosophy to guide administrative decision making, that sends a powerful message that this is a valued orientation. The orientation then permeates the organization, filtering down from the organization's highest administrative echelons through its departments and units, eventually affecting what happens at the bedside between nurse and patient. It becomes the organization's

> When the leadership of a unit, department, and institution adopts a strengths-based management approach, they send a powerful message that SBC is the orientation of care.

climate, its culture. It also gives nurses an opportunity to experience and feel how a strengths orientation can empower.

Nurse Catherine Oliver, in her newly created role as Clinical Practice Consultant of a major hospital merger, was given the task of harmonizing the care between two palliative care units at two different hospitals with the goal of creating one clinical unit operating on two different sites before the new hospital building was built. The two hospitals that were merging were the Royal Victoria Hospital (RVH) and the Montreal General Hospital (MGH) to become part of a five-hospital merger and create a new entity known as the McGill University Health Center. The unit at the RVH had been a pioneer in the field of palliative care. When the merger between these two hospitals began, it had been established over twenty-five years ago and was recognized internationally as a leader in palliative care, whereas the MGH unit had been in operation for just over five years. Although both units were experienced in palliative care, the MGH unit was considered by the RVH site to be the "new kid" on the block. Until the merger, both hospitals had prodigious and illustrious histories, and both enjoyed international reputations based on their impressive records of medical and nursing accomplishments. The MGH, with the newer palliative care unit, had been founded in 1821; the RVH, with the older palliative care unit, was the newer hospital, founded in 1893. These two hospitals had developed their own cultures, ways of doing things, rituals, routines, and distinctive identities. Although both were McGill University teaching hospitals, they were like siblings: Both prided themselves on the quality of their nursing departments. They were competitive and had enjoyed a healthy degree of rivalry, yet at the same time they had enjoyed a long history in which their nursing directors had worked collaboratively, supporting and encouraging the other.

Catherine's first thoughts when given the task of merging these two units was *"Where should she begin?"* She asked herself, *"How does one bring together the groups and have them work in a fashion that is not competitive, that is conducive to excellent patient/family care, that continues clinical growth, and that remains open to new ideas? Because the field of palliative care is very much whole person care and holistic."*

Catherine began with her own nursing orientation of focusing on strengths: *"The thing that helped me was that I knew both the units and the hospitals and could draw on their strengths."* Guided by her value and a concern for patient/family-centered care, she had several goals in mind: *"My goal was that clinical practice not suffer, that the care of patients and families whose loved ones were dying not suffer while we were going through an internal merger. And to assist the staff as much as possible to remain focused on the patients and the families."*

Catherine began the challenging process of merging the two units by meeting with the staff nurses of both units and bringing them together as one group, acknowledging what was at stake and beginning where the nurses were at: *"Each morning I spent with the group . . . we would talk about what we were scared of losing, what we were certain we wanted to maintain, what was the best of who we were, and would then sit around and brainstorm about how we were going to do it as a group."*

During these discussions, the group members focused on their values and the importance of being guided by them. As Catherine explained, *"We would discuss concretely—'Well, if this is our goal, if this is what we value, if this is what we as a group see as our strengths, then what will we do in order to create it; what do we need to do?' . . . And coming up with a common vision of what palliative care nursing was, and what the philosophy of palliative care was, drawing from those two quite distinct traditions, one being very lengthy and the other being quite young."*

Catherine gave the group a framework, called the *Forming–Storming–Norming–Performing*, a four-phase process model that was designed to help units make the transition from two units to one. As Catherine explained, the second phase, storming, was the most difficult: *"When they were storming, the group needed to know that that was part of the process and we needed to get through [it]. And everyone feels really good when they get together and 'Wow, isn't this great?' However, when they start to recognize their differences and start to argue and bicker, [they start in with] 'She's doing this' and 'She's not doing this' and 'I don't know how.' So it was important to give them a context of what was going on. I told them 'No, we're not going to stay here, and maybe we need to establish some ground rules for how we're going to get through this storming period.'"*

Besides establishing rules, Catherine played up each unit's strengths during this storming phase. She described how focusing on strengths changed the climate and the quality of the discussion: *"We asked the questions 'What were their strengths?,' [and] 'What were the things they were most proud of?' This was another way of looking at perhaps what they wanted to maintain and what they wanted to move into the future. To use another language, we were in effect 'co-constructing' a future. And we had to deal with the instrumental issues of common pieces of paper and protocols. I mean, there was a whole bunch of stuff that needed to be dealt with which we would do there, but there was more to the philosophical aspect of who we are as palliative care nurses and what did we value, where we are going to, what we were going to do, and how concretely we would do it."*

In the process of identifying their strengths, the groups discovered what they shared in common, those things that could bind them, rather than the differences that could divide them: *"I think it was important to hear the others say it, so that the values were common, and they would normally use specific examples. The more there was a sharing of patients, the more they could see what they were doing. They could identify the commonalities. They could see that they were all moving in the same direction."*

Over time, each group came to recognize strengths in individual nurses. They understood that they did not all have to have the same strengths; instead, they could have strengths that complemented each other. In listening to each other, they came to respect the knowledge and skills of the other. As Catherine recounted, *"They heard and they observed over time as they worked together that a particular nurse was really, really good with complex families. If we had someone with a complex family then this could be the nurse who went in to care for them. Or that this nurse was really good with chest tubes or whatever it might be. And that's part of forming and creating the team—it is about knowing that not everyone is created equal but that different people do have strengths in different areas."*

Identifying, understanding, and appreciating each other's strengths, as a unit and as individual nurses, allowed the nurses to articulate their goals and how these goals could get accomplished. Perhaps most important, it showed how working with strengths gave the team new hope, opened new possibilities, and created new opportunities. Together, they could blend their expertise and evolve into an even stronger entity, stronger than either unit had been separately. Through working with each other's expertise, they identified practical ways to move forward. By focusing on the positives, they came to realize what was possible. The merger was not without its bumps and detours, but in the end these two groups came together, made decisions, and took actions, bound by a common vision they had created together. They could see that as a group their power resided in their combined skills, capacities, and capabilities to move the enterprise forward. This was because their leader, Catherine Oliver, adapted her nursing framework of SBC into an orientation of strengths-based leadership to guide her actions and keep her focused, working in collaborative partnership with the nurses.

Key Summary Points

- Underlying nursing practice is a set of values, beliefs, and attitudes reflected in nurses' theoretical perspective and their social imaginings of how things could be. This theoretical perspective, which has been developed, elaborated, and refined through practical experiences, guides nurses' judgment, decisions, and actions.
- Because of nursing's long history and relationship with the field of medicine, nursing has at times adopted the medical model to guide their practice, in particular in the absence of a clearly developed and articulated nursing theoretical perspective.
- Nurses need to develop their own theoretical perspective, based on a set of core values, beliefs, and attitudes and in light of scientific evidence and clinical wisdom acquired through experience.
- A theoretical orientation and its underlying values can guide action at all levels of an institution and agency, from the highest administrative echelons to the management of a unit and can communicate to nurses what is appreciated and important about nursing.
- A well-articulated theoretical orientation enables nurses to understand and appreciate the range, variation, and complexity of their work rooted in traditions of caring and caregiving to promote health and facilitate recovery and healing. It gives nurses the knowledge and tools they need to nurse and the language to communicate not only what they do but also the importance of their work. It gives nurses their unique identity. SBC is a nursing perspective that fulfills these requirements.

Values Underlying Strengths-Based Nursing Care

3

LEARNING OBJECTIVES

After reading this chapter, you should be able to:

- Identify the assumptions underlying Strengths-Based Care
- List the eight core values of Strengths-Based Care
- Describe how each value is conceptualized
- Describe how each value guides Strengths-Based Care

Values underlie everything a person does in his personal and professional life. A person's value system guides decisions and shapes behavior and actions. Nurses subscribe to many values, and these values are often interconnected and together form a coherent and consistent worldview.

Consider Nurse Heather Hart's values and how her values come together to create a coherent nursing orientation that guides her behavior and actions with her patient, Ellen. In every nurse's career, there are those patients who leave an indelible impression, never to be forgotten. For Heather, Ellen was one of those special patients.

Ellen was a young woman, a mother of four, whom Heather nursed for six months on the palliative care unit until her death. Even before Heather met Ellen, she was already impressed with her. As Heather recalled: *"The little bits I had been told about her impressed me immediately even before seeing her. She was thirty-eight years old. She was the mother of four children who had been diagnosed with ovarian cancer ten years before. Right away a little flag went up for me: This is a young woman who has some fight in her and some will to live because that's a pretty devastating diagnosis, and to still be here ten years later, well, that was very impressive. This information made me wonder 'Who is Ellen?'"*

Ellen had been admitted to the unit while Heather had been away on vacation. It was the way Ellen greeted her that impressed Heather: *"She greeted me with a 'Hi. Welcome. Nice to meet you'—I was kind of the newcomer and she was welcoming me back to my unit. I saw some spunk, some life, some really positive energy coming out of this woman who was really, really ill. This was my first encounter with Ellen."*

Ellen was considered a "challenging" patient by many of the nurses. As Heather explained, *"None of the other nurses wanted to be her nurse every day, because of Ellen and the care she required. Ellen had a very complicated and complex abdominal dressing that could take an hour to an hour and a half to change. Because Ellen was very clear about how she wanted things done, when they should be done, and how they should be done, she was considered by some nurses to be demanding and somewhat inflexible."*

Despite these warnings, Heather decided to *"jump in"* and asked to be assigned to Ellen as her primary nurse.

In listening to Heather describe Ellen's various turning points in her journey and how she responded to Ellen, Heather's nursing values are revealed. It is these values that guide her decisions and are reflected in her nursing. As each value underlying Strengths-Based Care (SBC) is described in this chapter, I return to Heather's nursing of Ellen.

SBC is an approach that guides nurses in everyday practice and is based on a set of assumptions about health, person, environment, and nursing: the four elements that comprise nursing's meta-paradigm or core knowledge (Fawcett, 1984; Kim, 2010). Recall from Chapter 2 that *assumptions* are those ideas that are taken for granted or accepted as truth without the need to provide proof because they are derived from evidence and experience.

WHAT ARE THE UNDERLYING ASSUMPTIONS OF STRENGTHS-BASED NURSING CARE?

As summarized in Table 3.1, at the core of SBC are the following assumptions that relate to health, person, environment, and nursing:

- Individuals, families, and communities aspire to and are motivated to better health and healing
- Persons have the capacity to grow, transform, and self-heal
- Each person is unique. People's uniqueness is reflected in their responses to health and healing challenges and how they both physically and mentally respond and react to clinical interactions and therapeutics
- People function as an integrated whole
- People create their own meaning to understand themselves and make sense of their environments and experiences
- Inherent in all things, from cells to citizens to communities, reside potentials and strengths
- Problems, weaknesses, vulnerabilities, hardships, and suffering are part of the human condition
- Strengths are required for health and self-healing
- Within each person resides the power to self-heal. This power is in itself a strength
- Strengths enable people to adapt to different environments and cope with life experiences to meet a wide range of health challenges

- People reside in environments that range from healthy to toxic
- Environments contain powerful forces that select for specific strengths or deficits that will determine how a person survives and grows or succumbs and withers in that particular environment
- Nursing exists to care for individuals, families, and communities to help them achieve health, facilitate recovery and healing, alleviate suffering, and cope with problems
- Nursing works with people and their environments to select for and develop strengths to promote health and facilitate healing
- Nurses, by their presence and actions, are part of the person and family environments. They also create environments to enable healing

TABLE 3.1

Nursing metaparadigm and assumptions underlying SBC

Nursing Metaparadigm	SBC Assumptions
Health	Individuals, families, and communities aspire to and are motivated to better health
Person	Each person is unique Each person functions as an integrated whole Each person has the capacity to grow, transform, and self-heal People create their own meaning to understand themselves and their environments Inherent in all things, from cells to citizens to communities, reside potentials and strengths Problems, weaknesses, vulnerabilities, hardships, and suffering are part of the human condition. Strengths are required for health and healing Within each person resides the power to heal. This power is in itself a strength Strengths enable people to adapt to different environments and to a wide variety of health challenges
Environment	People reside in environments that range from healthy to toxic Environments contain powerful forces that select for strengths or deficits
Nursing	The field of nursing exists to care for individuals, families, and communities, to help them achieve health, facilitate healing, alleviate suffering, and cope with problems Nursing professionals work with people and their environments to select for and develop strengths to promote health and facilitate healing

VALUES UNDERLYING STRENGTHS-BASED NURSING CARE

These assumptions give rise to eight core values and beliefs about health, person, environment, and nursing that underlie SBC:

1. Health and healing
2. Uniqueness of the person
3. Holism and embodiment
4. Objective/subjective reality and created meaning

5. Self-determination
6. Person and environment are integral
7. Learning, readiness, and timing
8. Collaborative partnership between nurse and person

It is important to keep in mind that these values are highly interrelated and work together to form a comprehensive and coherent value system that finds expression in SBC.

Value 1: Health and Healing

Health care practitioners share a common focus of practice: health and healing. Despite this shared focus, the way they work to promote health and facilitate healing varies among the different health care professions. The differences are related to their conceptualizations of health and healing; what they see to be their role, mission, and mandate in the health care system and to society; and how they see themselves meeting their professional obligations (Kritek, 1997). Even within the same profession, there may be significant differences in the way one nurse cares for a person compared to the way another nurse works with that same person. Have you ever asked yourself why this is the case? Part of the answer lies in their different theoretical perspectives (as discussed in Chapter 2) and their ways of thinking about health and healing.

Conceptualizations

A. Health
There are many different ways of conceptualizing health (Smith, 1981). The most widely accepted view is to consider health relative to illness, that is, as the absence of disease. In this conceptualization, as the severity of the illness increases, the person's health is diminished. This idea can be illustrated with an hourglass. Think of the top of the hourglass as health and the bottom of the hourglass as illness. What happens when you turn an hourglass over? The health diminishes and the illness increases. One can then say that the person is not healthy. If a nurse subscribes to this view of health, then restoring health requires a focus on treating the disease or condition. When a person is considered healthy, it means that the disease is cured, the symptoms have been alleviated or are under control, and the person is better able to function and return to her normal activities.

Strengths-Based Care's conception of health

SBC's conception of health is inspired by the writings of Florence Nightingale, the McGill Model of Nursing (Gottlieb & Rowat, 1987), and knowledge of human development (Gottlieb & Gottlieb, 2007). Nightingale (1860) defined health in the medical sense, as an aspect of disease, as well as in the developmental sense, a process of becoming as the person grows and develops. She also believed that health was a learned response as well as a learning process. According to Nightingale, disease was an opportunity to promote health through the acts of restoration (healing), learning, and empowerment.

Nightingale believed that human beings had the power to promote and restore health, to learn from their experiences, and to prevent "dis-ease" by working with human nature and the environment. As MacDonald and Nightingale (2008) wrote,

> Health is not only to be well but to be able to use well every power we have . . . Man has to learn how circumstances regulate and modify human nature, to learn what circumstances develop and exercise human nature aright. (p. 311)

If one expands on and updates Nightingale's ideas of health in light of current scientific understandings one sees that health is multifaceted and takes its definition from the context or situation of the patient's condition and cultural environment. Health is conceptualized in SBC as a separate and distinct entity that coexists with disease (Allen, 1977, 1981). This means that, regardless of the seriousness of the person's disease, health is always present in some form. When there is illness or disease, health is influenced by and influences the illness experience; that is, health is within illness and illness is within health (Gottlieb & Gottlieb, 2007). "The nurse's role is to promote health, in particular during illness and traumatic events".

Nurse Margaret Eades, one founder of a cancer rehabilitation program, described health as a goal of nursing: "Cancer rehabilitation is viewed by many as an oxymoron, but it is not. It is helping the person live with a disease. Most chronic diseases like cancer, diabetes, and epilepsy cannot be cured, but they can be controlled. We can help people resume some normalcy and some healthy living, so they can grow and live beyond their condition."

Health is about creating wholeness. Health involves the development of the person's capabilities, capacities, special gifts, and competencies; in other words, the strengths he uses to enable him to survive, cope with, adapt, and function in the world and many lifeworlds in which he lives that are made up of multiple environments. Strengths—that is, qualities, competencies, and capacities—develop over the person's life span as that person dwells in and interacts with his many environments and experiences his many lifeworlds (see Chapter 4 for a full description and discussion of strengths). Health involves the way individuals and families (as well as communities) come to understand and know their many life-worlds, the way they choose to dwell and live in them, and how they develop their full personhood as they strive to find purpose and create meaning in living. An individual's many aspects become increasingly coordinated and integrated as he grows and develops into adulthood and throughout his life span.

Health also develops as a person deals with illness. Think of the actor Michael J. Fox, who has been diagnosed with Parkinson's disease. While his body deteriorates, he deepens as a person by being engaged with his family and devoting his life to finding a cure for Parkinson's disease. Thus, his health is a reflection of his own becoming that is ever present, even in the face of a debilitating disease.

The word *development* is often used interchangeably with *becoming, evolving*, and *growing*. Health is not development per se; instead, health emerges from, and is a reflection of, development of an integrated self (Gottlieb & Gottlieb, 2007). Health involves being able to

- Rally and recover from insults at the biological and behavioral level and, in the process, learn and change from the experience (Audy, 1971)

- Integrate various inputs to optimize functioning
- Effectively regulate arousal levels (physiological, emotional, cognitive); develop secure attachments, meaningful connections, and relationships; and cope effectively with expected and unexpected life events (Gottlieb & Gottlieb, 2007)
- Use internal and external resources appropriately and effectively to meet life challenges
- Have purpose and find meaning in one's life
- Use disruptions caused by illness, traumas, and hardships as opportunities for growth and transformation.
- Find ways to express one's unique personhood and creativity through developing capacities, competencies, and skills (Gottlieb & Gottlieb, 2007; Newman, 2008; Parse, 1999; Reed, 1997)

To summarize SBC's conception of health:

- Health is about creating wholeness, whereby the person develops capacities and competences to live life and deal with life's challenges. Health also is about how the many aspects of a person become integrated to enable her to be a complete, unified entity who finds meaning and purpose in living (see section titled "Value 3: Holism and Embodiment")

> Health exists at all times even when the body succumbs to disease, injury, and disability.

- Health is present and exists at all times even as the body succumbs to disease, injury, and disability
- Health is revealed at times of stress, when things are difficult, not easy
- Health is multifaceted and emerges from and is a reflection of development
- Health exists within illness and illness shapes a person's health
- It is in experiencing and living with illness and other life-changing events that people learn about themselves, their significant relationships, and the world in which they live. In the process of learning, they discover their own personhood and humanity and use what they have learned as opportunities to transform and further develop themselves and the world in which they live
- Health is dynamic, changing, evolving, and expanding. It is a person's inner spirit, her core strengths on which she calls to get the most out of living life as well as to meet life's challenges
- Health is a person's ability to adapt, cope and, most importantly, rally from insults. Insults can be biological, emotional, or situational. Rallying occurs through mobilizing and capitalizing on existing strengths, developing potentials, and turning deficits into strengths (see Chapter 10 for a full discussion of working with strengths)
- Health is when all aspects of the person—including the physical body, mental thoughts, emotions, spiritual awareness, attachments, social relationships, and the ability to regulate and cope—work together to make the person feel complete and whole

Now, consider the story of Texas-born Rabbi Ronnie Cahana, whose congregation took him and his family to Montreal, Quebec, Canada. In the prime of his life, at age 57, he suffered a debilitating brain stem stroke that left him quadriplegic. In reading the newspaper story, as told in Exhibit 3.1, reflect on why the reporter considers Rabbi Cahana "the healthiest and happiest person he knows." Compare your answer with the SBC indicators of health.

EXHIBIT 3.1

Reflect and connect *The healthiest person I know: The "Blinkischer" Rabbi*

By Gil Troy, *Canadian Jewish News*, August 15, 2011

On July 15, Ronnie Cahana, the 57-year-old rabbi of Congregation Beth-El in Montreal's Town of Mount Royal, suffered a massive stroke in his brainstem. He now lies immobilized in the Montreal Neurological Institute, unable to talk, walk or even wave. Yet, his mind is intact and his spirit is soaring, and from his hospital bed, Rabbi Cahana is teaching his devoted congregants, his loving family and the rest of us, about the soul's power and Judaism's deeper meaning, even when we lose the physical, the material. "I live in a broken place," he said when stricken, "but there's holy work to do."

Rabbi Cahana's body is in trouble. A ventilator and other tubes do for him what most of us do naturally. Nevertheless, he may be the healthiest—and happiest—person I know. "Emotional paralysis is far worse than physical paralysis," he preaches. "To live humanly is to believe in the pure and the profound. To live...is to choose the blessing over the curse. I choose blessing and feel blessed."

Before the stroke, this gangly, 6'2 Houston-born rabbi was the least Texan, and the most unconventional Conservative rabbi, I knew—I befriended Ronnie and his amazing wife, Karen, decades ago. A dazzling personality, both vital and ethereal, as well as a passionate Jew and perpetual seeker, Rabbi Cahana has never done small talk. He makes even the most casual interaction intense and intimate. Watching him with his congregants and his family is wondrous. His "How are you?" is never perfunctory. Rather, it's a sincere probe, asking whether you're getting the most out of your life, nurturing fulfilling relationships while benefiting from the kind of profound interaction he enjoys with Judaism and God.

Visiting the bedridden rabbi, you brace for heartbreak and emerge uplifted. He mouths words—or laboriously blinks them out. When no one can read his lips, he closes his eyes, and someone starts reciting "a, b, c ..." He opens his eyes at the desired letter. The "Blinkischer Rebbe," as Karen calls him, blinks out stirring weekly sermons, greeting congregants from his "subterranean world," urging them to use the blow he sustained to experience life and Judaism in new dimensions. "I know the end will be good," this rabbinic Stephen Hawking insists. "I did not lose anything. I gained."

All summer, Rabbi Cahana has bathed in his extraordinary family's love and laughter—he and Karen have five fabulous children, ages 14 to 23. Karen says it's hard to despair when he's so positive, when he delights in "feeling" every prayer

(continued)

EXHIBIT 3.1 (*Continued*)

for him, "visiting" with his late father, renewing his relationship to Judaism and God by painstakingly re-learning each mitzvah[a] (good deed—commandment by God), bringing new meaning to each commandment.

Every weekday morning, he puts on tefillin (phylacteries) at the same time his congregants do. "Finding spiritual paths in the hospital while vulnerable and fragile," he blinked to them, provides "a great delight of the day... I hear the tone, rhythm, the light banter, music and join you. I know our sounds and I listen to your voices. Our prayers are good and honest, and God looks favorably on the kind."

Currently, he can only wear the head phylacteries[b] This, he calls "the most healing of privileges. The retzuot [straps] course through the whole body... from the mind. Crown encircles the cranium. In the holiest of holies, the spirit, which we believe lies contiguously off of Hashem's (God's) holy knot, sits on the brainstem to heal, to repair, to purify the world."

Rabbi Cahana continues to progress. In fact, he has already progressed much faster than the doctors predicted.

[a]MITZVAH: Commandments of how to live a moral life that includes acts of kindness and all good deeds believed to be divined or inspired by God. Judaism has 620 such commandments.

[b]PHYLACTERIES: Little black leather boxes containing prayers worn by religious Jews during weekday morning prayers. One goes around the head, held by a leather strap whose knot falls in the back of the head, the other on the left arm, close to the heart.

Source: Reprinted with permission Gil Troy and *The Canadian Jewish News*

Reflect and Connect Instructions:

1. Why does Gil Troy consider Rabbi Ronnie Cahana to be "the healthiest person he knows"? Compare your answer with SBC's indicators of health.
2. How would Rabbi Cahana's health be rated from a deficit model or health as the absence of disease?
3. Using SBC indicators of health, describe which ones are present in Rabbi Cahana.
4. What are the advantages of working with this conceptualization of health in nursing Rabbi Cahana?

B. Healing

Nightingale saw healing as a reparative process regulated by the laws of nature. By discovering the laws of healing, she believed nurses could participate in the restorative process through acts that supported the person's innate mechanisms of healing (Dossey, Selnaders, & Beck, 2005).

Healing is part of the human condition because it involves suffering and anguish (Egnew, 2005; Mount, Boston, & Cohen, 2007). Healing implies that something has been broken, damaged, or maimed. We talk of healing a wounded body, a broken heart, and a destroyed soul. Healing is a response to suffering and the need to repair, rebound, and renew. As such, it has been associated with themes of wholeness, integrity, narratives, finding new meaning, and transcendence through spirituality (Egnew, 2005).

Nurses have conceptualized healing in different ways, but common to all definitions is the notion of wholeness (McElligott, 2010). Healing involves acts of becoming whole (Cowling, 2000; Kritek, 1997). McElligott (2010), by way of a concept analysis of the nursing literature, theoretically defined healing as "a positive, subjective, unpredictable process involving transformation to a new sense of wholeness, spiritual transcendence, and reinterpretation of life."(p. 257). She went on to operationally define healing as "the personal experience of transcending suffering and transforming wholeness resulting in serenity, interconnectedness, and a new sense of meaning" (p. 258). Healing requires that the person become aware of how healing takes place and then to actively engage in his own healing. Healing is not only a noun, but also a verb and, as such, involves many biological, psychological, cognitive, and relational processes to repair, restore, renew, redefine, regenerate, and rehabilitate. Healing may or may not involve curing; instead, it mainly involves conserving energy and redirecting that energy to repairing the damage caused by the disease, injury, insult, and treatment with the goal of restoring wholeness. Thus, nurses can measure healing by observing the patient's state of serenity, interconnectedness, and new level of meaning.

Health care professionals often focus on one part of the person as a way of healing the whole, yet healing begins with an appreciation of the whole and how the different parts of the person (i.e., mind/body/emotions/spirituality) are interrelated and interconnected. (The idea of whole or holism is elaborated in the section titled "Value 3: Holism and Embodiment").

Dr. Balfour Mount, a physician and pioneer in palliative care, described his process of healing in his quest for wholeness following several reoccurrences of cancer. Mount defined healing as involving "a process of opening, slowing, centering, trusting, and accepting. This process leads us away from preoccupation with all that has been lost to a clearer recognition of the potential that remains." Healing also requires letting go, experiencing the present, freeing oneself from past fears, or from fears of the future. Mount reminded us that healing may not always involve curing the disease; instead, healing is how a person comes to understand and live with the illness and develops other aspects of the self. Mount's personal experience is described in Exhibit 3.2.

Now let us return to Heather and how she conceptualizes health and healing.

VALUE 1

Nurse Heather Hart's Care of Ellen as Reflected in Health and Healing
Note that in Heather's description of Ellen (p. 56–57), the first thing that she commented on is not Ellen's medical history with cancer or her symptoms but rather on Ellen, the person. Heather asks herself *"Who is Ellen?"* Moreover, what Heather first notices is Ellen's health despite her illness when she said, *"I saw some spunk, some life, some really positive energy coming out of this woman who was really, really ill."* Heather is attuned to Ellen's special qualities that define Ellen's personhood, in other words, her strengths.

EXHIBIT 3.2

Personal experience *I Believe*

Balfour M. Mount
© CBC Radio—This I Believe, June 18, 2007
www.cbc.ca/thisibelieve

I believe in healing. I am not speaking of physical healing, a person can die healed: what I mean by "healing" is a shift away *from* anguish and suffering, *toward* an experience of integrity, wholeness and inner peace. The ultimate *goal* of healing is more effective service to others and to the global village of which we are temporary trustees.

My thoughts have been shaped by multiple personal brushes with death—a plane crash; two cancers and all that followed those diagnoses; a heart attack; the deaths of loved ones; my work as a cancer surgeon; the privilege of caring for the dying over the last three decades. Paradoxically, the message emerging from these experiences has been about *living*, not dying. The psyche, it would seem, has an intrinsic tendency toward healing, a will to wholeness, as it were.

I believe healing, like love, celebration, awe and ecstasy, happens in the present moment, free from ruminations about the past and fears for the future. It involves letting go, a leap of faith, "diving not drowning" as Carl Jung expressed it. ALS patient Philip Simmons called it "learning to fall." We fall *from* head, *to* heart; *from* egoism and defense mechanisms, *to* forgiveness of ourselves and others. We may thus come to glimpse the staggering potential of our essential selves and experience an awareness of the *healing connections* that provide meaning, hope and a sense of an inner peace.

I believe healing connections happen at four levels: a sense of connection to self; connection to others; connection to the world perceived through our senses (as with music, or the grandeur of nature); and connection to ultimate meaning, however perceived (God, the More, the Cosmos). While my experience of the first of these—connection to self—is slowly unfolding, I have, throughout life, been enriched beyond measure through each of the other domains. In spite of this, I have too often felt trapped by circumstances —stuck with the "Why me?" "Why now?" "What if?" questions of life. It is at such times that I am humbled by Viktor Frankl's comment following his liberation from Auschwitz, "Everything can be taken from a man but one thing: the last of human freedoms—to choose one's attitude in any given circumstances, to choose one's own way."

I believe my challenge is to open with acceptance to each moment; to listen to my intuition; to develop self-reflective skills; to be more gentle with myself; to think small; to give up illusions of control; to recognize that we are all in the same boat; to celebrate. If Frankl can find life worth celebrating in Auschwitz, chances are *I* can find reasons to celebrate.

(continued)

EXHIBIT 3.2 *(Continued)*

I believe healing involves a process of opening, slowing, centering, trusting and accepting. It involves recognizing the potential that remains, in spite of all that has been lost.

Finally, **I believe** that I must take up the journey toward healing anew each day. The renowned Jewish scholar, Hillel, put it succinctly, "If I don't do it, who will do it? If I don't do it now, when will I do it?"

C. Relationship between health and healing

Health and healing are both about wholeness. Health is about creating wholeness, whereas healing is about restoring and discovering wholeness.

Wholeness is the integration and coordination among the various aspects of a person, including the physical, mental, emotional, and social aspects of the person that work together to achieve coherence and completeness. Wholeness is when a person feels in balance, in harmony, and experiences a level of wellness that allows for optimal functioning. From conception to death, the focus is on developing all aspects of the person: his physical, cognitive, mental, emotional, social, and spiritual domains of functioning (Gottlieb & Gottlieb, 2007).

> Health and healing are about wholeness. Health is about creating wholeness, whereas healing is about restoring and rediscovering wholeness.

While healing, the person learns from the experience and, in the process, achieves a new level of health. Healing allows the person to experience a calmness and serenity, even if it is just for the moment. Health and healing are akin to what happened to Humpty Dumpty in the classic Mother Goose rhyme :

> Humpty Dumpty sat on a wall,
> Humpty Dumpty had a great fall;
> All the king's horses and all the king's men
> Couldn't put Humpty together again.   (*The Dorling Kindersley Book of Nursery Rhymes*, (2000).)

Before Humpty Dumpty fell off the wall, he was whole—healthy. Then catastrophe struck, and he fell off the wall. He required treatment to repair his shell. "All the king's horses and all the king's men / couldn't put Humpty together again." Let's imagine that, with the help of a SBC nurse, Humpty found the energy to put himself back together again!

Let us also assume that the effort of putting Humpty back together, to restore wholeness, most likely involved acts of self-healing, such as balancing activity and rest, promoting sleep, engaging in exercise, eating well, promoting relaxation, and reducing stress; in other words, any activity that promotes and supports the body's innate reparative processes. The body's reparative processes include, among many other things, boosting the immunological system, improving cardiac and kidney functioning, improving functioning of the mind, and so forth. It also involves attending to the emotional, mental, and spiritual to help patients make sense of what has happened to them in their quest to find new meaning and purpose.

Arthur Frank (2002), a sociologist and himself a patient, related his experience of being first diagnosed as having sustained a heart attack at the age of 39 and then, 15 months later, with testicular cancer. He wrote about his experiences with illness and its effects on himself, his family, and his life. Before the diagnosis, he had achieved a certain level of wholeness (health). He was a relatively young man who led a busy life, fully engaged in living. Once diagnosed, he experienced a wide range of emotions: fear and frustration with a body that seemed to be breaking down, fear of dying, anger for having his life disrupted, and a sense of vulnerability that something else could happen. Being ill disrupted his routine, altered his relationships, and caused him to reflect on the meaning of his life. During treatment, his life was suspended as he directed his energy to dealing with chemotherapy and its debilitating side effects. During and following treatment, he redirected his energy toward healing—not just restoring and repairing the damage that had been caused by his heart disease and his cancer and its treatment but also on renewing his body, mind, soul, and relationships. The act of restoring wholeness required a great deal of his energy and, in the process, he learned about himself and his will to live. He profited from this experience, learned about his own strengths and limitations, and about those people around him. He also discovered what really mattered to him.

SBC requires that nurses have knowledge and skills of health and healing that go far beyond an understanding of health that is merely the absence of disease. When nurses value health and healing in terms of wholeness, they are in a better position to promote health by creating wholeness, and to facilitate healing by restoring wholeness.

Value 2: Uniqueness of the Person

Everyone knows that no two people are alike, and yet there often exists, particularly in the health care system, a tendency to treat everyone as if they were the same. Each individual has her own special qualities and inner spirit that defines her unique personhood. Each individual occupies a special niche in his family and community that no one else can fill. In other words, each person is irreplaceable. What makes a person unique?

No two people, even identical twins, have the same genetic makeup (Fraga et al., 2005). It has always been assumed that identical twins (i.e., monozygotic twins) are clones of each other because they come from the same fertilized egg (i.e., zygote), yet monozygotic (identical) twins are indeed different. They may look alike, but both have their own unique character and personality (Harris, 2006). Part of what accounts for these differences is the influence of environment and unique experiences on a person's genetic makeup.

From the moment of conception until death, people are shaped and being shaped both by their genes (i.e., their *genotype*) and by their multiple environments. Environment interacts with genes to produce an individual's *phenotype* (i.e., the actual person). The environment, on the other hand, is influenced by a person's genetic makeup. All parents will tell you about the unique characteristics of their newborn infants. They know which baby was calm and which was hyperreactive, which baby liked to be cuddled and which stiffened to the parents' touch, which baby was outgoing and which was shy.

Researchers have established that these temperamental characteristics are genetic and will affect how an infant reacts to her environments and how parents are affected by the child's behavior (Plomin, 2009). Children who have difficulties regulating their emotions and are behaviorally difficult to control often have parents who show elevated levels of distress and resort to harsh parenting (Deater-Deckard, 2009). Therefore, parents, siblings, family members, peers, teachers and others in the person's social environments are influenced by that person's personality and genetic makeup (Bouchard, 2009).

In addition to the interactions between an individual's genetic-based characteristics and the environment at the whole-organism level are those that take place at the cellular and tissue levels. These interactions between cells and tissues, and their microenvironments (also known as *extracellular environments*) help determine the phenotype of cells and tissues. The term *microenvironment* refers to the fluid that surrounds cells and tissues, which is made up of water and chemicals.

Consider how a person's reproductive tissues develop. If, during the development of reproductive organs, the level of extracellular sex hormones is too low, then the person's sex organs will fail to develop properly, and the person will be infertile. Moreover, the microenvironment is in turn influenced by the external environment. If a person's diet lacks fat, then that person will not be able to produce adequate amounts of sex hormones (i.e., estrogen and testosterone). This will result in low sex hormone levels in the extracellular fluid that could affect the growth of certain tissues and organs such as reproductive cells.

At the whole-person level, all people have their own unique experiences and special circumstances that affect the course of their lives and, consequently, how they grow and develop and the individuals they become. Within cultures and different societies, individual differences are due to genetic variability and genotype–environment interactions (Arnett & Tanner, 2009). Moreover, people's lives are transformed by different transitional events (Meleis, Sawyer, Im, Hilfinger, & Schumacher, 2000; Schumacher & Meleis, 1994). These events have been classified into four types of transitional events: (a) developmental and life span events, (b) situational events, (c) social and cultural events, and (d) health and illness events.

Developmental and life span events are expected and are usually biologically driven. They include puberty, pregnancy, childbirth, menopause, aging, and death. *Situational events* are unique to that individual. They can be events or experiences that the person chooses, such as the partner they select or the college at which they choose to study, or they can be chance events. *Social and cultural events* are experiences that are affected by the social and cultural milieu in which the person grows up and develops. One example of a social and cultural event is immigrating to a new country. Finally, *health and illness events*, including accidents and trauma, can profoundly affect and change a person as well as those involved in the person's life. An encounter with a serious illness, or living with a chronic condition, often changes how a person views his body and its limitations (Frank, 2002). Because illness is a

> Transitions create opportunities for developing strengths because new competencies and skills are acquired.

"family affair," the person's illness can affect others' reactions to him, which in turn affects how the person copes with his own illness.

Transitional events are usually transformational, altering the course of a person's life. They are opportunities for developing strengths, including new competencies and skills. The way a person deals with the challenges inherent in any transitional event determines the course of that person's uniqueness. A person's uniqueness is also shaped by the historical times in which she lives—the social, political, and economic events that influence decisions and determine the nature of opportunities (see the section titled "Value 6: The Person and Environment Are Integral").

Another reason why no two people are alike is that each individual experiences various life environments very differently. Even individuals in the same environment are said to have "nonshared" environments (Dunn & Plomin, 1990). Consider siblings growing up in the same household with the same parents. It was always assumed that these children had the same experiences, even though they were different biologically. However, this assumption has proven to be false. Parents grow and develop; therefore, a second-born child has a very different set of parents than an older sibling because the parents are older, and thus more experienced, when the second child is born. Even identical twins are likely to have parents who relate to them differently because both twins have hundreds of genetic and nongenetic variations that define their individual personality, character, and strengths. Thus, a person's uniqueness is an expression of the interaction between her genetic, biological features and her environments based on the principles of nature via nurture (Gottlieb & Gottlieb, 2007).

These same ideas apply to the family. No two families are alike; each is made up of unique individuals, and together they create a specialized family identity with its own shared meanings, experiences, and strengths.

The health care system is designed to treat people in standardized, prescriptive, rigidly defined ways in which the prevalent principle of care is based on the premise that "one size fits all." This is evident in nursing care plans and medication and treatment regimens. This approach to care is clearly inconsistent with our knowledge of the biology and socialization of the person. By discovering and working with strengths, the unique features and qualities of the individual and family are revealed. Thus, SBC is a more effective and responsive way to honor each person's uniqueness and to provide people what they need for their own health and healing.

> The current health care system is prescriptive with a "one size fits all" approach to care, In practice, "one size fits no one" because everyone is unique.

Value 3: Holism and Embodiment

The current U.S. health care system is organized around body systems. In every hospital there are divisions labeled *cardiology, urology, neurology,* and so forth. This organizational structure extends to how some clinicians care for patients. Some nurses have as their main focus the diseased body part or symptom, not the person. Others view the patient as a person who just happens to be ill with a disease. Their focus of care should be on the person, on understanding his condition, and how he is dealing with it. When nurses reduce a person to his body parts—namely, tissues, organs, and systems—they "disembody" the person and thereby separate the person's body from his personhood. This worldview is often referred to as *reductionist*. Alternatively, clinicians can view the person as a whole, whereby parts of the body and the various body systems and domains of functioning are highly integrated. This worldview, in which the person is viewed as embodied and in which there are deemed to be no boundaries between mind and body, is commonly referred to as *holism*. Below, I briefly describe the reductionist view to illustrate how this view affects the way a nurse cares for a patient. Holism and embodiment comprise a different set of values that necessitates a different approach to nursing.

Conceptualizations

A. Reductionism and disembodiment

In looking at a patient through a reductionist lens, the body is viewed as an object that can be diagnosed and treated. The body is divided into organs and systems (*anatomized*), examined for how the organ or system functions (*physiologized*), and understood in terms of the biochemical reactions that take place at the cellular level (*biochemicalized*; Sakalys, 2006). For example, a patient may be seen as having a set of kidneys (anatomized), with an imbalance in kidney input and output (physiologized) and high creatinine levels (biochemicalized). Looking at the patient through through this lens, a nurse may focus solely on alleviating or treating the symptom, whereas the patient focuses on how the symptoms/disease affects her life. To continue the example, a woman may be distressed that she cannot urinate because she interprets this as a sign that she could die. Or consider a woman who experiences depression or anxiety following the removal of her breast because of a malignant tumor (cancer). A nurse could use medications to help the woman deal with her anxiety and not investigate further as to what may be contributing to this anxiety. On the other hand, this woman's anxiety may be due to any number of concerns, such as dealing with the actual treatment and its side effects of nausea and hair loss, or grieving the loss of her breast, that serves as a reminder that she has breast cancer and could die. She may also be dealing with the reactions of her partner, who is reluctant to look at her body, or she may be upset by her children's withdrawal from her for fear of losing their mother. It is as if the nurse and the patient are dealing with two different bodies and are concerned with different issues.

Reductionism not only divides the body into organs and systems but also divides the person into four different selves: (a) the biological self, (b) the psychological self, (c) the social self, and (d) the spiritual self. Clinicians commonly talk about treating the physical, emotional, social, or spiritual aspects of a person, and medical regimens are often prescribed to treat one of these areas without consideration of how all these aspects of the person make up the whole (Lloyd & Dunn, 2007). The case I just described is a good illustration of how the whole is indeed greater than the sum of its individual parts.

Another characteristic of reductionism is that it separates the person into the mind and body, which are treated as separate and distinct, unrelated entities. When body and mind are separated, this is commonly known as the *disembodied mind*. According to this view, the mind and the body are disconnected (Carnevale, 1995). The mind can exist without reference to what is happening in the body, and the body can be treated without considering how bodily changes affect the mind or even the development of brain structures. Disembodiment involves a distancing of the person from his body. A nurse caring for a patient with a broken arm may refer to the arm as "that arm," not "your arm." When nurses ask patients solely about their body parts, such as "How is your heart today?" rather than "How are you today? Any changes in how your heart is?" they are engaging in disembodiment.

Disembodying patients negates their personhood and fails to recognize how body, mind, and soul are one. Can there be a situation in which disembodiment is beneficial? There are situations when patients use disembodiment as a coping strategy to deal with overwhelming distress and pain. Morse and Mitcham (1998) discovered that patients who experienced agonizing pain as a result of severe burns coped by using disembodiment. Their study is described in Exhibit 3.3. When used as a coping strategy, disembodiment may in fact reinforce embodiment. When the patient's pain is under better control, he will be more likely to experience a better quality of life. He will be able to heal better as his being redirects resources to healing. Think of how much better a person sleeps when his pain is under control. Energy, a resource, is directed away from dealing with pain and toward sleeping. It is during sleep that tissues repair themselves and healing occurs.

The majority of health care professionals practice from a reductionist perspective—they reduce the person to his symptoms, separate organs from body systems, body systems from the person, and the person from his illness experience. In other words, they manage the person as a collection of disconnected parts, reduced to one or two narrow dimensions rather than as an integrated whole.

The alternative is to value the person as an integrated, embodied whole human being.

B. Holism and embodiment

Holism is premised on the belief that the person is a unified, indivisible whole and is more than and different from the sum of his parts (Rogers, 1970). In other words, a person cannot be understood just through examining his cells, tissues, organs, or systems. These structures may tell the nurse something about the organ or how the system is functioning, but each structure (i.e., cell, tissue, organ, or system) does not reveal to the nurse very much about who that person is and what makes him unique. As Martha Rogers (1970), an early nurse theorist and first proponent of a unitary concept of the person in nursing, pointed out, "No one mistakes a pancreas or digestive system for a man" (p. 47).

Embodiment means that the mind and body are one and work together as an interrelated, integrated whole. At the same time, there are two prevailing perspectives on holism and embodiment: (a) situated cognitivism and (b) phenomenological. Each seeks to answer the following question: What is the relationship among brain, mind, and body?

Situated-cognitivism view. Many people assume that the brain and mind are one and the same. This is not the case. They are related but are not the same. The body affects the functioning of the mind, and the mind affects and directs how the body functions. Dr. Daniel Siegel (1999), a psychiatrist, neurobiologist, and founder of the area of study called *interpersonal neurobiology*, has devoted his life to understanding the mind and its role in human development. He has argued convincingly, drawing

EXHIBIT 3.3

Empirical study   *How do signals of disembodiment help patients deal with extreme pain due to agonizing injuries?*

The Problem
Research literature discussing embodiment has yet to address the many and multiple modes of disembodiment.

The Issues
When patients exhibit disembodiment after experiencing agonizing injuries, what are the linguistic signals they use and why?

The Study
An analysis of six burn patients who had experienced agonizing injuries revealed reference to their own body parts using depersonalized language (i.e., *it, the, this*). To understand the reason for this, five potential explanations were explored to understand the use of disembodiment language. These included (a) as being due to loss of sensation, (b) as being due to loss of ability to control the affected part, (c) as learned from physicians, (d) as a means to protect the self in an agonizing situation, or (e) as a means of controlling overwhelming pain. These different explanations for the use of linguistic signals of disembodiment were assessed by comparing burn patient interviews with interviews of patients who differed by significant characteristics (i.e., patients who had spinal cord injuries, transplants, or myocardial infarction).

The Findings
The use of disembodying language by burn patients points toward a special human capacity to maintain the integrity of the self during prolonged agonizing experiences.

The Bottom Line
Patient narratives enabled the identification of the presence or absence of disembodying language and located its use when the pain was most intense. This study suggests that, in instances of excruciating pain, patients disembody in order to remove or distance the pain from the self.

Source: Morse & Mitcham, (1998).

on the latest scientific evidence, that the mind is an entity unto itself. Although the mind cannot be seen under a microscope, it does exist, because it defines a person's personhood. The mind affects, and is affected by, all human interactions and a person's interpersonal relationships. The mind is related to the brain inasmuch as all human interactions and connections create the physical structure of the brain. The brain's neuronal connections and structure are shaped by interpersonal experiences, the nature of human connections, and the quality of relationships (Siegel, 1999). In turn, a person's memory, emotion, the ability to regulate one's emotions, internal representations of the environment, and the like affect the functioning of the mind and define the person's reactions to, and the quality of, her existence and experiences. Siegel identified three principles that govern the mind and its interrelationship with the brain and body:

1. The mind emerges from a flow of energy and information between various parts within the brain (brain areas communicate with each other) and between brains (one person connecting with another person).
2. The mind is created within the internal neurophysiological processes (bodily experiences, including illness) and interpersonal experiences (i.e., relationships with others).
3. The structure and function of the brain are determined by experiences, in particular human relationships, that shape the genetically programmed maturation of the nervous system (p. 2).

The mind is formed through the person's earliest social experiences, primarily the quality of attachments and how an infant's basic needs are met. The mind is structured and altered by bodily experiences. Body and mind communicate and are connected through intricate and elaborate sets of neurological networks by means of biochemical transmitters that are found in the central nervous system, of which the brain is the command post. Scientists have found that a person's experiences can cause changes in brain structure and the way it is wired. A case in point is how researchers have found that individuals who were severely abused as children were found to have undergone alterations to the development of their limbic system, the area of the brain responsible for regulating emotions and memory (Teicher, 2002). As adults, they had difficulty regulating their emotions and experienced feelings of depression, irritability, and hostility.

Another example of situated-cognitivism embodiment was demonstrated in a study of the effects of mindfulness meditation on the brain and immunological functions. Individuals who took an eight-week meditative program showed alterations both in brain function and immune function compared with individuals who did not take this program (Davidson et al., 2003). The individuals who engaged in mindfulness meditation showed significant increases in both antibodies and brain function in response to an influenza vaccine. What is particularly interesting is that changes in the immune system were not directly related to exposure to a biological agent but were instigated directly by the brain. The implication of this research is that developing mental strength can facilitate healing by stimulating the immune system.

Phenomenological view. The second perspective of embodiment is the phenomenological view. A person who takes the phenomenological view tries to understand the person's *lived experience*—in other words, how that person experiences an event and what it is like to live with its aftereffects. This event can be living with an illness, dealing with the death of a child, or just living life day by day. The person lives and experiences an event as a whole, not as a body or as a mind. This view of embodiment is espoused by Dr. Patricia Benner, the renowned nurse theorist, whose ideas of caring are premised on the concept of embodiment in which the body and the mind are both "knowers" (Benner & Wrubel, 1989). Benner and Wrubel offered the following example to illustrate this idea: An individual comes upon a situation that his mind registers as potentially dangerous. His body often is the first to register and signal danger before he is consciously aware of what is happening. His heart begins to race, a knot forms in the pit of his stomach, his blood pressure shoots up, and he breaks out into a cold sweat. Both body and mind "know" and signal danger. Another example is the case of Naomi, suffering from ovarian cancer, who needs to give a urine specimen prior to chemotherapy. Naomi required ten cycles of chemotherapy, and with each treatment she had a more severe reaction to the accumulated effects of chemotherapy. The first time Naomi was asked to give a sample of her urine, she had no problem producing the specimen. By the fourth cycle, Naomi began to have more difficulty urinating. She could only produce a few drops. It was if her body knew what was to come. Her body was rebelling, refusing to cooperate. This may have been her body's way of trying to delay or avoid another chemotherapy treatment.

Holism and embodiment is about completeness and integration. It is achieved when all aspects of a person are working together in harmony. It focuses on how one area of a person's life affects other areas. When there is discord in a family, the patient may react viscerally and physically, as was the case of Marty.

Nurse Frank Carnevale, a former head nurse of a pediatric intensive care unit and pain consultant, tells of nursing a 12-year old-boy, Marty, who suffered from severe intestinal ulcers. Frank was asked to help Marty manage his uncontrollable and uncontrolled pain. In the course of getting to know Marty, Frank learned that Marty's parents were going through a bitter divorce.

As Frank related, *"One day, after working through some relaxation exercises with Marty to reduce his pain, I asked him: 'How are you? What's making you feel better? What's making you sad?' He said that he had been wanting to tell me something but was too shy to do so. And I said to him, 'You have my confidence, I will respect your privacy, don't worry.' Then Marty spoke at length about how awful, absolutely awful, he felt about what was going on between his mother and father. He went on and on about how much they fought in front of him and that he knew that it made his tummy worse because he was so upset. He was demoralized about his body and was so discouraged."*

Marty understood holism and embodiment. He understood that the emotional distress from his parents' divorce was registering in his gut and that his pain was affecting his parents and the way they responded to him.

Embodiment is the integration of body and mind shaped by the various social and cultural situations in which the person lives and, in particular, by the person's social relationships and connections (see section titled "Value 6: The Person and Environment Are Integral"). People express their innermost selves through their bodies. Think of how much the fashion industry spends on dressing the body. According to this industry, cosmetics and clothes are ways people express their individuality and communicate to others who they are. People judge others on the basis of appearance. An individual's mood is affected by her perception of how others think she looks and how well she herself thinks she looks. Consider the expression "I feel good when I look good." It is physical appearance that affects how people feel about themselves, how they relate to others, and how others in turn relate to them.

It is through understanding holism that nurses can identify a person's specific strengths. As Martha Rogers (1970) stated, "Only as man's oneness is apprehended is it possible to identify man's distinctive attributes" (p. 44). What she meant by *attributes* are here called *strengths*.

The field of nursing embraces the idea of knowing the whole person; however, as nurses attend to specific body parts (e.g., inserting a catheter, starting an IV) or alleviate symptoms (e.g., managing pain), they need to be aware that the person responds with her whole being. Nurses can understand the whole person often through caring for her parts, but they can care for the parts only if they keep the whole person as their focus of care (Newman, 2008). Let's return to Nurse Heather Hart's care of Ellen to understand how this value is reflected in Heather's nursing of Ellen.

VALUE 3

Nurse Heather Hart's Care of Ellen as Reflected in Holism, Embodiment

Heather gained insight into Ellen and learned more about who Ellen was when Ellen revealed how changes in her body affected how Ellen's husband related to her and how she saw herself. Soon after Heather met Ellen, Ellen asked her to take a picture of her with another nurse. Heather described what happened: *"As I was about to take the photo, I said 'Say cheese', and Ellen said, 'No, I think we should say sex.' There was this crazy moment, and what came out of Ellen's mouth really surprised me. She said, 'I haven't had sex in three years—not since my colostomy. My husband couldn't handle it.' I just sat with her for awhile, and I said, 'How has that been for you?' And she talked about how it had been and how it hadn't been good and the* [emotional] *pain* [it had caused her]. *"*

Ellen never talked about what was happening to her, and so the other staff members on the unit assumed that she was incapable of looking into herself. Heather continued: *"What I saw was a young woman with some insight into her situation who did have the capacity to look at her pain. She wasn't talking about it or sharing it a lot, but this suggested that maybe I was going to be privileged to learn about who Ellen was and what she was going through. This was an opening to make a connection with her in a little deeper way."*

Value 4: Objective/Subjective Reality and Created Meaning

There is a joke that every married person lives in three marriages: his marriage, her marriage, and what outsiders see as their marriage. There is some truth to this. There are many realities, and each person has his own perspective that affects him. The person arrives at certain understandings or meanings of the situation, which are then woven together to create a narrative to explain what is happening or has happened to them. Narratives weave together different events that are linked in meaning, interpretation, and explanation. They help integrate disparate threads and events in a person's life to create a coherent story. A person creates a narrative in order to make sense of the world and decide what is important and what is unimportant. As David Brooks (2009), an op-ed columnist for *The New York Times,* reminded us, "Among all the things we don't control, we do have control over our stories." Later in this column he wrote that "The most important power we have is the power to help select the lens through which we see reality" and that this reality is reflected in the way a person creates and re-creates storylines and then constructs and develops his narrative. The narrative that the person creates in turn shapes his behavior and the choices and decisions he makes.

This same idea also applies to health care providers who view the world through their own lens and can create their own stories about their patients if they are unaware of the patients' own stories. These ideas are commonly referred to as *subjective reality* and *created meaning*.

There also exists *objective reality*, which is derived from that which can be observed, measured, counted, and verified (Helman, 2007). Objective data contribute to objective reality and include blood analysis, urine testing, radiography readings, psychological assessments, and so forth. These are invaluable sources of information used by clinicians to help them arrive at a diagnosis. These data play a significant role in helping them grasp the clinical significance of a symptom, make a clinical judgment of what is significant and important to attend to, and make clinical decisions.

Most health care practitioners have traditionally valued objective data over subjective data. In fact, most assign more weight to objective data than to what the person says or believes (i.e., subjective data). Up until recently, subjective information obtained from the patient was considered to be a "black box," hidden from view, and, therefore, of little interest or consequence. If the information a person gave could not be directly observed, measured, and verified, it was considered less valid and of little importance or value compared to information that could be objectified and verified. Many health care practitioners believe they can accurately diagnose and treat a problem solely by relying on information obtained through clinical testing (e.g., blood tests, imaging data, x-rays) with minimal consultation of and cooperation from the patient.

In contrast, another school of thought believes that objective data are limited and limiting because they provide only part of the picture. If information does not include what the person is experiencing and how he is experiencing the event, there can be little understanding of the nature of the problem. In this school of thought it is important to ask a person about his experiences, not only to understand the problem but also to develop a treatment plan that fits. In fact, in some circles the pendulum has swung to the other extreme, where some scientists and practitioners believe that objective reality and truth is a mirage. They argue that objective data do not exist because such data, even those produced by the most sophisticated technology, still have to be interpreted. In other words, interpretation is a subjective act that is carried out by another person and must be filtered through her subjective lens and is dependent on her knowledge and prior experiences.

SBC values both objective data and subjective realities because each provides the nurse with different pieces of information that, when put together, create a more complete picture of the person. Nurses draw on knowledge from the basic and medical sciences, which value objective data; from the applied and human sciences, which value both objective and subjective data; as well as from the humanities, particularly philosophy, which involve a search for meaning and capture the essence of the human experience (Polifroni, 2011). It is a blending of the knowledge from the sciences and humanities in the search for understanding of the whole person, and together with the person and his family's experiences during health and traumatic life events, that contribute to the development of nursing science. Because of the nature of nursing, nurses require knowledge from many disciplines that can shed light on and give understanding to many different realities. A great deal of a nurse clinician's work is trying to figure out the problem by understanding the person and family within the context of their lives. Nurses engage in investigative detective work to arrive at a clinical grasp of the situation on which to base clinical interpretations, make clinical judgments in order to make informed clinical decisions (Benner, Hooper-Kyriakidis, & Stannard, 2011).

Conceptualizations

Subjective reality and created meaning

Every person has his own belief systems and personal experiences and has developed a perception of situations that form the basis of what he believes to be the truth. These perceptions then construct his realities. One of the most important movements in the past century has been to reconsider the question "What is reality?" (Wright & Bell, 2009). Zukav (1979) summarized what he believes is involved in creating reality:

> Reality is what we take to be true.
> What we take to be true is what we believe.
> What we believe is based on our perceptions.
> What we perceive depends on what we look for.
> What we look for depends on what we think.
> What we think determines what we take to be true.
> What we take to be true is our reality. (p. 328)

Every human being also needs to make sense of their lives and what is happening to them. In short, they need to create meaning. One way they do this is by constructing a narrative, a story about themselves, their lives, and their experiences, that makes sense to them (Liehr & Smith, 2008; Siegel, 1999). It is this narrative that serves to bridge perception, thought, and emotion. Thus, a person's story becomes her reality that affects how she then feels, thinks, reasons, and what she subsequently says and does. Because people's reality is expressed through their narratives, these narratives provide nurses a window into their patients' perspectives and how and what they are experiencing (Charon, 2001; Mattingly, 1998). Nurses need to ask themselves and their patients, "What does that look like to you from where you are at?" as a way to begin to enter the person's world (Frank, 2004).

There is a growing appreciation that subjective reality is a powerful influence that affects behavior and plays a central role in person-centered, whole-person care (Sullivan, 2003). People continuously interpret what is happening to them and around them, from moment to moment and from experience to experience. The need to create meaning takes on even greater importance when a person has to cope with difficult and negative events, such as illness, trauma, disability, loss, and death. It is the person's subjective reality that a nurse needs to understand if the nurse is to provide care in ways that are sensitive, meaningful, and responsive.

The role of the narrative in subjective reality and created meaning

Nurse Virginia Lee, who works with newly diagnosed cancer patients, understands that she needs to listen to the person's story because it is that story that will reveal who that patient is and what he wants. As Virginia explained, *"I learn from my patients' stories and interactions. They're the source of knowledge and wisdom because they've lived through it. I haven't gone through it and I need my patients' testimonials to tell me what their story is about. And each and every story is so unique because of their unique person-alities, their disposition in life, where they've gained these sources of knowledge, whether it's from family or from their business . . . it's just a wealth of information when they tell me their life story."*

People create meaning through complex processes that involve understanding and interpreting present events in light of past experiences and acquired knowledge. This process is similar to what nurses go through in arriving at a clinical understanding of their patients' situations. One way of creating meaning is by interpreting the unfamil-iar and relating it to something that is familiar or already known. Consider the famous poem that tells of six blind men who did not know what an elephant looked like, told in Exhibit 3.4. Each man felt a different part of the elephant and interpreted, on the basis of his own past experiences, the part of the elephant he was touching. Therefore, the three men all arrived at a different conception of what an elephant is. In much the same way, people attach meanings on the basis of their prior experiences and how they perceive a situation (Mattingly, 1998).

Another way to understand an experience is when the person dwells on the expe-rience and relives her story. In the course of telling her story, the person may come to experience the event differently and understand the situation in a new light. Each time she retells her story, she may come up with a new interpretation to explain the events and what happened. It is when people are fully engaged in telling their story that they create new meanings and insights into what they have experienced and are experiencing. Consider a woman who recounts the joy she experienced in giving birth. Many years later, she recasts the birth experience as one of the major events of her life and reexperiences the emotions and feelings of awe or trauma experienced at that time. Or consider a woman who has lost her father in a car accident. In telling the story and reliving the experience, she can expand her awareness of what hap-pened and why it happened. The way a person comes to understand an event will either promote self-healing or delay it. The issue here is not whether the narrative is factually correct but whether the story makes sense to the person. The way a person makes sense of a particular situation is determined through the meanings they have assigned to the situation, the context in which their story unfolds, and their beliefs about what has happened to them. These factors contribute to how patients under-stand their illness and how they come to live with it (Wright & Bell, 2009; Wright, Watson, & Bell, 1996).

Factors influencing subjective realities and created meaning. The following story illustrates how two individuals who are exposed to the same situation can each draw very different conclusions about it:

> A shoe factory sends two marketing scouts to a region of Africa to study the prospects of expanding their business. One scout sends back an e-mail saying: *"SITUATION HOPELESS—NO ONE WEARS SHOES HERE."* The other scout writes back triumphantly, *"GLORIOUS BUSINESS OPPORTUNITY— THEY HAVE NO SHOES!"* (Zander & Zander, 2000, p. 9)

EXHIBIT 3.4

The blind men and the elephant

John Godfrey Saxe's (1816–1887) Version of the Famous Indian
Legend

To learning much inclined,
Who went to see the Elephant
(Though all of them were blind),
That each by observation
Might satisfy his mind.

The *First* approach'd the Elephant,
And happening to fall
Against his broad and sturdy side,
At once began to bawl:
"God bless me! but the Elephant
Is very like a wall!"

The *Second*, feeling of the tusk,
Cried, "Ho! what have we here
So very round and smooth and sharp?
To me 'tis mighty clear
This wonder of an Elephant
Is very like a spear!"

The *Third* approached the animal,
And happening to take
The squirming trunk within his hands,
Thus boldly up and spake:
"I see," quoth he, "the Elephant
Is very like a snake!"

The *Fourth* reached out his eager hand,
And felt about the knee.
"What most this wondrous beast is like
Is mighty plain," quoth he,
'Tis clear enough the Elephant
Is very like a tree!"

The *Fifth*, who chanced to touch the ear,
Said: "E'en the blindest man
Can tell what this resembles most;
Deny the fact who can,
This marvel of an Elephant
Is very like a fan!"

(continued)

EXHIBIT 3.4 (*Continued*)

The *Sixth* no sooner had begun
About the beast to grope,
Then, seizing on the swinging tail
That fell within his scope,
"I see," quoth he, "the Elephant
Is very like a rope!"

And so these men of Indostan
Disputed loud and long,
Each in his own opinion
Exceeding stiff and strong,
Though each was partly in the right,
And all were in the wrong!

What might explain why these two men interpreted the same situation so differently?

Personal, family, and social factors contribute to the way a person frames a situation and creates meaning. An individual's biological makeup (e.g., genetic factors that influence his constitutional disposition, such as temperament), his innate and acquired interests, his physical and mental health, his unique circumstances, and the quality of his relationships are some of the many factors that combine to affect how an individual experiences an event. The way a person experiences a situation and interprets it is also determined by that person's belief and value systems, knowledge, and the context and circumstances in which the event happens. Individuals perceive and interpret events through the lens of their cultural background as well as that of the prevailing political and social climate. These are just some of the factors that influence what individuals consciously or unconsciously select and attend to and that help determine how they will react and respond. The issue here is that individuals are not passive recipients but are active players in constructing meaning. Things take on a different significance and assume a greater relevancy at different times in a person's life depending on her understanding of what is at stake and what needs to be accomplished. As Benner (2011) wrote, "Imagination is created, in part, by a deep background understanding and knowledge based on situated possibilities and skillful practice" (p. 349).

Nurses require different types of information to develop a complete and comprehensive understanding of the whole person. Part of SBC is working with information considered objective that reveals what is biologically working and what is not. This includes information obtained from laboratory tests (e.g., blood analyses, urine analyses), x-rays, imaging (e.g., ultrasound), and so forth. It also includes discovering and uncovering people's beliefs, understandings, and perceptions of their situation. Once again, let's return to Nurse Heather Hart and Ellen and how Ellen created meaning to understand her children's reactions to her.

Nurse Heather Hart's Care of Ellen as Reflected in Objective/Subjective Reality and Created Meaning

Nurse Heather Hart related an incident when Ellen left the hospital for a weekend to visit with her family. Upon her return, Heather found that Ellen was very upset. The weekend did not go as Ellen had expected. Heather described what happened: *"Ellen told me 'all the kids did was watch TV all weekend,' and I had the sense that she wanted to connect more with them."* Heather went on to explain the different interpretations Ellen had to explain her children's behavior: *"I had been out of the house for five months and they developed a pattern of functioning without me."*

Heather continued: *"That was her thinking, and she talked about that. She also was aware of the change in her physical appearance. Ellen took the time to put on makeup and wear something nice. She would try to preserve some of her old, former, youthful appearance."*

Ellen's feelings and behaviors are directed by her interpretations and created meanings as she tried to understand why her children reacted to her in the way they did.

Value 5: Self-Determination

Self-determination refers to the value that people have the right to choose and act in accordance with their own thoughts, needs, and feelings (Taylor, 1991). Self-determination requires that the nurse respects another person's right to exercise her own free will to make choices on her own, without coercion. Self-determination also is about encouraging individuals to make decisions about issues that affect their lives in matters of health and health care (Lofman, Pietila, & Haggman-Laitila, 2007; Nordgren & Fridlund, 2001). When people have the power to make choices for themselves, they are more likely to follow their choices and to feel empowered and thus take charge of their own health and health care decisions.

> Nurses who value self-determination recognize the right of the person to determine the course of their own life and make informed choices about decisions governing their health and health care without coercion.

Conceptualization

Self-determination is what motivates people to take action and determines how they will invest their energies. Three requirements are necessary for self-determination: (a) autonomy, (b) relatedness, and (c) competence (Deci & Ryan, 1985). Deci and Ryan (1985) considered autonomy, relatedness, and competence to be basic needs that must be satisfied to varying degrees. The way a person's needs for autonomy, relatedness, and competence are met will affect the extent to which that person has the confidence to choose and exercise his own free will.

Autonomy refers to a person's ability to regulate and control his emotions and make life decisions that are in his best interest (Ryan & Deci, 2006). This means the patient wishes to have control over his own life, and having control means being able to choose what he thinks is right and best for him.

Relatedness refers to a person's need to connect with others. Humans are social by nature and express their need for one another through the connections they make, the relationships they form, and the bonds they create. Decisions are not made in isolation. People need to consider the impact that their decisions will have on others in their social network. The individuals in a person's social network also affect that person's decisions. Consider a woman who has a family history of breast cancer and is contemplating having prophylactic mastectomies for her own long-term survival as well as to help alleviate the anxiety of her children, who fear she may eventually die of breast cancer.

Competence refers to "a condition or quality of effectiveness, ability, sufficiency, or success" (*Oxford English Dictionary*). People need competence to meet their goals. They spend a significant amount of time in developing competence or avoiding feeling incompetent (Elliot & Dweck, 2005). An individual's need to feel competent often drives her decisions. Furthermore, a person who feels competent is more likely to have the confidence to make decisions or to be involved in relevant decision-making processes.

Self-determination is affected by context. In some situations, a person may feel freer to make choices than in other situations. When nurses share knowledge and power with their patients and include them as partners in decisions that affect them, patients feel that they are able to exercise their will—in other words, to act with self-determination. A Swedish study showed that when nurses withheld information from patients or made decisions about their care for them, patients often felt powerless and not in control (Nordgren & Fridlund, 2001).

In some situations, a person has limited control. In a unified mind and body, the mind represents the capacity for choice, whereas the physical body, when sick, often represents that which cannot be chosen (Frank, 2004). In other words, often a person cannot reverse his physical condition even if he wants to. A person cannot choose whether or not to have type 1 diabetes (which usually has juvenile onset with an inherited genetic component). What can be chosen, however, is the manner in which a person chooses to live his life with a chronic condition, disability, or deteriorating body. Consider Philip Simmons, who suffered from amyotrophic lateral sclerosis (ALS), a fatal, degenerative motor neuron disorder that leaves the person trapped in a body that does not function. Although Simmons may have wanted to halt or slow the deterioration of his body caused by the disease, this was not under his control. However, he was free to choose how to live with his disease, which he did, as related in his book *Learning to Fall: The Blessings of an Imperfect Life* (Simmons, 2002). In choosing how to live, Simmons transcended his condition and chose to live life on his own terms instead of living life according to how someone with ALS is represented in the scientific literature or being told by others how he ought to live (Frank, 2004).

Another factor that affects a person's ability to exercise self-determination is her emotional state and how others responds to her. This is well illustrated in a story told by Nurse Siobhan Carney, who was caring for Mrs. Connor, an executive of a large corporation. Mrs. Connor was described as a highly independent woman (autonomy), skilled at her job (competence), and enjoyed a close relationship with her only daughter (relatedness). Here was a woman who was used to making decisions, taking charge, and being in control in her personal and professional life (self-determination). This all changed when she was admitted to hospital for treatment of a brain tumor.

As Siobhan described, *"The diagnosis of a brain tumor was devastating to her and her only child. When I met Mrs. Connor, she was just starting chemotherapy. Her seizures weren't well managed and she was in a lot of psychological distress, feeling completely helpless. This was a woman who was used to being completely in control and now she was completely deferring everything to her daughter. She was very passive in both planning her treatment and even answering questions about her symptoms."*

SBC affirms the person's and the family's right to self-determination. Self-determination enables individuals to become more empowered by exercising greater control and taking more responsibility for their health, health care, and health care decisions that affect how they will live.

However, not all health care professionals subscribe to this value. Nurses whose practice is based on a traditional hierarchical model may believe that their role is to decide what is best for their patients (see Chapter 1 for a discussion of the traditional hierarchical model). These practitioners are generally motivated by a desire to do good, that is, to protect and safeguard their patient's well-being, even if it means limiting the patient right to determine her own future.

Self-determination does not mean that patients alone are responsible for making decisions and that nurses abdicate their role in this area. Nurses who value self-determination believe that decisions are best made when individuals and families are well informed. This requires that patients and families be given the knowledge and information about the issues, have an opportunity to examine different options, and consider the implications of potential decisions. Patients' right to self-determination begins when nurses get to know them as individuals, listen to their stories, understand their past and current experiences, appreciate their values and beliefs, and take into account their situation and the circumstances governing their lives. It is only then that a nurse can be a credible source of information, help raise awareness about other positions and options, support them, and advocate for their decisions.

Nurse Cindy Dalton related the story of Nathan, a middle-age man diagnosed with Parkinson's disease and his partner, Nancy, who was Nathan's main caregiver. As Nathan's disease progressed, he experienced greater difficulty swallowing. However, food had always been very important to Nathan. He enjoyed food and considered himself somewhat of a "gourmand." He refused to have his food pureed, even though he choked on his food several times a week, which required Nancy to perform the Heimlich maneuver. Nancy found this increasingly stressful and distressing. Nathan, in exercising his right to choose, did so at Nancy's expense. Cindy helped the couple explore Nathan's decision about his eating and the impact it was having on him and on Nancy.

As Cindy related, *"What happened eventually was [that] Nancy's distress over Nathan's choice of food became quite significant, and he started to see that he had to give up certain foods. His decision was affecting this couple's harmony. Also, he was losing a lot of weight and he was becoming quite weak because he was not eating enough. Nathan eventually decided to have a feeding tube inserted into his stomach. We had to look at the effect that his decision (of eating all foods) was having on Nancy and the toll it was taking on him. He was not eating as much and was putting himself at risk for poorer health outcomes and a decline in his quality of life because Nathan liked to be quite active. It was helping him to know what was most important to himself. Although he knew what was most important to him, by talking it out, he realized that it (his decision) was working against him."*

Thus, Cindy practiced SBC and promoted Nathan's self-determination by recognizing his needs for autonomy, relatedness, and competence and helping create conditions that developed and facilitated the meeting of these needs.

VALUE 5

Nurse Heather Hart's Care of Ellen as Reflected Self-Determination is presented in the continuing narrative of Ellen and can be found on pages 98 to 99.

Value 6: The Person and Environment Are Integral

Florence Nightingale understood that the quality of a person's environment held the key to his health and healing. Nightingale focused primarily on the physical environment. She recognized that attention to nutrition, ventilation, clean water, good drainage, and cleanliness were basic requirements for health and healing (Nightingale, 1860). The nurse's role was to prevent disease; however, once *disease* occurred, attention to the environment would facilitate the person's innate restorative and reparative processes of healing. Although Nightingale focused on the physical environment, she also understood the importance of the person's interpersonal or social environment, that is, the impact that family and the nurse can have on the person's healing (Dossey et al., 2005). She cautioned nurses to walk slowly, to not hurry for fear of upsetting or disturbing the patient (Nightingale, 1860).

Although our understanding of environments and their relationship to health and healing have expanded since Nightingale's time, her ideas that attention to the environment is crucial and central to nursing must remain an essential value guiding nursing actions today (Rafferty & Wall, 2010).

Conceptualization

It is surprising that just a few years ago some health care professions believed they could understand a person without studying that person in context, that is, in her own environments. This approach was called *context-stripping*. Today, most practitioners understand that human beings do not grow up, develop, and heal in isolation but do so within their many physical, cultural, and social environments (Borenstein, 2010). Moreover, it is important to understand the circumstance surrounding an event, its timing in relation to other events that have happened in the past or are concurrently taking place, other people's responses and reactions, and so forth. All these affect the person and family's reactions and behaviors. The situating of each concern and event in its proper contexts is called the *context principle*. When we talk of context, we refer to the many environments within which a person lives, namely, home, work, school, social, hospital, health care system, and the like. We also talk about *situated experiences*, that is, gaining an understanding of the specifics of a problem through situating it in its proper context.

People dwell in multiple environments. It is the transactions between person and environment that give rise to experiences. Experiences create the person's realities and affect how an event is lived; the feelings and thoughts that are evoked; and the decisions, behavior, responses, and actions that follow.

Environments and experiences

There is a growing appreciation of the complex relationship between the person and his environments. One of the most important insights is that person and environment are integral (Bronfenbrenner, 1979). This means that the person is an essential part of his environment and the environment is an essential part of the person.* Each influences and is influenced by the other. The term *transaction* is used intentionally instead of the more familiar word *interaction*, because interactions imply a unidirectional effect, whereas transactions are reciprocal in nature (Aldwin, 2007). For example, consider how a person copes with a stressor. The stress will induce the person to respond (i.e., cope), and this response will in turn mitigate or intensify the stress. Think of what happens when a person is given bad news. Some people may sit down, others may scream, and still others may faint. The way a person copes with good and bad events will affect how the event is subsequently experienced. One approach may temporarily dull the joy or pain (i.e., of the stress), whereas another may intensify it. The way the person responds will in turn affect another's responses to the event as well as to the person.

Internal environments. A person's internal environment is made up of cells, tissues, organs, and systems. Internal environments are partially under the control of an individual's genes and genetic makeup. Genes establish the basic properties of that environment, such as the pH level, the presence of chemicals such as enzymes and hormones, and both the metabolism and movement of these elements. If an individual's genes—that is, a person's DNA sequence—acquires a mutation (an alteration to the DNA sequence), this could result in environmental changes within the cells, tissues, and organs both in their structure (i.e., their anatomy) and how they function (i.e., their physiology).

Biological factors, such as infectious microorganisms, can also have an effect on an individual's cellular environment. Consider the invasion of a bacteria and virus and how they mobilize and alter an individual's immunological responses. When

---

*Environments include the internal, external, and the social and cultural milieus in which the person lives. A person dwells in multiple environments, often at the same time.

dealing with the physical body, variations in extracellular enzyme and hormone levels can also clearly affect the internal cellular environments. For example, when an individual is under stress, his sympathetic nervous system is aroused. One of the consequences of the activation of the sympathetic nervous system is that the person's digestive system will either shut down entirely, or slow down, as the body attempts to redirect energy resources to deal with the stress or crisis. The person's internal environment is altered, and food remains undigested because of changes in the enzymatic and hormonal conditions within the digestive system. Most individuals are unaware of the moment-to-moment alterations in their internal environments. All they may be aware of is that they are experiencing a stress response to some perceived crisis or threat.

External environments. The person's external environments are those environments that surround him. The external environment can be biological or physical in nature.

In biological environments, the individual comes into contact with another living organism, such as a bacteria, virus, fungus, and so forth. If the person is in a susceptible state whereby her immunological system is compromised, she may succumb to disease.

People are affected by and can affect their ecosystems, that is, the quality of air they breathe, the purity of the water they drink, the availability and quality of food they eat, the nature of their physical space, and the neighborhood in which they live. Each of these factors affects a person's health and the way a person responds to illness.

Social and cultural environments (interpersonal relationships). A person's social environment is made up of relationships, connections, and interactions, with family, friends, acquaintances, and strangers. Environments are multilayered. For example, consider the persons with whom nurses have the most contact with other than the patient, namely, the family.

Within the family there are three levels of influence: (a) individual relationships, (b) the relational level within a family, and (c) the family as a unified system. At the individual level, influence occurs when one family member's actions affect another family member. At the second level, individuals form relationships, such as spousal, parent–child, and sibling. At the third level is the family as a unified system whereby the system reacts as a whole (see Figure 3.1). Consider what happens when a mother gets sick. The husband may worry about his wife and feel very much alone or abandoned because she is unavailable to him (individual level). He may also have to take over her role in the family, by cooking, cleaning, and caring for the children. His relationship with his children may change as a result (relational level). The family as a whole may find that their family routine is altered. They no longer have dinner together. Some children may become more involved in family life, whereas others may retreat or withdraw, which in turn changes the family's dynamics and ways of relating (system level). These changes can alter people's social relationships and the way they experience an event.

Social environments also include interactions, encounters, and relationships. One person may not know another person but is influenced by the latter's behavior and actions. Think of a new mother who observes another mother hugging her infant. Although this other mother is a stranger, the new mother may spontaneously imitate this other mother's behavior giving her own infant a hug. Think of how

FIGURE 3.1

Levels of family influence.

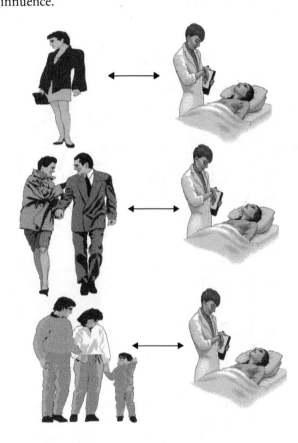

much people are influenced by what they read or what they see in the news and entertainment media.

Social environments can be ongoing, intermittent, causal, or transient in nature. Interactions can range from transitory, one-time encounters to relationships that have developed over a person's lifetime. The latter may often be deep, defining, and meaningful.

Social environments are nested within other social environments and are interconnected and interrelated. They may have direct or indirect influence. For example, the family is nested in work, community, and political/economic environments (Bronfenbrenner, 1979; see Figure 3.2). Bronfenbrenner's (1979) ecological system identified five systems of environmental influence that affect the person's development and functioning: (a) the microsystem, (b) the mesosystem, (c) the exosystems, (d) the macrosystem, and (e) the chronosystem. The *microsystem* is the one in which the individual or family immediately dwells that usually exerts the most influence. At the individual level, the family, school, peers, and neighborhood exert the most influence. The microsystem may change with various circumstances and as the person matures. The *mesosystem* refers to relationships and connections between environments as they impact the person's health and development. For example, the mesosystem explains how the person's workplace impacts

FIGURE 3.2

Urie Bronfenbrenner's multilevel environments affecting a person's development and health.

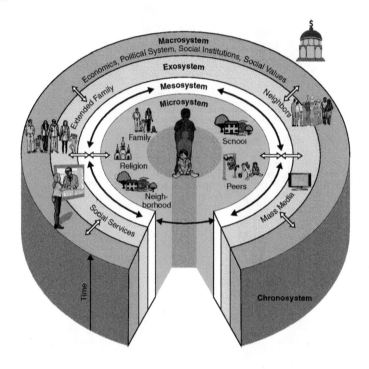

the family, which in turn affects its individual members. A mother who has lost her job becomes depressed. This in turn affects how she cares for her family. She may be less responsive to her children and husband and they in turn may become depressed or act out. The *exosystem* is made up of systems with which the person and family may have less direct or frequent contact (e.g., the legal system, the government, the health care system), but the workings of these affect the person nonetheless. The *macrosystem* describes the person's culture context. Cultural context refers to the ethnic, social-economic class, heritage, value system and the like that shapes a person's beliefs and identity. Macrosystems change over time and are recreated and reconstituted because of circumstances and experiences. Finally, the *chronosystem* involves the effects of the social-political-historical contexts and transitions that occur over the course of an individual's life span. It is concerned with how time changes the impact of an event.

Now let's consider how these systems work in concert. Think of a bedridden patient whose nurse ignores his call bells because the unit is understaffed. The patient, after waiting for a long time, becomes upset and frustrated and begins crying. When his wife visits, he yells at her (she is his microsystem). His encounters with the health care system and their staffing policy (mesosystem) affect how he treats his wife. His behavior might also reflect his level of anxiety and fear about his diagnosis. He may think he has a diagnosis that carries great stigma in his community (macrosystem). Coupled with this, he may not have delayed seeking help because he did not have health care insurance. In his country there is no universal health care coverage (exosystem). His reaction may in part stem from the uncertainty as he waits for the diagnosis. He is all-consumed with his illness. However, if the diagnosis proves to be of a chronic nature, his attitude and behavior will change over time as he learns to live with his condition, and his family learn how to accommodate and integrate it as an aspect of their lives so that it occupies less space and becomes less time consuming (chronosystem).

Social environments are cultural by nature. Culture is the fundamental foundation of human development and accounts for substantial differences between individuals (Arnett & Tanner, 2009). It comprises the total pattern of a group's values, beliefs, customs, art, technology, and ways of being and behaving that are transmitted and passed from generation to the next (Arnett & Tanner, 2009). Culture involves two dimensions: (a) ways of thinking and (b) ways of acting (Goodnow, 2010). All people grow up, develop, and are influenced by the cultural milieu in which they live. They in turn change the cultural environment through their ways of being and how they choose to live.

General principles governing person–environment transactions
Listed below are a number of principles about person–environment transactions:

- *A person's genotype or genetic makeup determines her responsiveness to environmental opportunities.* The person is genetically predisposed to select certain experiences in her environment over others. People will select opportunities that enhance their innate strengths (Scarr & McCartney, 1983). A person with athletic strength will more likely get involved in sports than a person who does not have such abilities.
- *There are three types of genotype–environment correlations, namely, passive, evocative, and active* (Scarr & McCartney, 1983). A *passive* environment is one in which the environment exerts an influence on the individual. This is seen during infancy, when biological parents provide a rearing environment that is affected by the infant's temperament. An *evocative* environment is when the person receives a response from his environment that is affected by his own behavior, such as when an angry patient evokes a hostile response from his nurses, and then labeled as a "difficult" patient. An *active* environment is when the person selects opportunities that are in keeping with his strengths, such as when a person is ready to learn and seeks out support groups to obtain information. Active environments can equally apply to a person's weaknesses, such as when an individual who is addicted to drugs chooses to be with other addicted individuals.
- *The person's biology, stress level, moods, and emotional states affect and are affected by her interactions with her environments.* For example, nurses who come to work in a good mood are more likely to be open and responsive to their patients.
- *Environments are modifiable.* A person's behavior can be affected by a change in the physical and social environments. Health care providers can be a powerful force in how a person deals with health challenges. It is within nurses' power to create health-promoting and healing environments through the relationships they create with the person, the clinical decisions they make, and how they attend to the person's physical environments. Nurses can have an effect on a person's behavior by modifying the physical environment, such as dimming lights

to promote sleep, and the social environment, by being fully present and attentively listening to their patient's concerns.

- *The environment and specific experiences of a person can alter a person's biological structures, such as his brain* (see section titled "Value 2: Uniqueness of the Person").
- *Some relationships are more influential than others,* depending on the history of the relationship, the quality of attachments, the nature of the connections, and the needs that a particular relationship fulfills.
- *Health behaviors are learned within the family environment.* Families are affected by a family member's illness and can affect the patient's recovery (Wright et al., 1996).
- *Social environments expand or contract as a function of age.* The earliest and most influential social environment on young children is the family. As children develop, their social environment expands. On the other hand, elderly individuals may experience a contraction of their social environments as they become less mobile and as friends become ill and die. Moreover, with age a person's passive environments can be replaced by evocative and active environments.
- *A person's reliance on her environment is related to her health, age, and vulnerability.* Consider a premature infant whose regulatory systems are not fully mature and therefore require greater environmental intervention to maintain temperature, cardiac, and respiratory functions (Hill, 1997).
- *Environments and experiences can be health promoting and support healing, or they can be toxic and detrimental to health.*
  - Health-promoting environments are most likely to happen when there is a goodness of fit, a concept on which I expand below.
  - Health-promoting environments also involve secure attachments and supportive relationships. These occur when a person feels safe with another person and can count on the other person for support. A supportive person is sensitive to and responsive to another's needs; often serves as that person's secure base; provides a safe haven, particularly during times of need and of stress; and engages in reciprocal and mutually satisfying exchanges (Snyder, Lopez, & Pedrotti, 2011). Supportive relationships are the foundations of good health and are essential for growth and transformation (Neufield & Harrison, 2010).
  - Health-promoting environments help in self-regulation through routines and rituals. They also help an individual to cope.
  - Health-promoting environments work with, capitalize on, mobilize, and develop individual, family, and community strengths and resources.
  - Environments also have the power to be nonhealing or even toxic (Neufield & Harrison, 2010). This is the case when the environment selects the person's weaknesses and deficits or fosters the development of deficits or puts the patient's safety at risk. Think of how peers or group pressure can encourage risk taking or destructive health behaviors. Consider how the hospital environment and the practices of clinicians can put patients at risk, such as when doctors are asked to work long hours or nurses are asked to work back-to-back shifts, thereby increasing the likelihood that errors will be made.

- *Environments are shaped by a person's strengths and can help develop those strengths.* Environments can support existing strengths and help a person develop the strengths that are needed for health and healing (see Chapter 10's discussion of working with existing strengths, developing strengths, and turning deficits into strengths).
- *Nurses are an integral part of a person's environment.* They can create healing environments to support a person's health and healing through their actions and interactions (Swanson & Wojnar, 2004). They can do so by working with the person's strengths rather than focusing only on problems, weaknesses, and deficits.

Goodness of fit

A health-promoting environment exists when there is a good fit between the person and their environment, that is, where there is a goodness of fit. Goodness of fit occurs when the person's capacities meet the demands and expectations of the environment. When this occurs, a positive transaction between the person and the environment occurs, and both person and environment are enriched, grow, and, in many cases, thrive. People thrive in environments that they find challenging because those environments encourage them to develop new capacities and skills—new strengths.

On the other hand, when the environmental demands exceed a person's capacities and are not supportive, the person may feel overwhelmed and frustrated, and then the interaction between person and environment is due to a poorness of fit. In their benign or mild form, these transactions neither cause trauma nor promote health and healing. In their most toxic forms, they may cause irreparable damage and, in some cases, even death. Consider what happens when a person has an infection. The immune system can manage the pathogens of most infections by containing, destroying, and eliminating them from the body. This is an example of goodness of fit because the response of the immunological system does not exceed the demands of what is being called for. An example of a poorness of fit is when an individual's immunological system is compromised and cannot respond to a pathogen (i.e., young, elderly, and/or chronically ill individuals) or in cases when the pathogens are so virulent that they overwhelm the person's immunological capacity to contain, destroy, or eliminate them. Consider what happens to families after the death of an infant. Some couples experience less marital intimacy, whereas other couples become closer (Gottlieb, Lang, & Amsel, 1996). The nature of this tragedy overwhelms some couples such that, in the midst of a mother's and father's grief, their relationship as a couple suffers.

Physical space can also affect the person's healing. Research has found that patients' moods are affected by the architecture and arrangement of the their physical space. Sunny hospital rooms expedite a patient's recovery from depression compared to darkened rooms (Beauchemin & Hays, 1996). Thus, a person and his social and physical environment are one, each shaping and being shaped by the other. Now reflect and connect on your own experience by thinking of those situations or relationships where there was a goodness of fit by answering the questions in Exhibit 3.5.

EXHIBIT 3.5

Reflect and connect   *Goodness of Fit and Poorness of Fit*

1. Describe a situation or an experience when you felt good about yourself
2. What made it a "good" fit? Describe what you brought to the situation and what was expected of you. How did your behavior affect the environment (others in the environment)?
3. Now describe a situation or an experience that frustrated you, made you anxious, angry, or feel like you wanted to leave.
4. Identify qualities in yourself and in the environment that contributed to the "poor" fit.

EXHIBIT 3.6

Personal experience   *Two physicians' ways of relating: A comparison*

Nathaly Gagnon, had been diagnosed with uterine cancer that required a total hysterectomy. In her follow-up visit six weeks after surgery, her surgeon, Dr. Shirley Johannes, delivered the news: *"You have Stage III cancer. You will be starting chemotherapy tomorrow."* She left without further comment. Nathaly felt that she had been given a death sentence. She felt her situation was hopeless and that she might as well just go home to die.

The following day, Nathaly sought a second opinion, from Dr. Gerald Batist. The first thing Dr. Batist did was look at her scan. He reviewed the scan in front of her: *"OK, let's see—lungs–clear…liver–clear…pancreas–clear…abdomen–clear…uterus has cancer, but now it is gone so that's clear too…no more cancer because there is no more uterus. You look pretty clear to me. Your lymph nodes don't look involved and if they are involved, it's miniscule. "*

Nathaly felt very much relieved and hopeful. As she said later, *"Dr. Batist made me feel like a renewed person. I don't feel that I have cancer, because I don't. I had it for one week, and then he cut it out of me before I even knew that I had it. I will begin chemotherapy as a precaution. I feel totally different from yesterday. Yesterday, I thought I was a dead woman, and today I feel happy and hopeful."*

One of the credos of all health care professionals is "do no harm." Unfortunately, some nurses and other health care practitioners can do harm through unkind acts, poor clinical judgment, and/or lack of skill that can compromise patients' safety, put them at risk, and cause them distress. Consider Nathaly Gagnon's following personal interactions with two different doctors following the surgical removal of a cancerous uterus as described in Exhibit 3.6. The first doctor, Shirley Johannes (a pseudonym) focused on the cancer diagnosis, and her medical follow-up treatment focused on deficits. In contrast, the second physician, Gerald Batist, an oncologist at the Jewish General Hospital in Montreal, Quebec, Canada, focused on the healthy functioning organs as well as the diseased organ that had been eradicated with surgery. This doctor's approach acknowledged both what was healthy and what was diseased. This is SBC in action. Dr. Johannes created in Nathaly a sense of despair and hopelessness, whereas Dr. Batist's sensitivity and strengths-based approach filled her with a sense of hope and renewal.

In SBC, nurses work with a person's internal, external, and social and cultural environments to elicit and maximize the person's strengths and resources to cope with illness and other physical insults. When patients know their strengths and can mobilize, capitalize, and develop them, they are in a far better position to recover physically and mentally and thus to be able to self-heal, and continue to develop to their fullest. Nurses, as part of their patients' environments, can influence patients' recovery through their nursing actions and the experiences they create. This influence can be both positive and negative, depending on how nurses interact with and care for patients and their families.

Nurses also need to be aware that patients and the workplace (e.g., interactions with colleagues, physicians, staff, hospital cultures, rules and regulations, etc.) are integral aspects of the nurses' environments and affect how they in turn relate to patients. These environments also influence nurses' own strengths, weaknesses, and vulnerabilities. Thus, nurses are a significant part of their patients' environments, and thus they can create, control, and modify those environments. Moreover, their nursing is influenced by their interactions within the workplace and the culture and climate of the institution or agency. Nurses who practice SBC recognize and reflect on how environments affect the quality of their practice.

VALUE 6

Nurse Heather Hart's Care of Ellen as Reflected in Person–Environment Being Integral
This value is presented in the continuing narrative of Ellen and can be found on p. 98–99.

Value 7: Learning, Readiness, and Timing

Human survival is dependent on what a person learns and how that information is used to enable the person to adapt, grow, and develop. From cells to citizens to communities, learning is at the heart of survival, change, and transformation. Learning begins at conception and continues throughout a person's life. Learning takes place at both the biological and behavioral levels to create the integrated, whole person.

Conceptualization

At the biological level, scientists are beginning to understand that cells can "learn" in order to adapt to changing conditions and to optimize functioning. At this level, learning involves establishing and pruning neurological pathways in the brain (Chechik, Meilijson, & Ruppin, 1999), regulating hormonal levels (McLachlan,

2001), and establishing immunologic and other defense and response systems (Lightman et al., 2001).

There are different ways learning takes place in the brain. For example, there are nerve cells in the brain, known as *mirror neurons* that can help people visually compare what they are currently observing with what they remember (Siegel, 2007). It was once believed that each part of the brain had a specific function and that if one part of the brain was destroyed the person would lose that particular function; however, scientists have shown that other parts of the brain can take over the functions of the destroyed part. This is referred to as *neural plasticity* (Collins, 2007; Doidge, 2007). These discoveries have shown how learning at the cellular level is reflected in behavior and how experience and training can alter the structure and function of the brain.

Learning also takes place at the *hormonal–cellular level*. Cells need to be stimulated in order to produce hormones. The more the cell is stimulated, the faster the hormone is released. Consider milk production in mothers. With a firstborn child, a mother has never produced milk before and it takes longer for her milk supply to be established. When her second baby is born, this mother's milk supply is more readily established. The sucking of the firstborn has "taught" the breast to release milk when the nipple is stimulated. The breast has "learned" that when an infant suckles, a message is sent by the hormone prolactin to the lacteal cells to release its milk.

Learning at the *immunological level* occurs as part of the body's defense system. When a person is exposed to various pathogens, the exposure elicits an immunologic defense system response that "remembers" different pathogens and then neutralizes and contains them before they spread very far. This is the basis of how a vaccination works. A person is exposed to an attenuated form of a bacteria or virus that sensitizes the immune system to produce antibodies that destroy the pathogenic microorganisms that are responsible for the disease.

Social learning involves an increase in awareness of oneself as well as others and how the world operates. It is about experiencing previous happenings in new and different ways.

At its most basic level, social learning is defined as the acquisition of information, knowledge, and skills through experiences that lead one to acquire new understandings and develop new skills, capacities, and competencies to be able to adapt to changing circumstances and function in the world. Social learning is the result of person–environment transactions. People learn by observing others, imitating their actions and behaviors, reflecting and thinking about things (introspection and reflection), learning through trial and error, and making meaning out of experience and creating narratives (Bandura, 1997; Weber, 2000). Learning is reflected by changes in brain activity. The plasticity of the brain in making and remaking neuronal connections and creating neuronal pathways is the biological process that underlies social learning.

Many factors affect learning, including personal factors (e.g., the person's age, physical status, brain capacity, learning styles), and situational factors (e.g., the cultural context of transmitted values and beliefs, past educational experiences, opportunities for learning, availability of resources, and access to people and resources such as libraries in neighborhoods); however, there are three essential conditions that affect a person's learning (a) active involvement in the learning process, (b) readiness for learning, and (c) timing of learning.

Learning as an active process. I use the term *learning* rather than the term *teaching* here deliberately. Learning requires the person be an active participant, whereas teaching implies that the person can be more passive. In order to learn, a person needs to become engaged in his own learning process. The person *constructs*, or accumulates, a bank of knowledge to understand himself, his relationships with others, his many lifeworlds, and the universe in general. In other words, the person is the creator of his own knowledge (Murray, Wenger, Downes, & Terrazas, 2011). Learning is always happening, because people are always experiencing new events and reflecting on them. They are continuously selecting, attending to, and interpreting that which is in their environments. It is these processes that enable people to understand and determine what is needed to navigate and function in a particular environment. When people become invested in their own learning, they can direct what they need to know and make better use of their existing knowledge and skills.

Active involvement in learning requires that a person pays attention to what is happening; selects what is relevant; is able to form and store representations (i.e., memory); and has the ability to regulate, plan, and execute a wide variety of actions (Byrne, 2007; Siegel, 1999). These functions—namely, attention, selection, memory, and perception—are some of the components that constitute a person's learning system (Siegel, 1999, 2007). A person's learning system is built to take advantage of experiences often created by interactions and relationships. The essential point is that the person is the architect of her own learning, and that it is this learning that enables her to cope with challenges, both big and small. For these reasons, it is important for nurses to appreciate how a person learns, in order to structure learning activities and learning environments that capitalize on and develop new strengths.

Readiness for learning. A person's readiness to learn is a critical component in learning and change. This is an idea with which everyone seems to be familiar, but it has been difficult to define, in part because the term *readiness* is used in several different ways. Readiness has been used to describe a state–"being in a state of readiness," such as "Are you ready?" Readiness has also been used to denote a process, such as "I'll be ready soon" (Dalton & Gottlieb, 2003).

Readiness is a prerequisite for change. Consider the familiar sayings associated with change or the beginning of a new action: "ready, set, go" or "ready, willing, and able" (Miller & Rollnick, 2002). In both sayings, the first word is *ready*. Without readiness, learning and change are difficult to bring about. Nurses need to consider their patients' state of readiness and how they get ready to change. They need to look for signs of readiness in their patients and work to help them get ready for change.

There are several precursors of readiness, including the biological (i.e., maturation), psychological and attitudinal (i.e., motivation, desire, and intent), and situational (i.e., cultural contexts, goodness of fit between person and environment).

Maturation is the sequence of changes that is often directed by preprogrammed genetically based factors that unfold at predetermined times. Maturation is influenced by opportunities for learning and practicing. Virtually all developmental tasks and skills, such as walking, talking, seeing, and hearing, are under genetic control and unfold at predetermined times when the person is exposed to specific experiences and opportunities to develop these capacities. Consider an infant's ability to sit. Sitting requires in part that the infant's nervous system has to be in a state of readiness; that is, certain areas of the brain have to be able to communicate with each other and send messages between the cerebellum (which is responsible for balance) and the motor cortex (which is responsible for muscle contraction and relaxation). No matter how much parents may try to get their infant to sit, if the infant's nervous system is not ready, usually because it is still in an immature state, the infant cannot and will not be able to sit.

The psychological basis of readiness is intertwined with a person's motivational system (i.e., desire for change). It is reflected in the following ways:

- People who believe they can do something are more likely to want to change.
- People are more likely to want to learn when they understand and appreciate the relevance of the information and the task at hand.
- Readiness requires a "can-do" attitude, or a degree of *self-efficacy*, a condition in which the person believes that she has the skills and competencies to accomplish a goal and can envision herself performing at a certain level to achieve a desired outcome (Bandura, 1997).
- Readiness involves both the intent to learn and a desire to invest in learning.

Nurse Charlotte Evans described the nature of collaborative partnership even in the end stages of life and the importance of readiness, learning, and allowing the patient to choose what is right for him. You may recall from Chapter 1 (see section titled "The Benefits of Strengths-Based Care") that Charlotte provided palliative care to Diane, who was suffering from ALS. Diane was totally paralyzed, unable to move, speak, or swallow, yet her mental faculties were not affected.

Charlotte described Diane: *"She participated fully in every decision that we made about her care because she was really an active participant in that, and that was so important to her. It was frustrating at times because we had certain ideas about what would be good for her and what we thought would really help her. And she would say, 'I'm not ready for that.' So we had to wait for her to come to a point where she would be ready for those interventions. And every step of the way she was with us and she'd say 'No, I'm not ready for that' and then the next day would say, 'Okay, I feel like I could do that today.' This was really a big learning experience for all of us—to realize that she had to be part of that process for it to work for her and for us."*

Time and timing. Learning is affected by time and timing.

Time can be thought of in terms of temporal time, that is, when an event occurs, the sequence of that event, and its duration. Time is important to patients' health and is a consideration in health care. Clinicians are concerned with understanding the chronology of events that preceded the onset of a disease and what happened once the first symptoms appeared. They often ask patients to reconstruct what happened. They are also interested in understanding the course of the disease—its progression or trajectory—to anticipate what might happen and what the person and family can expect. They are also interested in the length or duration of time, that is, how long the disease will last, how long a treatment takes, the peak actions of a drug (i.e., when its potency is at its greatest to have an effect), and the like.

Time is controlled internally by *biological clocks,* such as circadian rhythms and other chronobiologic factors. Biological clocks involve genetically preprogrammed processes that regulate many bodily functions including sleep–wake cycles, digestion, elimination, bone growth, reproduction, and so forth.

Time is also under the control of external time clocks. It is influenced by a person's age, cultural expectations, and norms, as well as by political, social, economic, and historical events. The *developmental antecedents*—that is, what happens before an event—and the consequences of life transitions, health and illness events, and behavior patterns vary according to when these transitions, events, or behavioral patterns happen in an individual's life (Arnett & Tanner, 2009). For example, a young girl of fourteen who becomes a mother will be affected quite differently than a woman having a child at age thirty-five. In terms of cultural context, adolescent pregnancy is more desired and acceptable in certain Asian countries, such as India, as compared to North America. Or consider what has happened in the Western world, as to the timing of when upper middle class and middle-class couples have their first baby. During the past fifteen years, some couples have been having babies in their thirties and even their early forties, unlike their parents, who had their children ten years earlier. Middle-class and upwardly mobile couples are postponing having children until their careers are well established and they believe they have the financial resources to support a family with a specific lifestyle. Economic and social factors are driving these decisions.

Timing refers to when change is most likely to occur. Timing requires an understanding of what is being changed and when change is most likely to be achieved (Gottlieb & Feeley, 1999). Individuals are most amenable to change and open to learning during periods of transition, critical life events, and stressful experiences because the status quo is no longer working and change is required to adapt or cope to the new realities brought on by these changing life circumstances (Meleis et al., 2000).

Nurses need to appreciate that every new experience, no matter how painful or difficult for the person and family, is an opportunity for learning about oneself, relationships, and how the world operates.

What are people learning? They may be learning about how to see a problem differently, feel less guilty about their responses to their situations, and are able to develop new understandings and ways of coping (Murphy, Taylor, & Townsend, 2001). It is in such situations that people need to uncover and discover existing and develop new strengths, such as new competencies and skills, to deal with the challenges. This requires that nurses create environments that help patients become actively involved in their own learning. It also requires that nurses look for signs of readiness in patients and those family members who want to be involved. When a person is not ready for a specific experience, it is important for the nurse to help him to become ready. Finally, this value requires that nurses be aware of time and the timing of their interventions so that they can support the person's natural ways of being and innate mechanims of healing. Being in tune with the person and maximizing learning requires an understanding the person and his strengths and potentials.

Consider how a family's readiness affected Nurse Lyne Charbonneau's work with a young couple, the Alonzos. Mrs. Alonzo had delivered an infant son at 24 weeks, preterm. He sustained several cranial hemorrhages but survived. Just as he stabilized, a nurse made an error that may have contributed to another intracranial haemorrhage. The staff members were unsure what effect these bleeds would have on this infant's long-term development. Lyne had developed a good relationship with these parents, but after the incident Mr. and Mrs. Alonzo withdrew from her and all the nursing staff.

Lyne understood this couple's need to distance from her, and she followed their lead. She recalled what happened just before the baby was discharged and the importance of timing: *"The baby got more stable, got bigger, got better, and at one point he was almost ready to go home when the parents took me aside on the unit, at the bedside, and the mom asked me: 'What does it mean [that] an infant is impaired? What exactly was the risk?' Even before that incident they knew that the baby would probably not develop normally. So I told them that this is something that we cannot really predict, we can only give statistics and I was telling them that usually I don't like to give statistics because it's just too general and I like to individualize information for a patient or a family. But still this is information that they wanted to have, so I gave them the information. I knew what it meant for them to ask that question. At one point, the mother started crying. What I remember questioning was how we should intervene depending on what parents want. I knew this family was very clear that at some points [during their infant's hospitalization] they were not ready to receive information; they were unable to ask. They were able to get information from books, on the Internet, or with us on the unit, but they were still not ready. It was changes in the status of their infant and after all [they had been through] they were able to say how they appreciated getting the information as much as the information was difficult to hear."*

Nurse Heather Hart's Care of Ellen as Reflected in Self-Determination, Person and Environment Are Integral, Learning, Readiness, and Timing

As Ellen's condition deteriorated, Heather related how the team was concerned by Ellen's refusal to talk with them about what she was going through:: *"The palliative care team has a lot of very good people, psychologists and music therapists and so on, and Ellen basically closed the door on them. She just wasn't interested. It troubled me in some ways because I thought 'Where does this end? How is the end (her death) going to look like for her? for her children, and so on?'"*

Heather decided not to bring up the subject of dying and death with Ellen. Then, one day, Ellen indicated her readiness to talk about her own death. Heather recounted how this event came about: *"Another patient whom Ellen had known quite well on the unit, died. On our unit we usually hold a universal prayer service and there were a lot of staff and family present. The patient was still in the bed. He had died in the middle of the night and Ellen was there, holding his hand during the universal prayer. I was completely taken by surprise. I had not expected that this would be the case. I just never pictured Ellen having the capacity or the desire to do this given her own pain and suffering."*

Heather recalled that after the service she wheeled Ellen back to her room: *"Ellen was a bit tearful and she was sitting in her chair. I sat on her bed and said,*

(continued)

'Are you alright? Do you want me to stay?' And she didn't say go or stay. Ellen was crying a little bit, and with Ellen you didn't push. I would never ask her, 'Tell me how you're feeling.' She might have said, 'There's the door.' So I just waited with her, and she cried and cried and it made me very sad. Ellen finally said, 'I won't get to see my children grow up and I won't know who they become.' I was just listening to her and I appreciated the depth of her despair and there again was a light on. Here was a little snippet of Ellen. She may have shut the door on the psychologist, and she shut the door on all the experts who could help her. She was not in denial. She understood what was happening to her. In all the darkness, in all of the pain or sadness, there was some little shred of hope or light [Heather's word for *strengths*] *that Ellen was working things through, in some way that she was not sharing but it was there."*

Heather waited for signs of readiness for Ellen to open up (Value 7: Readiness). She also knew that what she said and how she would say it would affect Ellen. Her timing was exquisite, honoring Ellen, her right to choose whom to talk to and what to disclose (Value 5: Self-Determination). Heather respected Ellen's right to determine whether she wanted to disclose her feelings about her impending death. In fact, she took her cues from Ellen and in so doing revealed just how attuned she was to Ellen when, after an emotional experience, she asked Ellen, *"Do you want me to stay?"* and not *"What are your feelings?"*, which may have forced Ellen to reveal something she did not want to or was not ready to say.

Ellen was deeply affected by her friend's death, which had triggered her feelings about her own impending death (Value 6: Person and Environment are Integral). Heather was also deeply affected by Ellen's suffering, which she continued to feel many years later. During the interview, Heather herself began to cry as she remembered Ellen, who had left a deep and long-lasting impression on her. It was in recognizing Ellen's strengths and caring for her to alleviate her suffering that Heather gained a deeper appreciation of Ellen, the person, and the importance of working with a person's "gifts."

Value 8: Collaborative Partnership

Although most practitioners understand that the nature of the relationship they form with patients and families is critical to the person's health and healing, few give more than a passing thought as to why a relationship seems to work with one person and family but not with another.

Conceptualization

There are two predominant approaches to the nurse–patient relationship: (a) the traditional hierarchical relationship and (b) the collaborative partnership (Gottlieb et al., 2006 see Table 3.2). Each approach is premised on a different set of values and beliefs about the nature of the nurse–patient relationship.

TABLE 3.2

Traditional hierarchical versus collaborative partnership forms of the nurse–person relationship

Comparison Criteria	Traditional Hierarchical (Paternalism)	Collaborative Partnership
Assumptions	The person needs to be taken care of by the professional The person is passive and not responsible for his care. The person lacks knowledge or the capabilities to understand and manage his illness or problems The professional possesses the knowledge and capabilities to manage illness and problems. The professional has the control and responsibility	The person is active and shares responsibility for his care The person has knowledge and capabilities that he can use to understand and manage his illness or problems or work toward his goals in ways that are meaningful to him
Focus	The person's illness, symptoms, or problems	The person's ability to be well, experience a high quality of life, and live in a meaningful way
Role of the nurse	The expert holds the knowledge and thus solves problems and makes decisions	A facilitator who encourages people to share their perceptions and expertise, to participate in joint decision making, and to develop the person's autonomy (i.e., ability to be self-directed) and self-efficacy Helps people more fully use their strengths and resources Has knowledge of people's illnesses and their selves
Role of the person	A passive recipient of professional's expertise	An active partner who plays an important role in setting goals and finding solutions that best fit the person
Nature of relationship	Characterized by the professional in the dominant role and the person in the subordinate role. There is a differential of power, and the relationship is asymmetrical	Is reciprocal and mutual; each partner gives and receives, and thus the relationship is more symmetrical or balanced Involves the continual negotiation of goals, roles, and responsibilities Both partners give up some autonomy because they value and trust the other's expertise. Both partners gain and grow
Goal setting	The professional determines the goals, typically based on the problem only	Goals are jointly determined
Evaluation	The professional assesses progress in achieving her goals for the person	The partners share in joint assessment of progress in achieving mutually determined goals
Expected outcome	The problem is solved or the person is considered noncompliant, thereby possibly being blamed for an unsuccessful outcome	The problem may or may not be solved, but the person's capabilities to manage current or future problems are enhanced. Joint responsibility is accepted for the outcomes.

Source: Reprinted with permission from Gottlieb, Feeley, with Dalton, (2006).

A. Traditional, hierarchical approach

The traditional, hierarchical approach to care is the dominant approach in the current health care system that governs the way practitioners interact with their patients. (This approach was described briefly in Chapter 1, when deficit-based care was compared and contrasted to SBC.) In this approach, the practitioners assume the major responsibility for determining the goals, the course of treatment, and the criteria for what they consider to be a desirable outcome. They are the experts and they "know-best." In this relationship, patients are expected to be more passive and follow the prescribed treatment regimens. It is a paternalistic model inasmuch as the professional assumes the "adult" role in the relationship and is more powerful and in charge, while the patient is expected to assume a more dependent, childlike role.

The traditional, hierarchical approach is described in its extreme form in Table 3.2. It will strike a chord inasmuch as it captures the essence of what often transpires between nurses and patients in their day-to-day encounters and interactions.

B. Collaborative partnership

SBC values a *collaborative partnership*, which is defined as "the pursuit of person-centered goals through a dynamic process that requires active participation and agreement of all partners" (Gottlieb et al., 2006, p. 8). A collaborative partnership is about *being with*, not about *doing for*, the person.

A collaborative partnership is nonhierarchical and lateral in structure because the nurse, the person, and the person's family are responsible for setting goals, developing a plan of care, evaluating what they are experiencing, resetting direction of their care and their lives, and celebrating when things go well. This approach recognizes that the person and nurse bring their own knowledge, skills, and experience to the relationship and that each partner has something to learn from the other. It is a relationship built on mutual respect and trust. Together, the person and nurse create a customized care plan that fits the uniqueness of the person and capitalizes and builds on the person's strengths. It allows the patient's voice to count as much as, if not more than, the health care professional's.

Consider how Nurse Virginia Lee described her role and the patient's role in developing a plan of care. To engage in a collaborative partnership requires that the nurse be fully present and engage in real, attentive, listening. As Virginia explained, *"What I learned is that [nurses] don't have all the answers but it's the patient that has the answers that are meaningful for them in their life context to help them cope with whatever adversity or illness that they're coping with. We always want to give information, [say] that we have the answers but what we need to do is sit back and listen attentively to what the patient has to say to us. It's placing their story in the context of their past, present, and future. As the person is telling me their story, the wheels in my head are turning. In my head I'm trying to place everything in some order to reflect back to them what I hear them saying. The patient then has an opportunity to say whether my interpretation is what it is or, 'No, that's not what it is.' What is important is engaging the patient in the process of reflection. They know what's happening in their life and what's going to fit their life and what will work in the future for them.... But the answer lies within them, the patient."*

The nurse's role is to create conditions that support the person's efforts to make decisions (Value 5: Self-Determination) and to assume greater responsibility that enable the person and family to heal and grow (Value 1: Health and Healing). The person and family are encouraged to be active partners in their own care and to work with the nurse to more fully understand their health issues (Value 7: Learning, Readiness, and Timing). The nurse is attuned to the person and family's available energy and sets the pace of their work together accordingly. They arrive at an understanding of what is possible, doable, and comfortable (see Chapter 9 for a fuller discussion of this).

The hallmark of a collaborative partnership is power sharing. Power sharing requires that each partner appreciate the other's strengths (Value 2: Uniqueness of the Person). For patients to share in power, they must believe that they have something to offer. They also must have confidence in their nurse's competencies and skills. When people discover their own strengths, they also discover their own power. In short, a collaborative partnership is about generosity and the willingness to share power. It is key to helping the person feel empowered. When people believe they have the abilities to accomplish their goals, they are more likely to take charge of their lives and their own health care.

The collaborative relationship facilitates the person to become empowered because it shifts attention:

- **FROM** focusing on deficits **TO** working with the person's strengths
- **FROM** doing for the person **TO** working with the person
- **FROM** focusing on disease and its treatment **TO** focusing on living and coping with challenges and adverse events
- **FROM** the nurse as teacher **TO** both the nurse and person as learners
- **FROM** measuring a set of specific outcomes **TO** allowing the person to determine their own goals and their own measures of success

VALUE 8

Nurse Heather Hart's Care of Ellen as Reflected in a Collaborative Partnership

Nurse Hart described her last days of nursing Ellen. The care she gave Ellen reflects the special partnership they had developed over six months and the abiding respect they had developed for each other. Heather recalled, *"It was a Wednesday, and Ellen had a very bad day. I thought she was going to die. She had uncontrolled pain and some delirium, and the medication that was given to her to calm her down, she became unresponsive. Before the family got there, I was alone with her. I took the picture of her four kids and tucked it into her arm and said, 'Now your children are with you and remember Ellen, you are with them too.' And I sat and sang to her because I just thought, 'There's nothing else I could do at this point.' I said goodbye and she looked very peaceful."*

Heather's action of slipping a photo of Ellen's children in her arms served to honor the trust that Ellen had placed in Heather when Ellen had shared with Heather her deepest sorrow and pain: leaving her children. However, Ellen did not die that day. She awoke from the coma before slipping back into a state of

(continued)

uncontrolled pain and delirium a day later. Heather recounted the final hours of Ellen's life and their last act of collaboration:

"I nursed her that night and I thought then, 'Oh my God, she is going to die as she's lived—fighting to the end.' We tried everything to ease her pain—massage, therapeutic touch, music—and nothing touched her or eased the pain. The only thing we had not started was a drip with a sedative. And Ellen, who I thought was unconscious, said, 'Heather, Heather, help, help stop the pain' and I said, 'Ellen, I have a drip, and if I start this drip you will go to sleep, and if you go to sleep, you are not likely to wake up. Do you want me to start the drip?' And she turned and looked me straight in the eyes and said, 'Stop the pain!' and I started the drip and she was able to let go and not fight with the medication. It was such a huge part of Ellen to fight and have control, but her body was completely beyond her control. Her pain was total pain. It was anguish and sorrow. It was spiritual pain that was physical pain. Even then I gave her the choice, and in hindsight I thought that was pretty good. I honored her directive right to the end. "

Theirs was a real partnership based on power sharing where both patient and nurse had a voice—where there was mutual respect, openness, and trust between them. As Heather recounted: *"I let her direct things, and mostly I would just be there for her. There was a trust that built up. She knew that I respected her and that I cared about her and who she was. I cared about what she was going through."*

Heather's nursing did not just happen by chance; it was Heather's way of being. It reflects who Heather is as a nurse—as one human being privileged to care for another human being. It is about those things that Heather believes in and considers important.

Heather's care of Ellen is what nursing looks like when nurses are guided by the values of SBC. Values become the benchmark against which to measure whether you, as a nurse, have made the right decisions. Values reflect who you are, how you want to nurse, and how you want to care for another in time of need.

Key Summary Points

- SBC is based on a number of assumptions about the health, person, environment, and nursing. From these assumptions eight core values are derived.
- The core values underlying SBC are Value 1: health and healing; Value 2: uniqueness of the person, Value 3: holism and embodiment, Value 4: objective/subjective reality and created meaning, Value 5: self-determination, Value 6: the person and environment are integral, Value 7: learning, readiness, and timing, Value 8: collaborative partnership.
- These eight values are interrelated and work together to form a comprehensive and coherent whole that underpins SBC. They inform the nurse about the person and family, what to focus on, and how to nurse them.

What Are Strengths? Characteristics of Strengths

4

LEARNING OBJECTIVES

After reading this chapter, you should be able to:

- Define what is meant by strengths
- Identify the language of strengths
- Describe the relationship between strengths and Strengths-Based Care
- Explain the relationship among strengths, potentials, resources, and resiliency
- List nine key characteristics of strengths and describe each characteristic

If you ask 100 people what their strengths are, you may be surprised by their answers. Most will have no difficulty answering this question. Some may tell you what they are good at and what they do best. Others may answer the question by telling you about their special talents that set them apart. Still others will tell you about qualities they have developed that have helped them cope with and overcome some difficult situations. And then there will be a small percentage of people who will shake their heads and will not be able to answer the question, either because they do not understand what you mean by the term *strengths* or because they believe they have no strengths. This last group would be wrong about themselves, because everyone has strengths. In fact, every person and every family has a large repertoire of strengths that they call forth every moment of every day to get the most out of life, deal with daily upsets and hassles, and cope with uncertainties and events that disrupt their lives. Such events can range from mildly annoying to catastrophic; they can be anticipated (e.g., dealing with the birth of a new baby) to unexpected (e.g., coping with the effects of a hurricane). They are events that expose the person's vulnerabilities and frailties, and it is by calling forth strengths or turning weaknesses into strengths that a person and family are able to cope and, in some cases, to become stronger and transform their lives.

Strengths define a person's and family's uniqueness. The way certain qualities are combined sets a person and family apart and defines their specialness. In uncovering, discovering, and developing strengths, a person and family come to define themselves and understand what they are capable of achieving and overcoming. These ideas extend to communities as well. Nurses need to know a person's strengths in order to understand how to capitalize and mobilize them in order to support the person during health and illness, and in times of suffering, recovery, and healing.

WHAT ARE STRENGTHS?

The word *strength* is an umbrella term that includes both the internal qualities of a person or unit (family, community) and the external resources available to them. The word *strength* has been used in many different ways, for example, to describe materials (*strong* or *weak, pliable* or *rigid*), to denote a virtue (*courageous* or *cowardly*), and to evaluate the likelihood of success ("*He has a strong chance of winning*"). What do these descriptions have in common? They all imply that strengths can be understood in relation to weaknesses or deficits; that is, if something is considered strong, this implies that it is not weak, and if something is deemed weak, then it cannot be strong. In people, strengths are *not* the opposite of weaknesses; they are a distinct and separate class of qualities, capabilities, competences, capacities, and skills that coexist with weaknesses. Knowing a person's weaknesses does not necessarily tell you very much about his strengths. The problem with defining strengths in terms of weaknesses is that it may blind the nurse to seeing patients for who they really are. It is not an either/or situation but rather a coexistence of both strengths and weaknesses.

Definition of Strengths for Strengths-Based Care

Strengths are a person or family's special and unique qualities that determine what a person can do and who she can become. They often define an individual's personhood and give expression to her humanity. Strengths are capabilities that enable a person to cope with life challenges; deal with uncertainties; and contribute to that person's ability to rally, rebound, and recover from all types of insults (e.g., illness, trauma, disability) and overcome adversities. People need strengths to meet goals, get the most out of living, contribute to health and well-being, and facilitate recovery and healing. In short, strengths allow people and families to live more fully in their environments, be present in their relationships and interactions, and engage in all aspects of living. They are invaluable sources of power and energy to help the person and family meet life's challenges, both big and small.

The concept of strength is often used interchangeably with *capability*. They include a person's assets, attributes, capacities, competencies, resources, skills, talents, and traits. Strengths can be biological, psychological, and social in nature.

Strengths are subjective—they are whatever the person, family, and health professional says they are. Sometimes, a nurse may label a patient's behavior as a strength, whereas the patient may view that same behavior as a weakness. Consider the example of School Nurse Lia Sanzone, who had a 10-year-old

> Strengths are invaluable sources of power and energy that reside in the person and can be called forth to meet life's challenges and develop opportunities.

girl, Alice, crying in her office. Alice cried as she described what it was like at home with her father, who had been newly diagnosed with cancer.

Lia described the situation: *"[There are] a lot of things that we as nurses read as a strength…What can be viewed as a strength by me will not necessarily be viewed as a strength by someone else. Take the example of…. Alice when I told her that crying was a strength. From Alice's understanding, crying was not a strength but a sign of weakness because you're not supposed to cry and make other people feel badly. That was her perception. I tried to change her perception based on my knowledge that it's okay to express your emotions. So it comes back to the same thing: If I view something as a strength, I then need to check that out with the person. For them to understand it as a strength, they need to perceive it as a strength. I ask them, 'What is your perception of this?'"*

Lia explained that changing a person's perception isn't always easy. She tries to understand why the person sees a behavior as a weakness by exploring that person's feelings about the behavior. Lia said, *"[I may ask], 'How did that make you feel?' And if they didn't feel good about it then I go back to the question 'Well, why not? How did you feel afterwards?'"*

Strengths may be expressed in different words and phrases. The latter often take the form of metaphors to communicate in a form of short-hand what is unique or special about the person and family. It is important for nurses to be attuned to a person and family's use of language and their choice of metaphors.

Language of Strengths: Descriptors and Metaphors

Language provides a window into a the way a person thinks, reasons, and experiences the world; about how he lives life, experiences the world, and functions in relationships. A person's language and choice of words reveal a great deal about what he is feeling and thinking. The way a person organizes his thoughts governs how he sees things (i.e., perceptions), which in turn affects how he behaves and the actions he takes (Lakoff & Johnson, 1980).

Descriptors and synonyms of strengths. Different words have been used to convey the meaning of strengths. The French word for strength is *le force*, a term that brings forth images of power, might, energy, and vigor. Disciplines and professions use different words for strengths. Positive psychology looks for the "positives" in describing a person. The business world talks of strengths in terms of capital, assets, energy, and resources. In the health care literature the word *strength* often is used interchangeably with *resiliency, energy,* and *personal resources.*

Some of the nurses who were interviewed for this book used the word *strengths* with their patients, clients, and families to describe their special qualities. Other nurses preferred such words as *light, gifts, uniqueness, abilities,* and *capacities.* Nurse Heather Hart captured the spirit of strengths in nursing when she said, *"I'm looking for the light, those little glimmers that make me think there's something there. I am looking for people's gifts of what they've got going for them."* Still other nurses avoid using the term *strength* with their patients, clients, and families initially and instead preferred to share with the person and family what they observed that impressed them.

Nurse Diane Lowden, a clinical nurse specialist who works with patients diagnosed with multiple sclerosis (MS), described her use of the word *strengths* in her clinical practice: *"When I ask people about themselves I don't usually use the word strengths. I usually talk about resources. I will ask, 'How do you work together as a family? What resources do you have? What enables your family to do the things that you can do?' And then, often I will reflect back to them at the end of an interview or throughout an interview, things that I see as strengths. It is then that I will tend to use the actual word 'strengths' with them. I will often say, 'I'm quite struck by how close a family you are. I'm quite struck by the strengths in your family.' And then I'll go and label some things that I see them doing that I see as strengths."*

Diane explained the effects on families of labeling a quality or behavior a strength. *"Families often feel devastated by their diagnosis, unsure of what to do, not knowing how to approach it, feeling very incompetent about their ability to manage the disease. Identifying their strengths and actually labeling them is helpful. It puts things from a place that is unfamiliar, unknown, foreign, and very scary territory to a place that they know very well—their own family. If a nurse can reflect that back to them, I think the family goes from feeling incompetent to competent. And you'll see that in the way they talk. The room gets lighter. Sometimes even their physical presence changes."*

Metaphors of strengths and weaknesses. A metaphor is "a figure of speech in which a word or phrase is applied to something which it is not literally applicable" (*Oxford English Dictionary*). People use metaphors to help structure their perceptions, understandings, and actions (Lakoff & Johnson, 1980). Metaphors are a shorthand way of communicating what the person is going through and what she can expect from the situation or from another person. For example, when you hear someone describing another person using the metaphor, "He has the constitution of a horse," what is that person trying to communicate about the other person? This metaphor generally means that the other person is strong and, by choosing this metaphor, sets up the expectation that the person will be able to overcome and recover from the disease, withstand the trauma, and weather the storm (another metaphor). Thus, metaphors play an important role in defining people's everyday reality and directing their reactions and actions. Patients often use metaphors to capture what they are experiencing. Andrew Durso is a 23-year-old young man who suffers from MS. He has chosen the metaphor of a "claw" to communicate to others what it is like to live with MS. Andrew's experience is described in Exhibit 4.1.

Reflect and connect on how the metaphors in Table 4.1 affect how you think, feel, and act in a situation or toward another person.

Examples of Strength Classification Systems

Health care professionals have developed different classification systems. The best known classification systems are diagnostic systems. Such systems are used to assign a diagnostic label to a group of symptoms or features based on a set of predetermined criteria. For example, the *Diagnostic and Statistical Manual of Mental Disorders* (DSM: American Psychiatric Association, 2000) is the classification system used to diagnose and label mental health disorders. Classification systems are designed to communicate complex conditions or disease through the use of a label. Thus, when a label such as *autism* or *schizophrenia* or *epilepsy* or *cardiac failure* is used, every trained practitioner can recite the relevant symptoms or features of that condition or disease.

Because different people value and need different things, there is no universal list or classification system of strengths that applies to everyone (Lewis & Burd-Sharps, 2010). Nonetheless, various health care disciplines have grouped qualities

EXHIBIT 4.1

Personal experience *Andrew Durso's MS Claw*

It's truly an evil disease, this MS of mine. I'm scared. I'm scared. I'm scared.

To put it in the right "frame," you need to know that my father was diagnosed in 1985, a couple of years prior to my entry into the world. As a teenager, I watched my father's disease progress—his own personal "MS claw" had a grip, though the speed at which his claw grasped him was entirely different. It was ten years before we began having to pick him up off the bathroom/bedroom/living room floor and help him get back to his feet. It was fifteen years before its talons began to break the skin and draw blood; that is to say, before he had completely lost his ability to walk. He now lives in long-term care, his MS claw never leaving him, its grip only ever tightening as we all look on, helpless, powerless, and impotent to do something, anything for him. This understandably really defined what my biggest fear was: that, one day, it'd be *me* being picked up off the bathroom/bedroom/living room floor. That, one day, it'd be me being grasped, clutched, left scarred and bleeding by my own MS claw. Then it happened. My biggest fear become reality. To my astonishment, the craziest thing happened: I dealt with it. And I continue to deal with it; as the claw tightens and loosens its grasp, I adjust. It never lets go. It has cut me several times. I can't walk. I can't type. I can't contain my bladder's contents. I have "difficulty" with romantic intimacy (I will allow you, to quote the Immortal Bard, to "take it in what sense thou wilt"—use your imagination).

Source: Andrew Durso, personal communication, Montreal, March 2012

TABLE 4.1

Reflect and connect: Metaphors used for strengths and weaknesses

Strength Metaphors	Deficit/weakness Metaphors
• "A light in a sea of darkness"	• "Reed swayed by the wind"
• "Strong as an ox"	• "Feet of clay"
• "Armed to the teeth"	• "Having a monkey on one's back"
• "To bear one's cross"	• "Achilles heel"
• "Seeing the world through rose-colored glasses"	• "A shadow of his former self"
• "Like a rock"	• "The wounds are deep"
• "Beating the odds"	• "The scars of war"
• "Roared to life"	• "On the brink of collapse"

Reflect and Connect Instructions:

1. Read the metaphors used for strengths (column 1) and the metaphors for weaknesses (column 2).
2. Select one metaphor from each column.
3. What do you think the metaphor means?
4. What is the metaphor's message?
5. If someone used this phrase to describe you, how would it make you feel?

into categories of strengths. The strengths they select are those that are needed to meet that discipline or profession's specific mission and fulfill its major goals. For example, positive psychology's main goal is a satisfying existence by promoting quality of life. Counseling psychology and early childhood special education have as their overriding goal the facilitation of growth by focusing on individuals' innate strengths to promote growth and development. Social work has as one of its primary goals the promotion of resiliency in the face of adversity. Nursing's main mission is health and healing. Even the alleviation of suffering, a major preoccupation of nursing, is carried out in the service of promoting health and healing.

Peterson and Seligman (2004) of the positive psychology movement developed a classification of six character strengths that are needed to live the good life. Each category is made up of a number of other strengths (see Table 4.2).

Counseling psychologists and psychotherapists have identified 10 categories of strengths to help psychologists assess clients' strengths so they can best help them in the counseling relationship (Smith, 2006). It is a preliminary list and is by no means exhaustive. Smith (2006) derived this list on the basis of what she found in the

TABLE 4.2

Classification of character strengths

Category	Definition	Specific Strengths
I. Wisdom and knowledge	Cognitive strengths that entail the acquisition and use of knowledge	• Curiosity • Open-mindedness • Love of learning • Perspective (wisdom)
II. Courage	Emotional strengths that involve the exercise of will to accomplish goals in the face of opposition, external or internal	• Bravery • Persistence • Integrity • Vitality
III. Humanity	Interpersonal strengths that involve tending and befriending others	• Love • Kindness • Social intelligence
IV. Justice	Civic strengths that underlie healthy community life	• Citizenship • Fairness • Leadership
V. Temperance	Strengths that protect against excess	• Forgiveness and mercy • Humility/modesty • Prudence • Self-regulation
VI. Transcendence	Strengths that forge connections to the larger universe and provide meaning	• Appreciation of beauty and excellence • Gratitude • Hope, optimism, future-mindedness • Humor • Spirituality

Source: Adapted from Peterson and Seligman, (2004).

TABLE 4.3

Ten categories of strengths for psychologists and therapists

Category	Specific Features
I. Wisdom and spiritual strengths	• Age-related: older people wiser, younger people foolish
II. Emotional strengths	Examples: Perseverance, insights, optimism, putting troubles in perspective, finding purpose and meaning in life, having hope, faith, love of life • Related to sound mental health
III. Character strengths	Examples: Integrity, honesty, discipline, courage, perseverance • Related to life satisfaction, happiness
IV. Creative strengths	Examples: Ability to appreciate art, ability to express oneself in writing, voice, and other art forms • Goes beyond novel and productive thinking
V. Relational and nurturing strengths	Examples: Ability to form meaningful relationships with others; ability to communicate; capacity to nurture, show compassion, cooperation, tolerance, empathy, forgiveness, love, and kindness
VI. Educational strengths	Examples: Academic degrees, educational attainment, informal education
VII. Cognitive strengths	Examples: Problem solving, decision making, ability to think and reason
VIII. Work-related and provider strengths	Examples: Secure employment, provide for one's family, generate wealth
IX. Use-of-resources strengths	Examples: Make use of social network, access to community services
X. Survival skills strengths	Examples: Ability to avoid pain, provide for basic physiological and safety needs • Related to health status

Source: Adapted from Smith (2006).

literature; it is shown in Table 4.3. Because strengths are deeply rooted in one's culture, psychologists are being encouraged to develop a universal classification system that will include strengths that apply to all cultures (Smith, 2006).

Saleebey (2008), a professor of social work, created the CPR mnemonic to catalogue strengths: *C* stands for competencies, capacities, and courage; *P* signifies promise, possibility, and positive expectations; and *R* indicates resilience, reserves, and resources needed to cope with adversity.

Walsh (2006), a social worker, identified three groups of family strengths—(a) family belief systems, (b) family organizational patterns, and (c) family communication processes—with which clinicians work in promoting family resiliency in the face of challenges and adversity (see Table 4.4). Consider the Sullivan family, whose infant son, Brad, required open-heart surgery to repair a serious heart defect. Nurse Devon Leguillette described the behaviors she noticed that she considered to be this family's

TABLE 4.4

Key strengths for family resilience

Family belief system	• Create meaning of adversity • Positive outlook • Transcendence and spirituality
Family organizational patterns	• Flexibility • Connectedness • Social and economic resources
Communication processes	• Clarity • Open emotional expression • Collaborative problem solving

Source: Adapted from Walsh, (2006).

strengths. Brad was in hospital for several months, and during this period Devon came to know the family very well. She accompanied the Sullivans through what she describes as a *"real rock and roll ride."*

Devon described the Sullivan family's strengths: *"Everything was [not] smooth, but what came to me about this family was that they had tremendous strength as a couple; because something like this can either make or break a couple. They had good communication. You can imagine: If a baby is in the hospital for two months it's pretty exhausting, never mind the fact that this mom just had twins. They were very flexible in their roles and the dad was very involved with the kids. They were able to move in and out of responsibilities. It was almost as if they had meetings every day to plan out the next twenty-four hours, how they were going to handle things. They were like a tag team—they took turns staying overnight."*

Feeley and Gottlieb (2000), professors of nursing, identified four categories of person and family strengths required for health and healing: (a) *traits* that reside within an individual or a family (e.g., optimism, resilience, openness, flexibility), which tend to be stable; (b) *assets* that reside within an individual (e.g., an intact immune system) or are available to the person and family (e.g., finances, supportive relationships); (c) *abilities, capabilities, competencies, and skills* that an individual or a family can develop through experience, acquiring information, learning, and practice (e.g., problem-solving skills); and (d) *a transient quality* that functions as a strength, which varies in intensity depending on the situation and circumstance (e.g., a person's level of motivation).

Leddy (2006), a nurse, identified seven "C" strengths that contribute to health, wellness, and well-being: (a) connection, (b) choice, (c) challenge, (d) capability, (e) confidence, (f) capacity, and (g) control. These concepts are used to promote healthiness in the way individuals find purpose and choose to exercise power. For example, power is needed to achieve goals. Power incorporates dimensions of challenge, confidence, choice, capability, and control. Challenge enables the individual to feel excitement and perceive opportunities in a given situation. Confidence helps the person to overcome and deal with obstacles. Choice provides the person with the freedom to choose from an array of possibilities, whereas control gives the person the power to control the amount and rate of change. According to Leddy (2006), nurses can promote healthiness by developing or working with these Cs.

Related Constructs Associated with Strengths: Potentials, Resources, and Resiliency

The word potential refers to something that is possible, as opposed to something that already exists. Potential exists when a person or situation has the capacity to develop into something different in the future. Potentials are precursors to strengths in that they do not function as a strength but can develop into a strength (Feeley & Gottlieb, 2000).

Clifton and Harter (2003) described a three-stage process of turning a potential into a strength: (a) *identification* of the potential strength; (b) *integration* of the potential that now performs as a strength into the person's view of himself, and (c) *changes* in a person's behavior that are based on the use of that strength.

The first step in the process is identifying a potential that can become a strength. Once recognized and identified, the quality needs to be labeled as a potential strength. Turning a potential into a strength requires that the person or trainer understand how to develop the potential. He also has to have knowledge of the potential and how it works as a strength. Once a potential has been developed into a strength, it then needs to be incorporated into the way the person views himself, that is, integrated into his self-concept. Finally, the potential, now performing as a strength, needs to be used to deal with a wide range of situations. The more the new strength is used, the more likely it will become an integral part of the person's repertoire of strengths. Consider the example of a family of five children, in which one teenage son shows an interest in helping his father learn how to perform home dialysis. After being trained in the various medical procedures and having an opportunity to practice them, the son becomes quite adept at performing home dialysis. He now sees himself as an important caregiver to his father and as an invaluable resource to the family. He has turned a potential—in this case, an interest in helping his father and learning the technical aspects of administering dialysis—into a strength.

Resources are assets, services, and opportunities that are external to the person and his family. They reside in a person's immediate environment and may be available when needed or called on. Resources may include finances, family relationships, religion, community, and the like. Resources can also be potentials until they are required. The person and family have to recognize their need for a particular resource, recognize who or what services are available to serve as a resource, know how to access them, and then use them to achieve their goals.

Resiliency is the ability to withstand, rebound, and recover from adversity and insults that challenge a person's physiological and psychological capacities (Jacelon, 1997; Walsh, 2006). The term *human resilience* refers to "the processes or patterns of positive adaptation and development in the context of significant threats to an individual's life or function" (Masten & Wright, 2010, p. 215). Resiliency is a concept that applies equally well to families and to communities.

There are several ways one can view resiliency in relation to strengths. One is to see strengths and resiliency as interchangeable. According to this view, resiliency is considered an inborn trait that enables a person to overcome adversity (Richardson, 2002). Thus, resiliency is a core personality trait or set of traits that serves as a building block for mental health and a protective factor against mental illness. Resiliency can also be a core feature that defines some families. It can be considered an inborn trait by virtue of how its members came together to create a loving, committed, and functioning unit to fulfill its needs and those of its members to meet life's challenges. When resilience is lacking, it can serve as a risk factor for and precursor to personality disorders (Skodol, 2010).

Another view is to think of resiliency as a process that develops as a person learns how to deal with adversity, minimize the harmful effects of traumatic life events, and eventually adapt (Fine, 1991; Masten & Reed, 2002). In the process of adapting to a challenge, a person develops new strengths. He may master developmental tasks and develop new competency skills (Masten & Wright, 2010). *Developmental tasks* are standards of behavior in different domains of functioning that are expected of individuals as they mature in a given culture and society (Masten & Coatsworth, 1998). On the other hand, *competency skills* refers to effective functioning in reference to expectations based on norms set down by a specific culture and society at a particular time in history (Masten & Wright, 2010). These ideas apply equally well to the family as well as to communities. By dealing with challenges and adversity, the family develops new family strengths. It does so in the process of fulfilling its family tasks and obligations. It also does so by developing new competency skills. As each family member develops, relationships within the family also change. Family relationships, namely, spousal, parent-child, and sibling relationships, develop and evolve in response to challenges. Roles, relationships, and responsibilities are often redefined that necessitate the learning of new skills. When this happens, the family's bank of strengths increases.

Resiliency is forged in the midst of adversity. It is an aspect of the human spirit that enables people to continue against all odds. It is in the process of navigating through life's challenges and the need to rebuild lives devastated by death, loss, illness, hardship, tragedy, and trauma that people discover their own strengths and develop new understandings, skills, and competencies (Walsh, 2006). When people have a large repertoire of strengths from which to draw, they become more resilient and are equipped to rally from insults more quickly. In short, strengths enable a person and family to take control and make good choices about their health and lives, and in the process of taking charge of themselves and their situations, they feel empowered. Terry Fox, a young Canadian hero, embodies these strengths. His story is told in Exhibit 4.2.

A similar process of empowerment takes place at the physiological level. The body becomes more resilient following exposure to harmful pathogens or disease. Consider how the heart compensates by setting up new circulatory pathways, referred to as *collateral circulation,* when there is an occlusion in one of the coronary blood vessels. Or think of how immunity is acquired after one has been exposed to a pathogen (e.g., through vaccination).

Strengths-Based Care (SBC) accommodates both views. Resiliency requires that the person and family already possess strengths, which they mobilize and capitalize on to deal with challenges and insults, and overcome adversity. In the process of dealing with these events, the person and family develop new capacities and skills and, as a result, become more resilient. Resiliency then becomes a strength that the person and family can call forth to deal with future physiological and psychological insults and traumas. With each successive challenge that the person and family successfully navigate, they learn about themselves, their environments, and the people in their different lifeworlds. These, in turn, are added to their repertoire of strengths.

EXHIBIT 4.2

Personal experience *The Terry Fox story: A profile in courage*

Terry Fox, a Canadian national hero, has inspired millions of Canadians and others worldwide with his courage, determination, and tenacity. In 1977, at age 18, after experiencing pain in his right knee, he was diagnosed with osteosarcoma, a form of cancer that starts at the knee and then works its way into the muscles and tendons. At the time, the only way to treat his condition was to amputate his right leg several inches above the knee. Three years after losing his leg to cancer, he decided to undertake a 5,000-mile run, running from coast to coast across Canada, to raise awareness and money for cancer research. This was unheard of at the time. In creating the Marathon of Hope, Terry's goal was to raise $1 from each Canadian citizen for cancer research. He began his Marathon of Hope by sending letters asking for grants to buy a running leg and soliciting sponsors to support his run despite the fact that he also suffered from a serious heart condition. Nothing was going to deter him.

Terry began his run by dipping his right leg into the Atlantic Ocean at St. John's, Newfoundland, on April 12, 1980. He intended to dip it in the Pacific Ocean when he arrived in Victoria, British Columbia. When he began his run, few had heard of him and what he was doing. After running for over 1500 miles, he finally was noticed. The media and the Canadian people began to track his run. Having completed 3,339 miles of his run, he began to experience breathing problems, and a chest X-ray revealed that his cancer had metastasized to his lungs. On September 1, 1980, after 143 days on the road, he was forced to stop his run. A Canadian national television network organized a nationwide telethon in the hopes of raising additional funds for the cause of cancer research. It proved so successful that $10.5 million were raised that day alone. By February 1981, $24.17 million had been raised, and Terry's dream of getting $1 from every single Canadian for cancer research had been realized. On June 27, 1981, Terry lapsed into a coma. He died the next day, at age 22.

Terry Fox's Marathon of Hope captured Canadians' imagination. He was proclaimed a national hero, and the annual Terry Fox Run events organized all across Canada, the United States, and in many other countries around the world, have so far raised more than $400 million for cancer research. Numerous magazine articles, books, and a movie have been made about Terry Fox, this Canadian hero. He has become a symbol of courage, vision, fortitude, and dedication.

What Is the Relationship Between a Strengths Perspective, Specific Strengths, and Strengths-Based Care?

A *strengths perspective* is the orientation or lens through which nurses view their patients and families. It reflects the nurses' values and guides their practice (see Chapter 2). Nurses look for *specific strengths* and work with those strengths to create with the patient and family their plan of care (see Chapter 9). In practice, SBC mobilizes the person and family's existing strengths and helps them develop new strengths to deal with problems and weaknesses and to promote health, recovery, and healing (for more detail, see Chapter 10). Using strengths in SBC means focusing on the following:

- Knowing the person and/or family, what is important and meaningful to them, and what they want to achieve
- Observing for and asking about what is working and what they do best
- Understanding that strengths can come in many forms and that strengths, in part, define the person and family's uniqueness
- Understanding that the person and family have potentials, strengths, resources, resiliencies weaknesses, and vulnerabilities.
- Appreciating that strengths are key to the person and family's health, recovery, and healing
- Helping the person and family recognize that they have the power to heal themselves (self-heal) when they respect and honor their own strengths and weaknesses and when they understand when and how best to use their strengths and to compensate for or minimize their weaknesses, taking into account the condition, circumstance, and context
- Understanding that nurses need to have or develop specific personal strengths in order to practice SBC. Nurse strengths are described, and approaches to develop them are discussed, in Chapter 5

> **CAVEAT**
>
> These ideas apply equally as well to communities.

Nurses who practice SBC understand that the issue facing them and their patients is *not* one of strengths *versus* deficits but of working with the person's strengths within the context of problems and deficits. Nurses and their patients and families may come to realize that problems and deficits can be opportunities for developing new strengths or refining existing ones. It is through discovering one's own strengths during adversity that the human spirit is revealed, renewed, and deepened.

Nurse Margaret Eades practices SBC in her work in oncology rehabilitation. She is constantly observing patients and assessing them for specific strengths in order to plan care. As she explains, *"I need to know the patient—who they are, what is important and meaningful to them. I need to understand this transition* [referring to change of health status] *where something has happened that has really derailed them. I bring that to the forefront, so that I can create the conditions to enable them to engage in their own care. I will use the ideas that they've given me to try to integrate it into my care with them."*

> It is during times of adversity that clients/patients/families/ communities discover their strengths and develop new ones. It is then that the human capacity for healing is revealed, renewed, and deepened.

Margaret described her work with Mr. Daly, who was referred to the follow-up rehabilitation cancer clinic to deal with his extreme fatigue during chemotherapy to treat his pancreatic cancer: *"Fatigue is a real thing. It's different from ordinary fatigue, and it doesn't go away very easily. The one intervention that makes a difference to fatigue is exercise. It increases the endorphins and makes a person feel better."* In working with Mr. Daly, the team discovered that he was an artist and wanted to return to his work. Margaret recounted her conversation with him: *"So here you are, you're an artist. In order to continue with your art, it takes energy. In order to have energy, we have some plans for you to do some physical activity* [exercise] *with the physiotherapist."* Margaret continued to explain the team's approach: *"It is about understanding the important role art played in his life (before his cancer) and bringing in the art as part of the plan to deal with his fatigue and lack of energy."* Margaret understands that the key to dealing with the patient's fatigue is not about handing out yet another medication or being prescriptive; it is about capitalizing on the things that are important to the patient, which the team has identified by talking to and listening to the patient and family—in Mr. Daly's case, his love for and interest in art—as a strength on which they can capitalize to plan the person's care, in Mr. Daly's case, to help him deal with the fatigue resulting from chemotherapy.

CHARACTERISTICS OF STRENGTHS

There are nine characteristics of strengths that nurses need to understand in order to know how best to use strengths to care for persons and families.

1. Strengths are developing entities
2. Strengths can be developed through learning
3. Strengths coexist with weaknesses and vulnerabilities
4. Strengths are related to goals
5. Strengths are defined by their context and circumstance
6. Strengths are multidimensional
7. Strengths can be depleted and replenished
8. Strengths are transferable
9. Strengths are personal constructions

1. Strengths are developing entities. People are born with both special traits, talents, and potentials that are unique to them, as well as general capacities that are common to all human beings to ensure survival and growth. Darwin recognized that an organism's ability to adapt to change was closely related to its survival. Thus, strengths are part of the human adaptation system; humans are biologically equipped to develop strengths (Masten & Reed, 2002; Smith, 2006; Watson & Ecken, 2003).

Recall from the definition of *strengths* provided earlier in this chapter that traits, talents, and capacities all can be potential strengths. For example, all humans have an inborn capacity to form relationships, yet there is wide variation in how people interact. Some individuals have high emotional intelligence and are able to connect more easily with others, whereas others are less socially adept and have difficulty relating (Goleman, 1995). The difference in social skills between individuals may be innate, inasmuch as some individuals have a gene that makes them more sociable and responsive to their surroundings. However, individuals can learn social skills by observing, relating, connecting, and interacting with others. In other words, they acquire skills through experiences and then, having opportunities to practice what they have learned. Consider how a person develops a talent such as music. The majority of humans are born with the capacity to hear and enjoy music, yet not all humans are musical or have the innate talent and singing voice of, for example, Celine Dion. Even Celine Dion continues to develop her musical talent through practice, voice training, and hard work.

Throughout a person's life span, from conception to death, humans develop new strengths and further hone and refine the ones they have. Strengths may express themselves in different forms at different ages. For example, courage (an important strength) may look very different in a 17-year-old than it does in a 70-year-old.

Other strengths have to be discovered or learned in the course of living and dealing with pain and suffering. Some people, when faced with an unexpected, catastrophic event, may discover a strength they did not realize they had. People will often say how surprised they were to discover aspects of themselves that they never knew existed. One example that comes to mind is the firemen who risked their lives to save people in the destruction of the World Trade Center's twin towers on September 11, 2001.

Strengths are governed by many developmental processes. The famed psychoanalyst and developmentalist Erik Erikson (1959) identified specific strengths that emerge from meeting and mastering challenges that occur at different stages in a person's life span. There are eight stages in the human life span, each with its own challenge that must be mastered for healthy ego development (i.e., the development of a healthy sense of self; see Table 4.5). Often, the stage is biologically driven and related

TABLE 4.5

Erik Erikson's (1959) eight developmental stages of and associated strengths with the successful resolution of the crisis of that stage

Ages and Stages	Developmental Challenges or Psychosocial Crisis	Basic Strengths
I. Infancy (Birth–18 months)	Trust vs. mistrust	Hope, faith
II. Toddlerhood (18 months–3 years	Autonomy vs. shame and doubt	Self-control, determination, will
III. Preschooler years (3–6 years)	Initiative vs. guilt	Purpose, courage
IV. School age (7–12 years)	Industry vs. inferiority	Competence
V. Adolescence (13–20 years)	Ego identity vs. role confusion	Fidelity, loyalty
VI. Young adulthood (the 20s)	Intimacy vs. isolation	Love, affiliation
VII. Middle adulthood (30s–50s)	Generativity vs. stagnation	Care
VIII. Old adulthood (50s and beyond)	Integrity vs. despair	Wisdom

Source: Adapted from Erikson (1959).

to maturation and timing. Erikson believed that the mastery of the specific challenge required that the person's daily interaction with others be of a certain quality. In the process of meeting that stage's challenge, the person develops important strengths. For example, the challenge in infancy is the need to trust. If a child's need for trust is met in infancy, that child will come to expect that when he requires help there will be a responsive person available to help him meet his need. This expectancy gives rise to feelings of hope, an important strength to possess. Failure to have basic needs met, such as when the infant's mother is unresponsive to his needs, gives rise in the infant to feelings of mistrust and an expectancy that the world is a hostile, uncaring place. Each developmental stage is an important benchmark in the person's journey of fulfilling their potential. Although Erikson proposed his theory in the 1950s, sufficient empirical evidence has now supported his ideas and the importance of these core strengths for a person's healthy development.

2. Strengths can be developed through learning. All strengths require some form of learning. Strengths develop primarily through a person's interaction with her environments. There are people who are "naturally" better in some areas than in others. All natural strengths (i.e., talents and gifts) still have to be developed through education, proper training, and opportunities to practice; otherwise, they will remain as potentials, either underdeveloped or entirely undeveloped unless they are developed. Consider Tiger Woods, who showed unusual athletic prowess at a very young age. His father recognized his talents when he was just a young boy and proceeded to develop and nurture them.

The same can be said for a personality trait. Individuals are born with different temperaments or constitutional makeups (Chess & Thomas, 1996). There are people who are born with outgoing personalities, such as the uninhibited, engaging child. On the other hand, there are children who from birth are cautious and inhibited. They feel apprehensive and anxious in new and unfamiliar social situations. These children are considered shy (Kagan, 1989; Kagan, Reznick, & Gibbons, 1989). The question that needs to be asked is whether shy children grow up to be shy adults. Not necessarily. Consider an outgoing child who is open to new experiences (i.e., a strength) compared to a shy child who is cautious and reserved and becomes anxious in new situations. Both children have a certain tendency or genetic predisposition to react to their environment in very specific ways; however, their behaviors or tendencies can be modified by experience. Shy children can learn to moderate their anxiety and overcome their fears when placed in unfamiliar situations by learning to regulate their emotions and developing new skills. They can do this by gaining insight and awareness into their own reactions and behaviors and those of others, developing more effective social skills, and learning new ways to cope. They can learn to control and compensate for their basic tendency of shyness.

Strengths are very much a reflection of a person's culture and are deeply rooted in that culture (Smith, 2006). Certain qualities may be viewed as a strength in one culture and a weakness in another. A particular strength reflects that which is valued in a particular culture or community. Individuals who excel at something or possess a capability or talent that is valued by their communiy often singled out for recognition, praise, and admiration and are often afforded special status. Consider the influence of culture in the development of autonomy. In general, the evidence indicates that children in the United States are encouraged to become autonomous individuals: to develop to their full potential, learn how to make their own choices, and all are considered equal in their right to pursue goals. These societal values are rooted in the economic, social, and political history of America. They are reflected in the way American children are socialized and in the child-rearing practices of their parents (Tamis-Lemonda & McFadden, 2010). Within a country as large and diverse as the United States, however, there are wide variations. There are subgroups within the country in which the emphasis on achievement, choice, and equality differ considerably. Every culture and environment have elements that enable or foster the development of certain qualities. They also create conditions that limit or thwart the development of other traits (Smith, 2006). Consider the role ethnicity plays in the development of specific strengths. Chinese and Chinese-American parents have a more positive attitude to the study of science than their American counterparts. They place greater emphasis on self-improvement, help children in their studies, and set higher standards when it comes to the study of science (Chen, 2001). Middle-class families tend to assign greater importance to educational achievement than working-class families. In families that place a high value on educational achievement, such as Chinese families, parents will encourage their children in their studies by becoming more involved in their children's education than their American counterparts.

Culture and values also play a role in the development of specific strengths through the institutions they create and the rituals they follow. Consider the values communicated within Jewish culture. Many Jews are taught from a very young age that they have an obligation to care for those who are less fortunate. Judaism teaches that it is a *mitzvah*, or moral obligation, to visit the sick and care for the less fortunate, including vulnerable individuals, strangers, widows, and orphans. Families form tightly knit units and are part of supportive and caring communities. Thus, children learn from a very young age by observing and experiencing acts of kindness that family, friends, and members of their community are important resources of support and help that can be called on both in times of celebration and during times of need. The ability to ask for support and use resources wisely is considered, in most families and communities, to be an important strength.

3. Strengths co-exist with weaknesses and vulnerabilities. Every person and family has both strengths and weaknesses. As Nurse Andra Leimanis explained, *"An individual is not all negative or all bad. . . . . some strengths may not be obvious; the nurse may have to dig a little bit, but they are there."*

At times, strengths and weaknesses may seem to be at odds with one another. At other times, strengths may counterbalance a weakness or prevent a weakness from becoming overwhelming. Let's continue with the example of the shy child. The child may want to play with the other children but may feel too anxious or socially awkward (weaknesses) to do so. He may go to his teacher for support (a strength—recognizes his need for support and seeks the appropriate help), who is attuned to his feelings and gives him a supportive hug. The teacher's presence and understanding serve to reduce his anxiety, which then allows him to join the other children at play. In hospitals, patients may be anxious when receiving a treatment; nurses can play an important role in alleviating their anxiety by staying with them during a procedure, holding their hand, or stroking their arm or shoulder gently. Once a patient's anxiety is better under control and the person is able to relax, he often is able to cope more effectively with the treatment. Jim Mulchahy, a former teacher diagnosed with end-stage lymphoma, made a YouTube video in which he describes the power of a nurse's touch in helping him get through a painful procedure (Jim Mulchahy: A Story of Care [YouTube], www.youtube.com/watch?v=dmjNiMHT8xo)

No person or family is immune to events that may cause undue hardship, pain, or suffering: Every person, at some point during her lifetime, is vulnerable. However, some people are better able to cope and recover from hardships depending on their inherent, innate strengths or acquired coping capabilities.

A focus on strengths is not about ignoring weaknesses or downplaying a person's vulnerabilities. Moreover, it is not about reframing problems and weaknesses in terms of strengths. It is not about whether the glass is half-empty (i.e., weaknesses) or whether it is half-full (i.e., strengths); instead, it is about understanding the whole. It is about finding strengths and recognizing that strengths coexist with weaknesses; about striking the vital balance between the two; and about understanding how strengths and weaknesses interact to promote health, recovery, and healing. A focus on strengths is about appreciating and discovering human strengths in the midst of problems and weaknesses and about how to work with strengths to mitigate vulnerability. Finally, a focus on strengths helps to uncover weaknesses.

Nurse Christina Clausen recognizes that a person possesses strengths and weaknesses and both are the focus of her nursing. She believes that strengths hold the key to helping people deal with their problems. It is in focusing on strengths that a person becomes less defensive and more open and is in a better position to deal with things that are not going right or that are not working. Christina explained, *"I think my way of looking is to understand people's weaknesses. It's often the approach of dealing with strengths first as the best way to get at weaknesses, for many reasons. People come to you and say 'This is what's wrong with me and, as nurses, we tend only to identify their weaknesses but can never to identify their strengths. I really feel that if I can make a positive approach in terms of helping them to identify their strengths, it allows them to accept some of the areas [of weakness] that might not be as easy. It almost gives them permission to go there; their defense mechanisms come down."*

> A focus on strengths is not about ignoring a person's weaknesses or downplaying vulnerabilities. Rather it is about understanding how strengths co-exist with weaknesses and learning how to use strengths to overcome weaknesses and minimize vulnerabilities.

Even researchers have maintained a deficit focus when studying phenomena while ignoring strengths. One of the few pioneering studies to focus on strengths and not just problems was one conducted by Marilyn Ford-Gilboe (2000) of single-parent families. She asked what the strengths of single-parent families were as compared to the strengths found in two-parent families. The findings of her study are reported in Exhibit 4.3.

4. Strengths are related to goals. Humans are by nature goal directed. They have the capacity to set goals for themselves and achieve them as they see fit (Ignatieff, 2000). Think of Sean, a 9-month old infant, who sees a red ball from across the room. His goal is to examine the ball. Motivated by curiosity, he is able to achieve this goal by crawling across the room. Thus, Sean exercises a new skill that he has been perfecting, namely, the act of crawling (strength), as well as inborn curiosity (another strength), to achieve his goal.

EXHIBIT 4.3

Empirical study   *A comparison of the strengths of single-parent and two-parent families*

The Problem
Although single-parent family life has become mainstream in many ways, knowledge about these families has been focused predominantly on the chronic problems they experience.

The Issues
1. What are the perceived strengths and weaknesses of two-parent families and single-parent families led by mothers who are separated or divorced?
2. How similar or different are these strengths by family type?
3. How do families explain the effect of self-identified strengths on their health status and health practices?

The Study
This study used a sample of 138 families (sixty-eight single parent and seventy two parent), recruited from a mid-size city in southern Ontario, a province in Canada. A subset of sixteen families were interviewed (families: seven single parent and nine two parent) to explore their experiences in greater depth.

The Findings
Although single-parent and two-parent families are different structurally, the nature and pattern of strengths were more similar than different. The strengths in both family types were that they were high on cohesiveness and closeness, optimistic, had open communication, and valued working together as a team. These strengths were used to help them cope with difficult situations and health problems.

The Bottom Line
These findings challenge stereotypical views of single-parent families that emphasize problems and vulnerability (weaknesses) and exclude a consideration of their strengths.

Source: Adapted from Ford-Gilboe (2000).

Various goals often require different sets of strengths. Different health care professions have different goals and therefore place emphasis on different sets of strengths.

For example, therapy conducted by advocates of positive psychology, with its goal of well-being, harmony, and living a balanced and good life, focuses on character and virtue strengths to meet these goals (Table 4.2, Peterson & Seligman, 2004). Wolin (2003), a social worker, identified seven "resiliency" strengths needed to deal with adversity, unexpected catastrophic events, or to survive violence and abuse. She stated that people need the strength of independence to provide for their physical and emotional safety, whereas humor (another strength) introduces lightness into an otherwise dark situation and is often required to recover from trauma.

Nurses on the other hand, look for biological strengths that support the body's innate mechanisms of healing and the person's and family's efforts to cope, repair, and restore following an insult—an illness, trauma, injury and the like. Consider the story told by Nurse Althea McBean of Mrs. Grill, a 69-year-old woman who suffered a cardiac arrest due to the blockage of a major coronary artery. She had major neurological damage, was being kept alive by a ventilator, and was not expected to survive. Althea noticed that Mrs. Grill always had a smile on her face even though the she was in a semicomatose state: *"I interpreted from her smile that she was determined to go on, no matter what."* Despite Mrs. Grill's poor prognosis, Althea saw the situation differently from the other members of the medical team: *"The fact that she had this magnificent smile is what got me focused on getting her through this traumatic event. This was an important strength."* Althea also felt that Mrs. Grill had a chance of recovery. She came to this conclusion because she saw that her age (biological strength) and previous medical history (biological strength) were working in her favor: *"The other strength she had was the fact that she was 69 years old and her only past medical history was that she had high blood pressure and high cholesterol, which were being treated with medication. And she was very functional. She didn't have a significant past medical history. She was very healthy."*

Althea continued to identify Mrs. Grill's current situation by looking for other biological indicators of strengths: *"The fact that she suffered the [cardiac arrest] and her vital organs were preserved and functioning; the fact that she was able to open her eyes, was starting to move, and her kidneys and liver were functioning, were strengths working in her favor."*

Thus, nurses need to ask themselves, as well as the patient and family the following questions:

- What is working or functioning?
- What does this person have going for them?
- What is the person's goal?
- What are my goals for the person?
- What would they want to see happen?
- What would I like to see happen to them?

Once these questions have been answered, nurses need to ask themselves, "What are the strengths that the person requires to meet this goal?"

There are times when neither the goal nor the strength is obvious. Consider 5-year-old, Anthony who was in the hospital for two weeks for undiagnosed seizures.

During his time in the hospital, Anthony began to throw temper tantrums. It was often unclear what precipitated a temper tantrum. Some nurses reported that Anthony was a well-behaved little boy, whereas others described him as "difficult," "uncontrollable," and "impossible." The nurses began to systematically record when Anthony had a temper tantrum; what events preceded a tantrum, who was his assigned nurse at the time, and the like. What they found surprised them. They noted that Anthony threw tantrums with some nurses but not with others. With the nurses Anthony liked, he was good as gold, the "perfect" patient—a well-behaved little boy. With nurses whom he did not like, however, he was "horrid." They then determined that Anthony's goal was to control his environment through his temper tantrums. On the surface, having a tantrum is not normally considered a strength; however, in this case, Anthony's temper tantrums could be considered a strength. He used a tantrum to maintain control over his environment.

Nurse Emilie Gauthier explained how strengths are the tools nurses use to help people achieve their health goals: *"As nurses, we give patients the tools to improve their health. A strength is like a motor—it drives the person to their health goals. We talk about having a positive attitude as being a strength, being motivated is another strength, etc. These are all strengths that the person can use to help them with their health goals."*

5. *Strengths are defined by their context.* The context/situation or a specific circumstance often defines whether a particular quality is functioning as a strength or a weakness. A behavior can be labeled a strength only when it is viewed in context. For example, think of perseverance. A person who is obese and needs to lose weight requires perseverance to stay on a diet. In this context, perseverance is a strength. However, once the person achieves a desirable weight but continues to persevere on the diet and moves from obesity to anorexia, this strength then has converted into a weakness.

Both nurses and patients need to ask themselves questions such as the following: "Are their behavior or actions appropriate in the situation or for the circumstance?" If the answer is yes, then the quality or behavior is performing as a strength.

Nurse Cheryl Armistead recalled the role that context plays in defining whether a quality functions as a strength or weakness: *"Because I have seen in my practice that one can be a little overenthusiastic with our understanding of people's strengths and resources. . . . I think we have to remind ourselves that a strength of two weeks ago in today's context might not be considered a strength anymore. That's where we try to figure out the balance."*

6. *A strength is multidimensional.* Strengths are usually made up of many different qualities. These qualities can combine to create another strength.

Consider the strength of "responsive parenting." Kathryn Barnard, the renowned nurse scholar in the field of maternal and infant health, recognized that the foundation of healthy child development resides in the quality of the early interactions between caregiver/parent and child (the Barnard model is described in Sumner & Spietz, 2004). Responsive parenting is a critical component of healthy mother–infant interaction. Responsive parenting is a strength; however, responsiveness is made up of a number of other strengths, such as a mother's sensitivity to her infant's cues, attunement to the infant's distress, and so forth. Each of these qualities in turn involves many skills.

Consider what is involved in "sensitivity" to infant cues. First, the mother must know how to position the infant in such a way as to make eye contact. She needs to hold her infant close to her body to read the infant's subtle cues, recognize and respond contingently to these cues, and pace the amount and intensity of her responses to her infant's engagement behaviors. Thus, individual strengths combine to create a strength that comprises different dimensions. Nurses may focus on one strength as a way to develop a more comprehensive strength. That is why it is important for a nurse to appreciate the different dimensions of a strength. For example, a nurse may help a new mother learn how to become more responsive to her infant. She could do this, for example, by helping her learn how to read her infant's cues, by showing her how to position her infant so that she can see her infant's face more easily, and by enabling her to more readily identify and read her infant's cues.

7. A strength can be depleted and replenished. Strengths are finite. They need to be thought of in terms of a resource capacity. What I mean by *resource capacity* is that strengths can become depleted with overuse and may need to be replenished or recharged. This is because strengths involve energy. Think about what happens to a muscle when it is in continuous use: It eventually tires. The muscle cannot be in a constant state of contraction; it must be given time to recover before it can function effectively again. In this case, the muscle is depleted of adenosine triphosphate, the molecular form of energy used in cells that becomes depleted with excessive muscle contraction. Thus, muscle tissue has a finite and limited resource capacity.

The same principle applies to other strengths. Consider self-control, an important strength involved in self-regulation. Self-control is, as the term implies, a person's ability to exert control over oneself (Muraven & Baumeister, 2000), and it is used to deal with almost every aspect of daily living. Self-control is an important strength because it allows a person to delay urges, control emotions, make decisions, and follow medical/ lifestyle regimens, and the like. Think of the role self-control plays in eating. When the person feels rested, it is easier to exercise self-control. For example, when rested, a person may have an easier time resisting reaching for that extra piece of cake or having a second helping. However, when the person is tired, he may have more difficulty exercising self-control and may not be able to resist temptation.

> Strengths are finite and can become depleted. The role of nursing is to recognize when the person needs to recharge and replenish.

There are several key assumptions that affect strength's resource capacity:

- A person's strength resource capacity is affected by age, temperament, and gender. A young child tends to have less resource capacity than an adult. A tired child may be unable to control herself and have more "meltdowns," whereas a tired adult may dip into his reserves and persevere
- A strength's resource capacity varies from person to person
- A person's strength resource capacity is affected by context and circumstance. Pain, depression, and anxiety drain a person's resource capacity, leaving a person less able to mobilize and capitalize on her existing strengths to deal with stress

- A person's strength resource capacity can be replenished. A number of strategies can be used to replenish resource capacity, such as conserving or redirecting energy through rest, taking time out, removing stressors, and exercising. A change in circumstances or taking a trip also can help replenish resource capacity
- A person's strength resource capacity can be developed and expanded over time
- Nurses can help families understand their own resource capacity and develop ways to replenish depleted reserves

Nurse Cheryl Armistead described caring for Mrs. Bhutto, a young mother and recent immigrant to Canada. Her infant had failed to gain weight. Cheryl described this mother's resourcefulness and the lengths to which Mrs. Bhutto went to get her daughter the proper medical treatment: *"Mrs. Bhutto somehow was able to communicate her needs without formal knowledge of how the medical system worked [strength]. She had this ability to know her child, monitor her child's condition, and reach out and identify that there was something that she could do [strength].. She was also establishing herself in the community, developing a network of support and resources [strength].. But I think at a certain point the situation started to overwhelm her. Everyone has his or her limits. This is where it gets very interesting when we begin to look at strengths and resources. This mother had resources around her, but culturally it wasn't appropriate to ask her cousin to babysit. She was at a point where her baby was in the hospital for several weeks. Her other child needed to be cared for. Her resources and her energy became depleted. When I talk about strengths, one of the caveats I have is 'Be careful.' A person needs permission to say "Enough already—what worked in the past is just not sufficient now."*

8. A strength is transferable. Strengths are not situation specific; the same strength can be used in different situations. Peterson and Seligman (2004) found that strengths differed in terms of being *tonic* (constant) or *phasic* (waxing and waning depending on their use). Tonic-type strengths, such as humor or flexibility, are integral to a person. These types of strengths are not called into service to deal with one specific situation and then discarded but are ever present to be called upon as needed. They can be transferred from one situation to another. In contrast, phasic strengths (e.g., motivation) are called into service to deal with a particular situation. These strengths come and go as needed. They are more situation dependent and can be considered transient strengths (Feeley & Gottlieb, 2000).

Nurse Esther Leforet described how she worked with this characteristic of a strength in nursing with Mr. Richards, who was in cardiac distress. He was a fireman, and by knowing this information Esther was able to use it to help him calm himself down, *"Mr. Richards was used to dealing with life-and-death situations. He had done a lot of fighting; he had even fought in a war. When he was admitted with a heart attack, he had to be intubated. He had to have all these treatments, and he had to be repeatedly defibrillated after the heart attack because he had arrhythmia. I was able to draw from him the story of his dealing with high stress, life-and-death situations. He was able to remember that he had that kind of knowledge and this was just another one of those situations that he could deal with as calmly as possible, to remain calm in the face of possible repeated defibrillation, which he found is extremely uncomfortable. So he could draw on his past experience and I reinforced that so that hopefully he could draw on his strengths."* Esther helped Mr. Richards transfer the strength of knowing how to calm himself in his work as a fireman to calming himself during a difficult medical procedure (i.e., defibrillation).

9. Strengths are personal constructions. A strength is whatever a person says is her strength. Strengths lie in the "eyes of the beholder." A quality, characteristic, capacity or behavior is labeled as a strength often because a person has experienced how that strength contributes to her functioning and well-being. If a certain quality helps the person achieve her goals, she will identify that quality as one of her strengths. For example, if the person links her dedication to hard work with achieving what she has set out to accomplish, then she will include dedication and hard work on her personal list of strengths. If a child is told that he is lovable and charming and is treated as such then he will feel lovable and will internalize this quality into his self-concept. He will call forth this quality and use it to connect to others.

Because strengths are constructions that are based on a person's interpretation of a quality, some people will label a behavior a strength, whereas others may label that same behavior as a weakness. How can this be? At issue here is, first, what is perceived and then how the event or behavior is interpreted. The labeling of something as a strength or a weakness involves many processes, including selection, attention, observation, perception, interpretation, and creation of the narrative. All these processes take place on two levels: (a) the person and (b) the environment (i.e., their relationships). The interplay between the person's own behavior and how that behavior is interpreted by others determines whether the quality or behavior is viewed as a strength by the person herself and others whose lives she affects.

Consider the following situation, as told by Nurse Sharyn Andrews. An unemployed, single mother, Sally, decides to give her youngest child, age 7 years, to her sister to be cared for temporarily because she is overwhelmed and is having difficulty coping. Is she a neglectful, uncaring, selfish mother who is abandoning her daughter, or is she a sensitive mother who recognizes her own limitations in that she is unable to provide the quality of mothering her daughter needs? As Sharyn observed, many would label this woman as a "bad or selfish" mother. They likely would reason that "good" mothers do not give their children to another person to care for, even if just temporarily. Or do they? Let's reexamine this situation from a different mind set and a different set of cultural values. It is common practice for middle- and upper class parents to send their children to camp during the summer months or to after-school play activities, to hire babysitters, have full-time nannies, or engage in all of these practices. They do this for their children, but it also gives them a respite, time for themselves. Few people would label these mothers "bad or selfish." A culture or society in which one lives, sanctions what are acceptable ways of coping with burn-out (e.g., hiring nannies, sending a child to camp) and what are less acceptable or even nonacceptable ways of behaving (e.g., sending a child to live with an aunt). However, Sharyn discovered that Sally found herself overwhelmed, depressed, and incapable of caring for her daughter. She worried about "losing it" and harming her daughter and felt her daughter would be in a more secure and safer place in the care of her sister. Like the mother who hires a babysitter, Sally exhibited the same strength of recognizing her own limitation and taking actions that were in the best interest of her child.

Strengths can be visible or invisible, obvious, or in need of discovery. In some people, strengths are more obvious and more apparent than in others. Some people's strengths need to be recognized, uncovered, and discovered.

Why some nurses describe one behavior as a strength whereas other nurses interpret the same behavior as a deficit may be due in part to their knowledge of the person and family, the situation, the assumptions under which they operate, the values and beliefs they hold, and the way they interpret or explain a situation. Nurses need to be aware of the factors that are affecting their perceptions and interpretations in judging a quality or an action as a strength or a weakness.

Key Summary Points

- Strengths are a person's unique qualities and resources that define her personhood and contribute to her health and healing.
- Strengths can be biological, psychological, and social.
- Strengths are invaluable sources of power and energy that a person uses to meet challenges, both big and small. They contribute to how a person lives, makes decisions in his everyday life, and to the quality of his life. They also affect how a person and family rally, recover, and heal following an insult that has caused physical and/or emotional trauma.
- Three strength-related concepts are (a) potentials, (b) resources, and (c) resiliency.
- There are nine characteristics of strengths: (1) strengths are developing entities, (2) strengths can be learned, (3) strengths coexist with weaknesses and vulnerabilities, (4) strengths are related to goals, (5) strengths are defined by the context and circumstance, (6) strengths are multidimensional, (7) strengths can be depleted and replenished, (8) strengths are transferable, and (9) strengths are personal constructions.

Essential Nurse Qualities Required for Strengths-Based Care

5

LEARNING OBJECTIVES

After reading this chapter, you should be able to:

- Describe the relationship between nurse strengths and Strengths-Based Care
- Identify the four categories of essential nurse qualities to practice Strengths-Based Care
- Define each strength, its contribution to Strengths-Based Care, and the approaches to develop the specific strength

Up until now, the focus of this book has been on the person and family's strengths. Yet there are two parties in the nurse–person relationship, namely, the person/family and the nurse. Practicing Strengths-Based Care (SBC) requires that the nurse be aware of her own strengths, vulnerabilities, and weaknesses. This awareness extends to an understanding of how her behavior affects the person and family, and how their behavior affects her responses. This level of awareness is essential if the nurse is to be able to identify and develop strengths in another person. When nurses have a well-developed level of self-awareness, their nursing changes from a serendipitous, haphazard way of responding in a situation to one that is more mindful, thoughtful, conscious, and deliberate. In other words, the nurse has greater control over what she says and does and is aware of why she does what she does. This is an important part in the growth and development of a being a professional.

All therapeutic relationships require that the practitioner possess some degree of empathy and compassion. These are essential ingredients needed to help another human being, especially during his times of need. Empathy and compassion are starting points, but they are not enough. SBC requires that the nurse also have other essential qualities. These qualities have been grouped into four major categories of strengths:

1. Strengths of mindset
2. Strengths of knowledge and knowing
3. Strengths of relationship
4. Strengths of advocacy

CAVEAT

Although 11 strengths have been identified as necessary to practice SBC, keep in mind that these strengths are a basic list and should be considered a starting point.

Every nurse has many strengths. Some strengths are unique to their own personhood, and others will be developed over time. As a nurse learns, develops, and matures both personally and professionally, he will develop new capabilities of caring for another person. Furthermore, in the act of nursing, or while observing other skilled clinicians, the nurse will gain a deeper appreciation of his own qualities and the qualities involved in caring for another human being with skill, knowledge, dignity, and respect. These qualities will be added to the nurse's jewel box of strengths.

Before proceeding it is important to review the characteristics of strengths that I described in Chapter 4. These same characteristics that help to define a quality as a strength in a person obviously apply to a discussion of nurses' strengths. As you proceed through this chapter, consider the work of Nurse Catherine Gros with Marie and her mother, Linda.

Marie is a young woman in her 20s, pregnant with her second child. Marie has been diagnosed with bipolar disorder and schizophrenia and is hospitalized in a major mental health care institution. She smokes and takes drugs and is in an unstable relationship with the baby's father. After giving birth to her first child, Marie's first infant was taken from her by social welfare services and placed in foster care. Marie does not want to give up her second baby, the one she is now carrying. Catherine brings her own special qualities to the nurse–patient relationship, and it is these qualities, along with her values and strengths-based nursing orientation, that affect her work with Marie, Marie's mother, and the staff. Throughout this chapter, we return to Catherine and Marie to illustrate the different strengths that Catherine requires to nurse this family.

CATEGORIES AND SUBCATEGORIES OF NURSE STRENGTHS

I. Strengths of Mindset are the qualities that give rise to a set of attitudes, outlooks, philosophies, or values that affect one's way of behaving (*Oxford English Dictionary*). The specific subcategories of strengths in this category include

- Mindfulness
- Humility
- Open-mindedness
- Nonjudgmental attitudes (i.e., acceptance)

II. Strengths of Knowledge and Knowing are the qualities that are needed to acquire and use information. They give rise to new ideas and motivate the nurse to seek out new information about the person. The specific subcategories of strengths in this category include

- Curiosity
- Self-reflection

III. Strengths of Relationships are the qualities that are needed to connect with others and create and maintain a collaborative partnership. The specific subcategories of strengths in this category include

- Respect and trust
- Empathy
- Compassion and kindness

IV. Strengths of Advocacy are the qualities that are needed to protect, stand up for, and defend another person and family. The specific subcategories of strengths in this category include

- Courage
- Self-efficacy

CAVEAT

Also keep in mind that although each quality may be a separate strength, these strengths are highly interrelated and function interdependently. Think of the eleven strengths as forming a highly interconnected network. Many of the approaches to promote one particular strength will also help develop other strengths.

Strengths of Mindset

The term *mindset* relates to a certain way of thinking. A person's mindset is reflected in the attitudes and values that often affects a nurse's judgment and thinking and, consequently, his behaviors and actions. Mindset includes the specific strengths of mindfulness, humility, open-mindedness, and a nonjudgmental attitude.

Mindfulness

Mindfulness refers to a set of skills required to connect with patients and maintain caring relationships. It is a special type of awareness that involves paying attention to and becoming aware of and in tune with one's own physical, emotional, mental, spiritual, and cognitive (i.e., thinking) states in order to engage more fully with oneself and with others. Guy Armstrong, a meditation teacher, succinctly defined mindfulness as "knowing what you are experiencing while you are experiencing it" (cited in Germer, 2009).

Mindfulness requires that people take heed of what is going on around them rather than operating on automatic pilot. Thus, mindfulness, according to one of its founders, Jon Kabat-Zinn (1994), involves paying attention in a particular way "on purpose, in the present moment, and non-judgmentally."

Shapiro and his colleagues (Shapiro, Carlson, Astin, & Freedman, 2006), building on the work of Kabat-Zinn (1994), suggested that there are three components to mindfulness: (a) intention, (b) attention, and (c) attitude. This involves doing something on purpose, or with intention; paying attention to what one is doing; in a particular way, or with a mindful attitude. In short, it is about having a relationship with oneself (a self-relationship) so that one can better connect with and care for another person (Siegel, 2007).

Relationship to Strengths-Based Care: Mindfulness has been found to promote health and healing, improve well-being, reduce stress, treat depression, and help individuals find greater peace and harmony in their lives. Mindfulness is a necessary condition for the development of a therapeutic relationship between therapist/clinician and client. Wallin (2007), a psychotherapist, described the role mindfulness plays in creating the therapeutic relationship. His ideas apply equally well to the nurse-patient/client/family relationship. First, mindfulness enables a nurse to be more fully present in the moment and to be open to her patient rather than being physically present while at the same time being mentally elsewhere. Mindfulness is not letting oneself become distracted with something else. When a nurse is fully present, she is more likely to notice things that might otherwise have gone unnoticed. Second, mindfulness requires that the nurse be attuned to her own needs as well as to the needs of the person under her care. When nurses are attuned to and in tune with what they are experiencing, they are in a better position to separate out their own feelings from those of their patients. Third, mindfulness encourages acceptance. When people feel accepted, they are more likely to explore issues that are troubling them.

> Nurses are more likely to notice the person when they are fully present.

Approaches to promote mindfulness: Nurses can develop a set of skills to increase their own mindfulness. They can also use these skills to help patients become more mindful. These skills involve learning new techniques, and using them regularly until they become integrated into the nurse's way of thinking and her approach in practice. In other words, until they become *habits of the mind.*

There are two major approaches to develop mindfulness: (a) formal training and (b) informal training.

Formal path to mindfulness. The formal path requires special training in specific techniques designed to increase awareness of what is going on inside oneself and to become attuned to one's own bodily sensations, emotions and, to a lesser extent, thoughts. The most common techniques are meditation and yoga; both are designed to free the person from distractions by training the mind and body to focus on the here-and-now (Germer, 2009).

Informal path to mindfulness. The informal path involves performing simple exercises designed to increase awareness by helping focus on the here-and-now. They usually have three components: (a) stop, (b) observe, and (c) return (Germer, 2009).

1. *Stop* refers to stopping what you are doing in order to slow down and shift your attention to what is happening to you. Slowing down helps increase self-awareness
2. *Observe* what is happening by becoming a spectator–observer. This involves scanning your inner feelings, emotions, and sensations and then labeling them
3. *Return* to what is capturing your attention. Often, the mind wanders and changes focus

Jon Kabat-Zinn has developed a brief meditation to increase mindful awareness that can be viewed on YouTube as well as a series of mindfulness CDs and tapes (Kabat-Zinn, 2007; see, e.g., http://www.youtube.com/watch?v=xoLQ3qkh0w0 and http://www.youtube.com/watch?v=rSU8ftmmhmw).

Daniel Siegel, a psychiatrist and founder and director of the Mindsight Institute in Los Angeles, also has developed techniques to increase mindfulness. He has created an approach to improve mindfulness by training in his "wheel of awareness" (Siegel, 2010). Siegel's (2010) wheel of awareness includes becoming attuned to and tracking one's own sensations, observations, and concepts. Similar to any wheel, Siegel's wheel of awareness consists of a rim, spokes, and a hub. The rim contains the sensations, observations, and concepts; the spokes are the information gathered through a person's different sensory systems; and the hub filters, selects, and interprets the information (for a fuller discussion of these ideas, see the section titled "Clinical Grasp" in Chapter 7). Important here is the fact that any nurse can become attuned to her own internal experiences—that is, what is happening inside of herself—because what goes on inside the nurse affects how she reacts to and responds to particular experiences and, consequently, the actions she decides to take. Nurses need to continuously monitor their own internal bodily sensations and to be aware of how they are observing what is happening inside them and how their feelings or 'gut' reactions are influencing what information they are selecting to attend to and how the information is then being processed and interpreted. For example, in any given situation the nurse can stop and make note of her own bodily sensation, such as her breathing. She can ask herself, "Is my breathing normal, labored, rapid, shallow?" She can stop to observe the sensations she is having by becoming a "fly on the wall" and looking down on herself, asking "What am I experiencing, feeling at this moment in time?" The nurse can also increase her awareness by making sense of the experience, by getting in touch with what it all means, and by considering the salience of the information she is taking in by asking herself— "Why did I just do what I did?" What is important here is that nurses can and should train to track their own internal world and bodily sensation. Daniel Siegel refers to this as *internal education* and as the basis of mindsight training. "Mindsight" is a term he coined to describe the human capacity to perceive the inner workings of one's own mind in order to be more sensitive and responsive to another person.

Daniel Siegel offers web-based video lectures in mindsight training for the professional and the general public. His courses are available 24/7. (www.MindsightInstitute.com).

Humility

Humility is characterized by an accurate understanding of one's own unique qualities as well as one's own limitations (Tangney, 2002). It involves knowing what one knows and, just as important, what one does not know. Tangney (2002) identified humility's key features:

- An accurate (not underestimated or overestimated) sense of one's abilities and achievements
- The ability to acknowledge one's mistakes, imperfections, gaps in knowledge, and limitations
- An openness to new ideas, contradictory information, and advice
- The ability to keep one's abilities and accomplishments in perspective
- A relatively low focus on the self
- An appreciation for another person's contribution

Humility is the opposite of *arrogance*, the belief that one is better than another person. Arrogance serves to distance one person from another person from whom one can learn. In contrast, humility serves to connect one person to another (Templeton, 1997). Nurse Catherine Gros explained the attitude that underlies her approach to working with patients and their families: *"I have to enter into their world in order to believe it and be a learner. If you're the expert who knows what's best for [the patient and family], it may be insignificant. Ultimately, it's not going to affect you. But if you see them as a human being in all their complexity, in all their resiliency, [you] can learn from that, and people always amaze me. And it is very genuine. Who am I to tell this family what to do who has navigated this whole situation and [has] survived until now, and I'm now stepping in and telling them what they have to do?"*

Because of Catherine's humility, she often begins an encounter with the person and family by saying, *"I'm here to learn from you. This is really a difficult situation right now. I'm here. Tell me about that. What's going on for you, and how can I best help you?"* This was Catherine's mindset in her work with Marie and Marie's mother, Linda.

Relationship to Strengths-Based Care: Humility opens the nurse to learning from the person and others. Humble nurses know that they have expertise in some areas, yet they do not assume they are experts in what others need and aspire to (Barry & Gordon, 2009).

Humility is required for collaborative partnership. One of the core features of a collaborative partnership is the sharing of power (Gottlieb & Feeley, 2006), and this requires humility on the part of the nurse. An arrogant person enjoys having power and exercising that power over another person. An arrogant person communicates a "know-it-all" attitude and does not listen to others, in particular to patients. Dr. Richard, a professor of physiotherapy, was recuperating from back and prostate surgery in a rehabilitation facility. In Exhibit 5.1, he recounted an encounter he had with Dr. Lotus, who showed both arrogance and ignorance, and describes the distress this physician caused him.

On the other hand, a nurse who values collaborative partnership is aware of the inherent power in his position but does everything to share that power with the patient. His satisfaction comes not from the power exercised over another but from creating the conditions that helps other people feel empowered to take charge of their own lives and health care decisions.

Approaches for promoting humility: Humility is a quality that one can learn in various ways, including developing greater self-awareness, seeking out supportive

EXHIBIT 5.1

Personal experience *Professor Sam Richard*[a]*: Psychologically Harmed by an Ignorant and Arrogant Physician*

Sam Richard, a university professor in physiotherapy, was diagnosed with late stage prostate cancer. Before surgery, he decided to take a road trip, when his back "went out." His back pain never resolved itself and continued to deteriorate. His neurologist advised that he have an emergency disectomy to relieve the compression on his L-4 nerve, just 10 days before the scheduled prostatectomy. There were some complications following the disectomy, surgery, and the prostatectomy operation was lengthier than expected. This lengthy surgery further irritated the root nerve, leaving Sam weak and unable to walk. He required intensive physical and occupational therapies. He was transferred to a rehabilitation hospital. On the second day of his arrival, he was assigned a physician, Dr. Elizabeth Lotus. Dr. Lotus introduced herself and began by saying "Mr. Richard, I see you have prostate cancer with metastases to your spine," whereupon Sam, somewhat taken aback, corrected her: "These are two comorbid conditions, that unfortunately occurred almost at the same time." The following week, Dr. Lotus, during her weekly rounds, visited Sam with the news that he had a slightly elevated liver enzyme level. Without asking any questions as to possible explanations, she asked him, "Have you been worked up for metastases yet?" When she left the room, Sam was upset and and thought, "How dare she break down my defenses!" He decided to discuss the matter with her. He called Dr. Lotus in and introduced himself as both a patient and a fellow health care professional. He explained that, as a health care professional, using the word *metastases* was inappropriate particularly when the patient is not using it. *Metastases* is a loaded word and could increase a patient's distress. Dr. Lotus not only ignored what Sam was saying but defended her actions as being appropriate. Sam tried to explain that, as a patient, he felt vulnerable, and he reminded her that the first rule that doctors and all health care professionals were obliged to follow was to cause their patients "no harm." At this point, Dr. Lotus got up and abruptly left. Sam lodged a formal complaint and later explained to the hospital administrators that there was no place in the health care system for clinicians who are both ignorant and arrogant: ignorant when physicians—or, for that matter, any health care professionals—fail to read a patient's chart and acquaint themselves with the patient's history, and arrogant when the health care professionals fail to listen to what the patient is telling them.

[a]A true story. The professor and doctor names are changed to protect anonymity.

relationships and environments, providing physical care to a person, and finding a role model to observe.

Develop greater self-awareness. Nurses must gain deeper insights into their own strengths. Arrogance is fostered when one person exercises power over another and takes advantage of the other person, particularly when that other person is vulnerable, insecure, or has a low sense of self-worth. The need to exercise power is often a response to one's own feelings of insecurity or inferiority. Nurses need to understand the relationship between arrogance, insecurity, and self-worth. Thus, they need to attend to their own feelings of insecurity and self-worth by recognizing their unique strengths and limitations. When nurses acknowledge, accept, and embrace their own strengths as well as their limitations, they then can be more open to others.

Seek out supportive relationships and environments. Humility is fostered when a person feels safe and secure. Support from family, friend, and colleagues, particularly when a person feels stressed or is functioning under stressful conditions, will help alleviate anxiety and feelings of insecurity.

Give physical care. When nurses provide physical care, they often engage in acts of humility because patients entrust them with their bodies. Nurses need to become mindful of how bodily care is one of the unique aspects of their profession. Being connected to patients and ministering to their bodily needs can transform the nurse and, in the process, the nurse–patient relationship. One nurse who provided foot care to her patient was motivated to undertake a study of humility and its practice in nursing when giving physical care. This study is described in Exhibit 5.2.

Find a role model to observe. Another strategy that helps to develop humility is to observe a person who shows humility and who can serve as a role model (Kachorek et al., 2004). Often, the most accomplished people are the most modest and humble. Humble people accept both positive and negative feedback calmly, without overreacting. They tend not to interpret negative feedback as an attack on their own personhood but rather as helpful information.

A good way to understand this strength is to observe two individuals, one you consider humble and the other you consider arrogant, or to observe two events in which you believed a person behaved arrogantly and in another in which a person behaved with humility. You can also describe an incident involving yourself in which you believed you behaved arrogantly and another incident in which you showed humility (see Exhibit 5.3).

Open-mindedness

Open-mindedness is the willingness to actively seek out different ideas, to be open to diverse opinions, and to entertain different beliefs. It involves the ability to revise one's ideas and responses in light of different evidence (Peterson & Seligman, 2004b). It also involves being able to appreciate another's perspective and experiences.

Relationship to Strengths-Based Care: Open-mindedness is a prerequisite strength for entertaining and appreciating differences. It allows a nurse to more readily accept another person's way of being and doing and to see beyond the problem, to look for opportunities, possibilities, and potential solutions. Most significantly, open-mindedness promotes "good thinking," because it prevents snap judgments, premature closure, and drawing conclusions based on faulty assumptions, all of which can lead to poor clinical judgments and decisions (Benner et al., 2011).

Approaches for promoting open-mindedness: There are several way to promote open-mindedness.

Attentive listening through presence: Nurses develop open-mindedness when they learn how to listen to another person's perspective and opinions. Attentive or real

EXHIBIT 5.2

Empirical study *Humility and Its Practice in Nursing*

The Problem
To determine how important an act of humility is in helping nurses to connect with their patients.

The Issues
Symbolically, washing feet is an act of humility. Following the author's personal experience of transformation as a result of washing the feet of a terminally ill patient for whom she was caring, she undertook an exploratory study to investigate nurses' experience of washing patients' feet.

The Study
Seven postregistration student nurses (five women and two men) participated in this descriptive study by washing the feet of as many patients as they could over a defined period of time. They were then interviewed about the experience. The transcribed interviews were analyzed using the heuristic inquiry approach. (Heuristic inquiry is a way of discerning personal involvement in an activity).

The Findings
The results suggest that an intimate act of humility—in this case, washing another person's feet—can be both positive and participatory. During the act of washing their patient's feet, nurses reported feelings of happiness, relaxation, and lightness. They felt that while performing this act they were able to connect with their patients in a very special way. This special connection was reflected in their choice of words they used to describe the effect this intimate bodily act had on themselves and the responses it called forth in their patients. Their choice of language to describe the experience is similar to language used to describe humility.

The Bottom Line
Washing another's person feet is an intimate act and can help a nurse get in touch with feelings of humility. Humility is an important emotion for one person to connect in a meaningful way to another person.

Source: Adapted from de Vries (2004).

listening, rather than pseudolistening, occurs when a nurse is fully present to hear what the person says and when the nurse quiets her own personal internal dialogue (Dossey, 1995). In other words, the nurse listens attentively to what the person has to say rather than simply waiting for the person to stop talking so that she can express what is on her mind. To do this, nurses must leave their own thoughts and preoccupations aside and be fully present. This form of listening and presence is known as *being in the moment* or *mindful* (for a fuller discussion of authentic presence and attentive listening, see Chapter 8).

EXHIBIT 5.3

Exercise *Comparing Arrogance and Humility*

Reflect and Connect Instructions:

1. Select a person who you observed behaving arrogantly in a particular event and one who you thought behaved with humility. The person can be a friend, student, professor, colleague, clinician. You can also think of an event in which you behaved arrogantly and one in which you behaved with humility
2. Describe the specific following behaviors:

Behaviors	Arrogance	Humility
Body language		
Communication style (e.g., listening, talking)		
Giving information		
Responses to feedback		
Other		

3. Compare and contrast the two approaches.
4. What was the other person's responses?
5. If there were other individuals present, how did they respond?
6. If you described your own behavior, consider how you felt during the event and how you felt about yourself after the incident.

Presence can take three forms: (a) physical, (b) psychological, and (c) therapeutic (McKivergin, & Daubenmire, 1994). They are described in more detail in Table 5.1.

1. *Physical presence* involves "being there" for the person during the acts of giving body-to-body care. This happens when the nurse intervenes or provides care to the person, including routine care
2. *Psychological presence* is the nurse's "being with" the person. On this level, the nurse makes an emotional and mental connection with the patient and family using her interpersonal skills of empathetic communication. The nurse creates a milieu in which the person feels that the nurse can meet her needs for help, comfort, and support
3. *Therapeutic presence* is when the nurse connects to the whole person. This occurs when the nurse involves the patient in such activities as mediation and imagery.

Nonjudgmental attitude (acceptance)

Nonjudgmental means that a person shows tolerance for another person's beliefs, values, behavior, or perspective, by not condemning or being critical. Nurses have their own set of beliefs and values that may or may not differ from those of the person they

TABLE 5.1

Levels of therapeutic presence

Level of Interaction	Type of Contact	Skills
Physical presence	Body to body	Seeing, hearing, being there when giving physical routine care
Psychological presence	Mind to mind	Communicating, real listening, empathy, being nonjudgmental
Therapeutic presence	Spirit to spirit	Centering, meditating, connecting, using imagery

Source: Adapted from McKivergin and Daubenmire (1994).

are nursing. However, to be nonjudgmental, the nurse needs to try to understand the situation from the person's perspective (Gottlieb & Feeley, 2006).

Relationship to Strengths-Based Care: SBC is predicated on the belief that people hold different beliefs, engage in different lifestyles, and make different choices. Nurses may not agree with some of the person and family's beliefs, or subscribe to some of their lifestyle practices, but what nurses need to learn is how to respect other people's choices, particularly when they differ from their own. Nurse Monica Gallagher learned about what was involved in being nonjudgmental while caring for an infant who was dying from a rare genetic disorder. While this infant was dying, the mother, Mrs. Hallandale, discovered that she was pregnant and decided to abort this pregnancy because the fetus had tested positive for the same genetic disorder. In spite of their genetic history, Mr. and Mrs. Hallandale continued to try to have a family. After a few years, Mrs. Hallandale delivered twins, only to be told after the twins' birth that one of the infants also carried the fatal gene. The Hallandales decided to care for their second dying infant at home, going against what Monica believed to be the right decision.

Monica shared her beliefs about judging others: *"From this family, I learned not to be the parents. I learned to allow the family to make choices for their child regardless of whether I thought that I wouldn't do the same thing if I were in their shoes. This was probably the first family that I didn't really judge, but supported them in whatever decision that they made. Maybe I wouldn't have taken all of their choices the parents made, or even half of them. I really struggled and worked very, very hard at not being the family for this child and not thinking that I had to be the family."*

Moreover, in order to gain the person's trust, the nurse needs to see the person for who he is and find some common ground in order to connect. As Nurse Christina Rosmus explained, *"It's about meeting people where they are. It's about being nonjudgmental, knowing that everyone has something going for themselves, beginning with what they bring. It's about always looking beyond and seeing their positives even when overwhelmed by problems and deficits."*

Approaches for promoting nonjudgmental attitudes: Ignorance is the fuel that creates a judgmental and critical attitude. Often, individuals make assumptions about a person on the basis of hearsay and faulty or incomplete information. Impressions are taken as facts rather than derived from information and learning. Consider how the hijab, the head covering worn by some Muslim women, is viewed in different societies.

In some societies, the hijab is an indicator of female modesty and reverence, whereas in others it is viewed as a symbol of female subjugation and inferiority. The nurse's culture and the society in which she lives may color her views.

The following techniques can promote a nonjudgmental attitude.

Refrain from giving advice; listen instead. One important technique is to listen to people as they sort out their thoughts and feelings about a situation or when they are trying to decide on a course of action that is best for them. They have to live with their decision. Nurse Monica Gallagher discovered that the best thing she can do is to not give her opinion but to be present and listen as parents struggle to make decisions that is right for them: "*Give no advice, like none, ever. Again, [this is] something you learn not to do, you don't give advice. Just listen, let them talk, close the door, encourage them to close the door so they are not [distracted by the] environment—close the door and just sit and listen.*"

Look for additional information. Learning to be nonjudgmental is about withholding judgment. A nurse can develop a nonjudgmental attitude by not rushing to premature conclusions but instead looking for evidence that supports or refutes the person's and family's choices. This evidence is often found through listening for consistency as well as inconsistency in a person's story, seeking out different opinions, and examining the basis on which their opinions have been formed. A nonjudgmental attitude can also be fostered by reading widely and becoming better informed.

Get in touch with your feelings. A nurse may need to become more self-aware by getting in touch with her own thoughts, feelings, and reactions. She can ask herself, "What am I feeling?" She may further examine her feelings by asking herself, "Why am I reacting in this way?" and "Does this situation or person feel familiar?" Often, a patient triggers a memory and a reaction in the nurse that comes from her past. In these cases, the nurse can ask herself, "Does this person remind me of somebody I know or knew?" For example, the nurse may react negatively to a patient because that patient reminds her of her own sister with whom she has had a difficult relationship. There also may be certain patients or clients for whom the nurse has difficulty providing care. A nurse who has been abused in the past may have difficulty caring for abusive, bullying patients, or the nurse whose brother recently died from ALS may have difficulty caring for patients with multiple sclerosis because just watching them struggle to perform activities of daily living is just too painful a reminder of his own brother's suffering.

Learn how to mask surprise, alarm, or shock. Nurses need to first connect to their own emotions and responses so they can understand which situations upset them and which ones evoke feelings of anger, guilt, or shame. By linking the situations to their own emotional responses, nurses can increase their self-awareness and better prepare themselves to recognize situations that they find shocking or upsetting. In this way, a nurse can be prepared to better deal with such situations when the need arises in the future. Nurses usually have difficulties when the patient's problem concerns issues or involves behavior that the nurse finds to be foreign, repulsive, or goes counter to their own lifestyle choices, beliefs, and values. An inexperienced nurse may react with shock and surprise. With experience and increased exposure to different situations, nurses can learn, to mask surprise and adopt a more neutral stance when patients and families discuss intimate or shocking details about their lives.

Do not criticize, scold, or admonish. When people feel vulnerable, they may be overly sensitive to any critical remarks. Criticism is disempowering. Nurses need to be aware not only of the message they send but also of how they deliver the message. Nurses must think first about what they want to say, choose their words carefully, and share their thoughts and feelings only when they feel calm. They should ask themselves, "How do I communicate to the person that I accept them for who they are?"

Take the time to get to know the patient as a person. Judgments are often made in haste. A nurse is more likely to be nonjudgmental when he takes the time to get to know the person and family. There is a tendency to focus on differences between the nurse and the person rather than on what they have in common—their similarities. When the nurse chooses to look for commonalities, he will more likely be able to identify with the person and family. Commonalities bind, whereas differences divide (Caplan, 2008).

Nurse Amy Nyland described taking care of Ray, a young man who was readmitted to the hospital for epilepsy because he had refused to take his medication and to follow the prescribed medical treatment. The doctors and nurses were frustrated with him; in fact, they were angry at what they perceived to be a preventable situation. They considered his actions to be juvenile, an almost adolescent form of rebellion. Amy withheld judgment.

"When I first met Ray, I introduced myself, and I told him 'I'll be with you today, and if there's anything at all, I can be free today, please don't hesitate to call me.' I was just trying to say 'How are you doing?', and he said. 'Fine, fine.' A little bit later I came back and sat down and said, 'May I sit down?' We were just talking and in a very casual way when I said 'This must be really hard time for you' as [the medical team] were investigating, trying to figure out what was going on. And I asked, 'Can you tell me the story of the last couple of weeks?' And he did. I just listened and he told me about not taking his medication. I mentioned that a friend of mine had been in a similar situation and used to periodically stop and I said, 'Do you ever do this?' I said in my friend's case she was just fed up, and Ray nodded. [I told him that] she said 'I go on strike,' and then he sort of smiled. So he started talking about that, about why he chose not to do what he knew he was supposed to do."

Amy continued that she felt it was important to listen to Ray in order to understand why he made the choices he did. If Amy had judged Ray out of hand, like most of the other staff, she would never have understood why Ray made the decision not to comply with his medical regimen. Moreover, Amy now had an opportunity to explore with Ray what his condition meant to him, how he lived with it, what role epilepsy played in his life, and how his condition defined him.

Strengths of Knowledge and Knowing

The second group of strengths that are needed to practice SBC include the acquisition and use of information from formal sources (e.g., books, monographs, articles, the Internet) and from experience. Nurses need "to acquire habits, disposition, discernment, skills, and emotional responses of excellent practice" (Benner, 2003, p. 374). SBC requires that nurses develop not only knowledge but also learn a way of knowing.

Knowledge consists of concepts, theories, and ideas about an identified area of information, whereas *knowing* can be viewed as an individual's perception of the complexities of a particular situation and draws on one's inner knowledge resources that have been garnered through experience in living (Benoleil, 1987). Both are required to nurse. Knowledge and knowing require the following specific strengths:

- Curiosity
- Self-reflection

Curiosity

Curiosity refers to a person's innate or intrinsic desire for experience and knowledge (Kashdan, 2004). It is a strength that individuals possess in varying degrees. Curiosity is the capacity that enables an individual to adapt to changing conditions. It is through the strength of curiosity that people come to know themselves, their environments, and how to interact with and relate to others. Knowing is an essential quality in caring (Mayeroff, 1971). It is only when the nurse comes to understand and truly know a person that the nurse can be responsive and respond appropriately.

Curiosity is involved in acquiring both general and specific forms of knowledge. *General knowledge* refers to information about universal responses, whereas *specific knowledge* relates to the particulars about a person—that patient, that family, that community, and the like. For example, when the person cuts himself, there is a general inflammatory response (general knowledge); however, that person's inflammatory response is affected by the nature of the wound, the microorganism to which he was exposed, his age, the presence of other infections, and so forth (specific knowledge). General knowledge derives from a priori knowledge, which is known through scientific inquiry or is learned from books and other sources of information. Specific knowledge about the person is developed through exploration, experimentation, and discovery with the person or with those individuals who know her well.

Relationship to Strengths-Based Care: Curiosity enables a nurse to become more involved with the person and their situation, which in turn leads to greater discoveries and a deeper understanding of the person and his family. It is by delving deeper into a situation, and thus uncovering and making connections, that a nurse develops a greater appreciation and understanding of the complexities of the person's and family's situation.

Consider the case of Nurse Althea McBean, whose curiosity led her to understand her patient, Mr. Roberts, in a totally different light. Mr. Roberts had come to the emergency department experiencing what appeared to be symptoms of a heart attack.

Althea described the situation: *"He was very agitated and was refusing all medical attention, and he said, 'I want to get out of here. I've got to get home, I got to get out.' The other nurses had labeled him as 'uncooperative' and 'refusing all medical attention.' I approached him and said, 'Tell me what happened.' In describing his story, I learned that he was a dog breeder. He bred very vicious dogs for the police force. He lived alone, and he bred these dogs in his yard. He lived out in the country and felt he was the only one the dogs would allow near them. So he was very agitated because he wanted to get back to his dogs. He wanted to go to a hospital closer to his home where at least he could do some sort of arranging about attending to his dogs. I knew I needed to help him to bring his anxiety down. So I said to him, 'Okay, how are we going to address this situation? Now that we know what is causing your anxiety, how we can we resolve what is bothering you right now?' We considered all the options he could use to get help with his dogs and still receive treatment at the hospital. He turned and said to me, 'I am feeling better already.' He was visibly calmer."*

Althea got the story because she was curious. She refrained from labeling Mr. Robert's behavior and wanted to know why he was refusing medical attention.

When the nurse lacks curiosity, she may rely on a priori overgeneralizations and faulty assumptions to make decisions. She may fixate on a problem without understanding the problem fully. In both cases, this way of thinking often is responsible for poor judgment and tunnel vision.

Approaches for promoting curiosity: When nurses lack curiosity they run the risk of finding themselves bored and practicing nursing in a prescriptive way. It is a one-size-fits-all type of nursing where there is a lack of interest in the patients and the work becomes routine. It is in these situations that a nurse is most likely to perceive and treat the person and problem as one and the same. In other words, the patient is defined as the disease—The pancreatic cancer in Room 230. There are a number of techniques that nurses can use to develop curiosity.

Increase awareness of what is known and what is not known. When nurses are aware of what they know and what they do not know, they are in a better position to determine where to seek information. It is in the process of exploring that the nurse's interest may be piqued and may motivate her to want to learn more.

Create more open-ended learning experiences. Curiosity is fostered in environments that encourage exploration and discovery. When learning is based on interest and curiosity, exploration usually follows. Think of the nurse who is interested in yoga. She is more likely to learn the name of the different muscle groups involved in different yoga positions. An interest in yoga may stimulate her to learn more about the physics governing the leverage of muscles and bones and then to apply this knowledge to body alignment and lifting techniques when she is caring for patients. Nurses can develop curiosity when they see the relevance of knowing specific information and acquiring skills to meet personal and professional goals.

Learn to ask "why" questions. A basic need of all human beings is to understand and explain why things happen. It is this need to discover the causes of actions—that is, why things are the way they are—that fuels curiosity (Schuman, 2002). Children are consistently asking "why" questions. Nurses need to rediscover their innate curiosity and learn how to ask themselves "why" questions about their patients. "I wonder *why* Mrs. Brown won't take her medication?" "*Why* does Amy continue to engage in unprotected sex despite having had two unplanned pregnancies?"

Frame the situation as part of an unfolding story. Everybody's life is an unfolding story. People love to listen to stories because stories capture their imagination and tell about the human condition. In listening to stories, people learn something about themselves and their fellow men and women. Stories are more interesting than isolated facts. When isolated facts are placed in context and become joined in creating a story, they take on different meanings and significance. Begin to think in terms of stories. Every person and family that a nurse meets has a story to tell, a narrative about themselves and their lives that, when listened to, will often fascinate.

Now let's return to Catherine, the nurse who cares for Marie, the young pregnant woman diagnosed with bipolar disorder and schizophrenia, and her mother, Linda. Catherine described her interest in getting to know this family.

"I was really drawn to this family and just very curious about them. And I liked them. I enjoyed the time I spent with both the daughter and the mother, and so our interactions were very positive. And through those interactions I got a sense of what their goals were and where they were coming from. That's what we want to find out in any situation 'What's this like for you? What do you want? What's important to you?'"

By talking and listening to Marie and Linda, Catherine discovered just how important the pregnancy was to Marie and how concerned Linda was for her daughter's well-being: *"Marie was very excited about her pregnancy, and Linda, the grandmother, while worried, was clearly invested in this pregnancy and wanted things to work out well. So they had goals, both as individuals and as a family, around this pregnancy. Linda would tell me things like 'This is so bad for Marie. You know, her cousin was pregnant, and everybody was celebrating, and she had a baby shower, and it was a time of great joy, and Marie is so alone in this. Everybody thinks it's a terrible problem and everybody is ignoring it. They're not talking to her about it. It's a huge problem for everybody, and she must feel so alone in this and there's no one really to share her joy.' I could see that Linda was trying to share her joy. Here's a normal developmental life event that is usually celebrated in society but because you have a mental illness, all of a sudden, it becomes a problem".*

Catherine's curiosity helped her uncover some of the many dimensions of Marie's and Linda's lives and the family situation that was having an effect on them.

Self-Reflection

Self-reflection is the capacity to examine critically one's own thoughts, emotions, and actions as well as those of another person (Atkins & Murphy, 1993). It is a mode of operating that leads to greater self-awareness and, in turn, results in more deliberate, intentional, and purposeful ways of behaving both at the personal and professional levels. It is one of the most important ways that nurses can learn from their experiences to develop their own unique style of practice (Benner et al., 2011; Jasper, 2003). Professional practice is predicated on self-awareness and reflection and enable practitioners to make sense of practice, critically examine their practice, know their own limitations, make connections, and develop important insights that then become their guideposts to direct their future actions.

Self-reflection should occur before, during, and after an encounter with a patient. When nurses reflect before an encounter, they are trying to anticipate what could occur so they can be prepared to respond to any number of possible scenarios. When nurses reflect during an encounter, they are "thinking in action," and this thinking forms the basis for moment-to moment clinical decisions (Benner et al., 2011). Nurses also need to develop the habit of "reflecting-on-action," that is, reviewing and thinking after an encounter, thinking about what transpired, what went well, and what could have

> Professional practice requires the nurse to develop self-awareness, become reflexive, and practice mindfulness. When nurses critically examine their own practice, they develop greater self-awareness and awareness of others, can identify repeated patterns of behavior, and gain important insights to guide future nursing actions.

been done differently to make things better. Self-reflection contributes to flexibility of thinking and maximizes learning from experiences.

Relationship to Strengths-Based Care: Self-reflection is an important *habit of the mind*. It is an essential quality that nurses need to develop in order to practice SBC. Research has shown that reflection in and on practice is important to accomplish the following:

- Develop flexibility in responding to different situations with different persons and to tailor care to the person's and family's uniqueness (Schon, 1983)
- Increase awareness of one's own limitations and biases that may likely interfere with being open to learning about others (Jasper, 2003)
- Monitor the effectiveness of care and make the necessary changes and adjustments (Greenwood, 1998)
- Recognize negative feelings that might interfere with the nurse–patient relationship (McQueen, 2000)

Approaches for promoting self-reflection: Self-reflection is a deliberate act of thinking about the present situation or what has happened or will happen. There are many ways to develop self-reflective thinking skills; several are suggested below.

Engage in clinical discussion with colleagues. One of the most important ways to encourage self-reflection is to engage in clinical discussions with colleagues and peers. This can be accomplished through structured group discussion or a semistructured clinical conference with a person who serves as a resource. This person can be somebody who has experience and expertise; who can raise questions; give information; and identify what is salient, why it is salient, and the like. In both types of discussion forums members take turns presenting a clinical case from their practice. The process of preparing for a case presentation requires that the nurse reflect on the patient and the clinical situation, what he has observed, what knowledge he used to base his decisions and the actions he took. The nurse needs to provide the rationale for why he did what he did on the basis of the evidence. Evidence comes from empirical studies, personal knowledge, and prior experience with that particular patient and family or a similar group of patients, clients, and families. It is in the process of reconstructing the events and telling the "story" that the nurse has an opportunity to reflect on his own feelings and thoughts in response to what the person said or did. The nurse may use a reflective process form of recording to help him reconstruct the events that affected his responses (see Table 5.2). Discussing, examining, analyzing, questioning, and putting forth different interpretations are several ways to develop reflective skills.

Develop your own set of self-reflective questions. Nurses who are reflective practitioners have developed a way of thinking that becomes a habit of the mind—their way of being, thinking, and, consequently, their way of practicing. They have several questions that they keep in the back of their mind that they ask of themselves

---

TABLE 5.2

Self-reflective process recording

What the person or family said or did	What the nurse felt and thought	What the nurse said or did

routinely. All nurses need to develop their own set of reflective questions that they ask themselves before, during, and after every encounter. Dr. Judith Ritchie, a well-known Canadian nurse clinician and scholar, has developed her own set of self-reflection questions that she uses routinely with patients and has taught to countless of students and front-line nurses (see Table 5.3).

Follow a structured framework of self-reflection. Several structured frameworks are available to help nurses develop self-reflection skills. The most straightforward of these was developed by Borton (1970). It asks the practitioner to describe the incident or situation, analyze or interpret the incident in light of a theory, accepted knowledge or prior experience, and consider different alternatives and actions to deal with the incident or situation. Nurses are required to ask themselves three types of questions: (a) "What?" questions, which are aimed at describing the incident; (b) "So what?" questions, which help one analyze and interpret what went on; and (c) "Now what?" questions, which stimulate one to think of other possible actions (see Figure 5.1 for an expanded version of Borton's developmental framework of self-reflection; Rolfe, Freshwater, & Jasper, 2001). The following are examples of these questions:

- **"What?" questions, such as "What is happening?" and "What was I doing?"** These help the nurse to describe the experience, incident, or situation in detail
- **"So what?" questions, such as "So what more do I need to know in order to understand the situation?" and "So what could I have done that was different?"** These help the nurse analyze and interpret what went on. The nurse needs to draw on different sources of accepted knowledge, theory, and prior experience to help her make sense of this particular incident or situation
- **"Now what?" questions, such as "Now what do I do to make things better?" "Now what might be the consequences of this action?"** These help the nurse consider and evaluate other alternatives and actions in a thoughtful and deliberate manner

---

TABLE 5.3

Dr. Judith Ritchie's self-reflective questions

- What is going on here?
- Is this similar to something that I have seen before, or is this familiar—and, if so, what is it that is familiar?
- Have I seen or read about this before?
- How does this compare to *x*, and what's new?
- What more do I need to know?
- How do I know that I know?
- What do I need to do? Why?
- So what? What does this mean for the person? For the family? For organizing nursing on the unit (or in the organization)? For nursing?

Source: Dr. Judith Ritchie, Associate Director Nursing Research, McGill University Health Center, Montreal, Canada and Professor, School of Nursing, McGill University, Montreal, Canada.

Reflective writing: Use of field notes, a journal, or critical incident report. Another useful way to develop reflective thinking skills is through *reflective writing.* Reflective writing differs from other forms of writing in that its purpose is to develop deeper insights from experiences. It can also help a person order thoughts and feelings, prioritize, and sort out the salient from the less salient and the important from the less important.

The writing of *field notes* in the form of journaling, an activity that instructors ask of students, has been an invaluable tool for helping students develop their critical thinking skills. A journal has been found to be an important tool for organizing one's thoughts and ideas, getting in touch with one's feelings, increasing self-awareness, developing insights, and considering alternative ways of behaving. *Process recordings* help nurses reconstruct a critical incident in their practice. A critical incident can be a mortifying moment or an incident that went particularly well. The object of all three techniques in self-reflection (i.e., reflective writing, field notes, and process recordings)

FIGURE 5.1

A framework for reflexive practice.

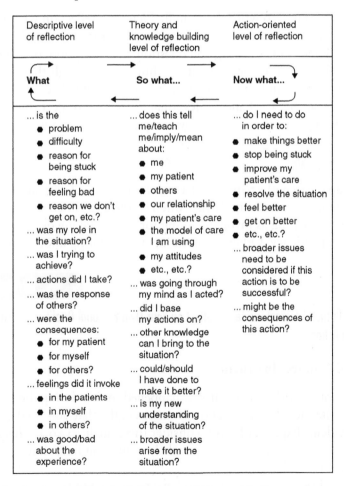

Source: Reprinted with permission from Rolfe, Freshwater, & Jasper, (2001).

is to understand, analyze, and learn from an event to improve practice. The important point here is that, in the act of writing, a nurse sets aside "thinking" time to reflect on his own behavior in practice. The following are a number of suggestions that help in reflective writing:

- Write in the first person. Use "I." This helps you to take ownership of the incident and become a participant rather than an observer
- Avoid using "They should have" statements. Once the incident has occurred, you can't change it and you can't change another's behavior (Jasper, 2003)
- Every entry should describe the incident, have an analysis or "reflection-of-what-transpired" section, and a space to raise and record questions in need of further exploration
- Set aside time specially devoted to writing. Get into the habit of writing, even if just for a few minutes every day or every other day. This will allow you to have a written record of your own development and learning
- Take time to review what you have written that day, or over the course of a week, a month, a year. Examine these writings in light of your educational objectives and reset your directions accordingly

Now take a moment to write about an incident and reflect on what made it a critical event. A critical incident is an event or situation that was significant. It affected you in some way such as by making you question an assumption, or call into question or reaffirm a belief, attitude, or value. It was important enough that it caused you to stop, question, reflect, and think about it. It is an incident that could have a significant impact on your personal and professional learning. Connect this incident to the strengths you brought to the situation, by completing Exhibit 5.4.

Strengths of Relationships

The third group of strengths required of a nurse is to connect with another person and create a collaborative partnership. Nurses often connect to patients through acts of caring. Some consider caring as involving doing for others, taking over, being the expert, and fostering dependency. Others view caring as promoting another person's growth

---

EXHIBIT 5.4

Reflect and Connect Critical Incident: Reflect on Your Own Personal Qualities (Strengths) and Link Them to Action

Reflect and Connect Instructions:

1. Write about a critical incident that happened to you during the past month.
2. Review the incident and identify your strengths that you used to deal with this incident. Explain why you consider these qualities your strengths.
3. In reflecting about how you responded, would you have done anything differently? If so, what?
4. What qualities would you need to have responded in this way?

through being with that person and creating the conditions in which the person can discover her own strengths and capacities (Mayeroff, 1971). This latter approach to caring is rooted in a deep respect for the separateness of another human being while at the same time fostering a connectedness that makes him feel safe and secure enough to open himself up to new possibilities for his own development and growth. It is this commitment to another person's health, recovery, and healing that is at the heart of SBC and requires that the nurse know how to connect with different types of people to form trusting relationships.

Many skills are involved in relationship building, but underlying these skills lie three essential strengths that a nurse must have or must develop:

- Respect and trust
- Empathy
- Compassion and loving kindness

Respect and Trust

The cornerstone of any relationship is respect, both for oneself and for the other person. Respect requires that one pays attention to oneself and to another's wants and needs. It also involves treating the person with deference, honor, and esteem (*Oxford English Dictionary*).

Respect allows a nurse to actively listen with an open, nonjudgmental mind; to accept differences in opinions and perspectives; to work out differences and find common ground; and to accept people for who they are rather than what the nurse would like them to be. Respect is communicated in the way the nurse meets the person's bodily needs. It is reflected in the tenderness with which the nurse touches and tends to the body (Vanier, 1998). Respect is also reflected in the way the nurse communicates trust in patients and their judgment. Respect and trust must be felt and communicated in ways that are authentic and genuinely heartfelt.

Nurse John Kayser told about Jane, a woman with whom he had worked for seven years to help her quit smoking. Together, they had tried every program, every trick in the book. Nothing seemed to work, until John encouraged Jane to join a group that put smoking cessation into the hands of God. During their work together, John learned that Jane was a religious person. They had finally hit on the right strategy. Jane finally gave up cigarettes. When I asked John why he hadn't given up on Jane sooner, he simply replied, "*She was a nice person.*" This answer did not satisfy me. When I asked John the question again, phrased in a somewhat different way—"*What did you see in Jane that made you want to continue to help her?*"—John replied, "*Her tenacity, her persistence. She kept coming back. How could I give up on her when she never gave up on herself?*"

Relationship to Strengths-Based Care: Respect is required to allow another person to grow. When a person feels respected, he is more likely to enter into dialogue, open up, and listen to another's opinion even when that opinion differs from his own. Respect incorporates elements such as being empathetic—providing autonomy, recognizing the person's individuality, and treating the person with dignity (Dickert & Kass, 2009).

Respect is an important prerequisite of trust. *Trust* is having faith and confidence in another person's decisions. Trust can be established only when there is mutual respect. Nurses show trust when they respect that patients will grow in their own way and in their own time. Trust means that the nurse allows the person to make mistakes and learn from them (Mayeroff, 1971). It is when the nurse trusts the person that the person comes to trust herself and her own judgment and develops confidence in the decisions she has made. This type of thinking and feeling, engendered by respect and trust, is at the heart of what is needed to become self-empowered.

Consider Nurse Lidia De Simone, who cared for Celeste, a single mother on welfare who was the sole caregiver of her severely disabled child. Lidia came to respect and admire Celeste, and it is this admiration that strengthened their relationship: *"What I respected was that she was caring for a very disabled child. She had . . . many opportunities to leave that child in the hospital but never did. Although Celeste did not live in poverty, she was very close to it. She lived in a basement apartment that was dark and dingy. She had no freedom, absolutely no freedom. She didn't have a lot of family support and not a heck of a lot of friends, because she didn't have the opportunity to go out and meet people. She was really stuck at home. What I respected about her was that, in these two rooms, in this very narrow, very abridged life, she was a full person. She was a whole person. She was a complete person. She wasn't critical—she wasn't angry. She had all the qualities you would want a human to have. She cared, she was interactive, she was alert, and yet her existence was in these two rooms."*

Approaches for promoting respect and trust: Respect is an attitude that is reflected in one's behavior. Respect permeates all aspects of one's being. There are a number of ways to develop respect.

Respect for oneself and trust in one's own judgment. Nurses are more likely to respect another person when they respect themselves. When nurses feel secure and comfortable with themselves, they are more likely to be open to others. Respect comes from acting out of conviction rather than behaving in ways that please others. Respect for oneself means having integrity; being honest, sincere, and genuine; and behaving in ways that are authentic (Sheldon, Davidson, & Pollard, 2004). Nurses are more likely to act out of conviction and with integrity when they behave in ways that are consistent with their values and beliefs. To do this, they need to get in touch with what is important to them and how they want to nurse.

Care about the person while caring for the person. Year after year, nurses continue to be the top ranking professional group most trusted by the public. In fact, a Gallup poll on honesty and ethics revealed that 84% of Americans rate nurses' honesty and ethical standards either high or very high (Gallup, 2008). This survey of trust applies to nurses as a group; however, individual nurses still need to gain the trust of individual patients. Patients are more likely to trust their nurse when they feel that their nurse cares *about* them while caring *for* them (de Raeve, 2002).

Trustworthiness comes from being cared for by a competent and skilled practitioner. Patients trust nurses who meet their physical and emotional needs based on knowledge and with skill. They also tend to trust nurses who treat them with respect and preserve their dignity. Nurses who take the time to get to know a person and family are more likely to earn their patients' respect and gain their trust.

Engage, don't be avoidant or distance yourself. Respect is communicated when the nurse is authentically present and fully engaged. There are many reasons why nurses may want to avoid a particular patient. Nurses need to get in touch with their own feelings so that they can manage situations and patients with whom they feel uncomfortable or even threatened. For example, if the nurse feels threatened by a person, she needs to assess how realistic is the threat. If the threat is real, then she needs to get the help she needs to nurse that person. If a nurse wants to avoid the person because she lacks knowledge and skills, then she needs to understand that she does not need to have all the answers immediately. What people often need from their nurse is simply their presence, not for somebody to "fix" their problems. Nurses have many opportunities to create a special connection with their patients when they follow them over time and weather the patient's crises with them.

Gentleness and respect for the human body. Nursing is one of the few professions that involve caring for the human body, tending to basic bodily functions, and giving physical care (e.g., bathing, backrubs, wound care, foot care). Nursing care involves coming into the person's personal and private space and dealing with situations that are potentially embarrassing (Wolf, 2009). Patients often find themselves in positions of dependency, relying on strangers to meet their most basic and intimate needs. They often feel frightened and compromised when they are at their most vulnerable, particularly when dealing with uncertainty: an unclear diagnosis, an unpredictable prognosis, or unknown disease trajectory. They all too often find themselves in strange environments such as hospitals, clinics, or intensive care units, that exacerbate their fears and insecurities. However, nurses can make patients feel comfortable both physically and emotionally in the following ways:

- By communicating respect for patients in the way nurses interact with them
- By protecting patients' privacy
- By preserving patients' dignity in the way nurses touch a patient's body and handle his bodily functions. A nurse who is embarrassed will often communicate that embarrassment, which could evoke feelings of shame in the patient

When the nurse preserves her patients' dignity, respects their privacy, and cares for their body with gentleness, then she conveys respect and engenders trust. Consider the case of Mrs. Norton, whose veins were very fragile because of repeated needle punctures. Her nurse, Cynthia Tulsa, recognized this and knew there was another nurse on the unit who was more skilled than she was at taking blood. Cynthia asked Mrs. Norton permission to ask the other nurse to take her blood. Mrs. Norton was very appreciative. She interpreted Cynthia's gesture as an act of kindness and caring. Cynthia was willing to put her own pride aside to minimize Mrs. Norton's pain.

Be truthful and reliable. The majority of health care professionals see their role as the professional who protects the person and family from harm. Many professionals believe their role is to shield people from bad news. Nurses need to find a balance between protecting the person while at the same time being transparent and truthful. Patients and families come to trust and depend on the nurse when the information they are given is truthful and reliable. This does not mean that nurses have to be blunt. They need to be gentle and responsive in how they give information and to be careful that the language they use communicates hope even when they are delivering bad news.

Trust is also established when a person knows what to expect. A nurse will gain the person's trust when he knows the nurse can be counted on. The little gestures often prove to be most significant. For example, if the nurse tells the patient that she will return in 20 minutes, and does so, the patient soon recognizes that the nurse is dependable. Conversely, nurses who do not follow through, who say one thing and do another, or cover up for a colleague, will in a very short period of time lose that person's confidence and with it his respect and trust.

Empathy

Empathy is recognized as the cornerstone, the most essential ingredient one must have in order to care for another person. Empathy is an essential element of compassion, caring, and respect. According to Carl Rogers (1992), founder of humanistic psychotherapy, empathy is the ability "to sense the client's world as if it were your own but without ever losing the 'as if' quality" (p. 29). The as-if quality is when the practitioner understands what the person is experiencing "as if" he, the practitioner, were experiencing it himself (Walsh, 2008). Empathy is relational. In other words, empathy involves knowing another person—her thoughts and feelings. This level of knowing can occur only within a trusting, mutually respectful relationship (Batson et al., 2002).

Relationship to Strengths-Based Care: Empathy bridges the divide between nurse and patient. It enables the nurse to gain some understanding into the patient's world and how he is experiencing it (Charon, 2001). This in turn helps the nurse gain insights into the person's strengths and weaknesses. Moreover, empathy plays an important role in a person's health and healing. Research has shown that when nurses show empathy toward patients, patients report less distress and decreased anxiety and report being more satisfied with the care they are receiving (Yu & Kirk, 2008).

Approaches for promoting empathy: Empathy is a strength that can be learned, improved, and refined through conscious effort and with practice (Walsh, 2008). The following techniques can help the nurse become more empathic.

Assume the posture of another person. Actors try to imitate the behavior, posture, and voice of the individuals they are portraying in order to understand who those individuals are and what might have motivated them to behave in the ways that they did. Nurses can use this strategy to help them understand what their patients may be experiencing. Thus, assuming the physical posture or mental attitude of another person by imitating them may help nurses appreciate what their patients may be feeling and experiencing. It is important to imagine how you would think and feel if you were in the other person's place. A more advanced form of imitation is *perspective taking*. Perspective taking is a capability that most children develop by the ages of four or five.

It requires that the person de-center from herself and try to imagine what it must be like for the other person by adopting that person's perspective. This technique can help raise nurses' awareness and sensitivity only when they begin to genuinely consider what the person is going through. Recently, a nurse colleague told me that, back in the 1980s, when she interviewed for a position as staff nurse in a large psychiatric facility, part of the hiring process was to spend five days on the unit as a patient. This part of the hiring process was to help prospective staff gain a deeper appreciation of the patients' hospital experience.

Nurses should never assume that they know what a person is experiencing. Only that person can describe her own experiences. Nurses need to avoid using such statements

One person can never completely imagine what another person is experiencing because each person feels and lives an experience in unique, individual ways.

as—"I know how you must be feeling." and "I know what you are going through." Instead, the nurse should phrase the question thus: "It is difficult to fully understand what you are going through. Please, tell me about what you what you are experiencing."

Compassion and Kindness

Compassion and kindness are fundamental ways of behaving toward another human being, in particular when dealing with another person's suffering. Compassion is a way of expressing one's own humanity (Post & McCullough, 2004) and is the foundation of kindness (Germer, 2009).

Compassion is the emotion evoked by the suffering of others and an acknowledged awareness of their suffering (Cassell, 2002). It is often accompanied by a desire to alleviate or at least mitigate suffering.

Compassion is a strength that allows one person to connect to other people to help ease their pain and suffering. Doing so requires knowledge of suffering. Suffering is a state of severe distress that threatens the integrity of the person.

Compassion and kindness are based on the belief that others, when in need of care and comfort, need to be treated gently. They also require that the nurse be able to identify to some degree with the sufferer in order to act in that person's best interest. It is when the nurse does not identify totally with the sufferer, such as if she distances herself from the person, or ignores or is oblivious to another's pain, that she can exacerbate their suffering by being unsympathetic, unkind, inattentive and, at the worst, abusive.

Compassion and kindness should be embodied in every caregiving act. Compassion is communicated in the nurse's tone of voice; facial expression; and gestures, such as in the way the nurse touches and attends to the person. For example, when a patient has been incontinent, the way in which the nurse deals with the situation should communicate compassion and mitigate the person's embarrassment and feelings of shame and guilt. A nurse who acts with compassion is sensitive to patients' feelings, seeks to preserve their dignity, safeguards their privacy, and attends to their needs.

Relationship to Strengths-Based Care: Compassion is a strength that acknowledges the whole person, his uniqueness. Compassion means that the nurse sees the person as a human being and not as an object. When nurses treat the person as an object, reduce her to her diagnosis rather than treating her as a human being, the danger is that the nurse can become indifferent to another person's suffering (Cassell, 2002). Compassion also enables the person to experience her own situation in a different light. When people are treated with compassion, they are more likely to view a negative situation as an opportunity for learning rather than as a failure or a disaster. In other words, compassion helps to soften the impact of negative events.

Approaches for promoting compassion and kindness: Compassion and acts of kindness are integrally tied to empathy and helping. Compassion, therefore, can be fostered by improving empathic responses as well as by teaching helping skills. The following are additional techniques to develop this strength.

Develop self-compassion. An important strategy for helping nurses develop compassion for another person is to first develop compassion for oneself. Self-compassion involves three basic components (Neff, 2003): (a) self-kindness, that is extending kindness to oneself in the same way he would show kindness to another person who is in need or in pain; (b) common humanity, that is, recognizing that what he is experiencing has been experienced by most people at one time in their lives, to some degree; and (c) mindfulness, that is, holding one's pain in balance with other things that are going on in one's own life. Thus, self-compassion requires the nurse to move from "mental work to heart work" by becoming more mindful and in tune with their own thoughts and feelings and more tolerant and accepting of themselves (Germer, 2009).

Self-compassion begins when nurses become attuned to their own needs, feelings of inadequacy and failure, and personal sufferings. It continues when nurses learn to like themselves and to accept feelings for what they are, without labeling, interpreting, and judging themselves too negatively or too critically. Nurses can use many of the informal paths to mindfulness described earlier in this chapter to deal with their own negativity and to help develop self-compassion and self-acceptance.

Ask the person to tell you about his suffering and what he is experiencing. Nurses are more likely to be compassionate when they can understand and identify with the person's pain and suffering. Nurses need to recognize another's distress, be sensitive to his suffering, share in his experience, and provide comfort measures (Burnell, 2009). Because suffering and distress are so subjective and are experienced in very unique ways, it is important that nurses ask patients to tell them about their experiences. A nurse may simply say, "Help me to understand what you are going through." The nurse then needs to take the time to listen to the patient's answer. He can then acknowledge, absorb, and respond more fully to the person's distress.

Strengths of Advocacy

An essential role of nursing is to serve as the person's advocate. Although patients and families are encouraged to take responsibility for their own health care, they often find themselves vulnerable, lacking knowledge of the health care system, and feeling overwhelmed when they are in crisis or in need of help (Benner, 2003). They have to rely on nurses to protect them and help them navigate through a complex health care system that often is strange and unknown and often feels intimidating. To advocate on behalf of patients and families requires that nurses protect, stand up for, defend, support, and plead on behalf of the person and family. Advocacy is the opposite of paternalism (Gadow, 1990; Minicucci et al., 2003) and is an important

> Patients and families find it difficult to navigate a health care system that often feels strange and intimidating. They need a guide, coach, supporter, and advocate. Nurses play these roles when they protect, stand up for, defend, and support patients and their families.

characteristic of collaborative partnership. Nurses are most likely to want to advocate for a person when they believe the person's right to have a say in decisions affecting her care has been violated or when her opinion has been negated, ignored, or discounted.

Advocating on behalf of a person often involves pleading for something different and changing the minds of people in positions of power. Advocating requires the nurse to have the following strengths to fulfill this role:

- Courage
- Self-efficacy

Courage

Courage involves standing up for one's beliefs and fighting for what is right even in the face of opposition (Peterson & Seligman, 2004c). It involves taking risks, overcoming or at least containing one's own fears, persevering, and acting with integrity. Doing the right thing often takes courage because it often entails doing something that is not easy.

There are different forms of courage, namely, physical, moral, and vital (Lopez et al., 2003).

Physical courage involves putting oneself physically in harm's way to save another person. Physical courage is when health care professionals put the safety of their patients above their own self-interest, as when caring for patients with potentially deadly infections, in war zones, and during natural disasters. During the 2003 SARS epidemic, 200 nurses contracted the disease in Taiwan while caring for patients, and four died from this virulent, pernicious virus (Lee et al., 2005).

Moral courage involves standing up for one's beliefs, fighting for what is right in the face of being rejected, screamed at, and intimidated. Nurses who do this are often called *whistleblowers*. A whistleblower is an informant who exposes wrongdoing within an organization in the hope of stopping it (http://www.wordnetweb.princeton.edu). Margaret Haywood became a whistleblower when she filmed the abuse of elderly patients in a geriatric hospital in England in the hope of stopping it (see Exhibit 5.5). Nurses display moral courage every day when they advocate for their patients despite opposing opinions from other health care staff.

Vital courage is the perseverance through a disease or disability when the outcome is uncertain or ambiguous. It is about accompanying people through difficult times by encouraging them, giving them hope, and helping them to find meaning and purpose in living. Patients' courage often is an inspiration and motivation for nurses to have courage, and vice versa. Patients and nurses give courage to one another. Dr. David Burt, at 37, father of two young children, was stricken with ALS, a degenerative, motor neuron disease for which there is no cure. Within a year of diagnosis he had lost all motor function, including his ability to speak and use his tongue and lips. David was able to communicate only through moving his eyes and blinking. He spent two hours a day dictating his thoughts and experiences to his nurse, Shirley Brown. This took place during the 1970s, when there were no aids to help David communicate. Each evening, Shirley would sit near David's bed as he communicated by blinking what he wanted to say. This was no easy feat. David "dictated" what was in his mind; Shirley took the dictation by going through the alphabet. When she came to the letter of the word David wanted, he would blink.

EXHIBIT 5.5

Personal experience of moral courage *"Whistleblower" Nurse Margaret Hayward*

Margaret Haywood, age 58, was found guilty of misconduct at a hearing of the Nursing and Midwifery Council in central London, England, and then subsequently removed from the nursing register. Although she admitted breaching patient confidentiality, she also said that she had agreed to film for the BBC undercover, inside the Royal Sussex Hospital in Brighton, to highlight the awful conditions on the wards. The footage from her hidden camera was shown in a BBC Panorama program "Undercover Nurses," screened in July 2005.

The divorced mother of three, who had been a nurse for more than 20 years, agreed to work on the program and took shifts at the Royal Sussex Hospital between November 2004 and May 2005. The hospital, which at the time had the lowest rating from British health care regulators and a £8 million ($14 million USD) deficit, had received a number of complaints before filming started.

Concerns about standards of care were raised in the British House of Commons after the program was broadcast, and Sussex University Hospitals National Health Service Trust issued a public apology admitting to "serious lapses in the quality of care." But the Nursing Midwifery Council's fitness-to-practice-panel ruled yesterday that Mrs. Haywood had prioritized filming over her obligations as a nurse and had therefore breached patient confidentiality.

Mrs. Haywood, a grandmother of seven, now works for a private care home. She admitted to the charge of breaching confidentiality, even though all patients on the program gave consent after they were filmed. She had told reporters after the verdict that she would be "devastated" if she were struck off the nursing registry. "I've worked so hard. Nursing is my life. I'm devoted to it and I'm passionate about what I do. I think it's a case of shooting the messenger. I admitted breaching patient confidentiality but I did not expect them to conclude that my fitness-to-practice had been impaired."

Source: "Whistleblower" Nurse Margaret Hayward Struck Off (Nursing Registry)" (2009).

And so it was that David recorded his thoughts and inner experiences—by methodically identifying each letter of each word. Words were joined with other words to painstakingly form sentences that then became paragraphs, and paragraphs, pages—all of which began with a slight movement of his eyes. During his three-year ordeal with ALS, David dictated hundreds of pages that captured his experience, what it was like to live in a locked-in bodily state with a mind fully aware, sharper than ever, more lucid, sensitive, and intact. Through all this, David never short-circuited his thoughts. He dictated full sentences. He retained his sense of humor and, through his actions and way of being, came to express his humanity and humanness. He had always been a kind and compassionate man. He continued to be a kind and compassionate man, never one to complain or wallow in self-pity and always concerned for others. These are the choices he made. This is how he chose to live his life. David, who faced a dreadful disease in the prime of his life, showed unbelievable courage, and this courage inspired others. David drew strength from Shirley and her courage. Despite the odds, the terrible prognosis, and downward trajectory of this disease, David and Shirley faced the future together: Each drew strengths from the other's courage. Theirs was a special nurse–patient relationship, a special friendship forged in the face of adversity.

Courage is a strength that is made up of several other character traits, including bravery, persistence, integrity, and vitality (Peterson & Seligman, 2004a).

Relationship to Strengths-Based Care: Courage is the fuel that enables both the nurse and the person to take charge and to feel empowered. Recall from Chapter 3 that SBC values self-determination, and self-determination requires that nurses show courage in advocating on behalf of others.

Approaches to promote courage: At the most basic level, the lack of courage to act is often rooted in fear, an emotion that stems from some real or imagined threat to one's physical self or sense of selfhood. Fear can stem from many sources, such as fear of bodily harm, fear of embarrassment or looking foolish, fear of loss of self-esteem, and fear of being criticized or rejected. Fear evokes a physiological response (e.g., dry mouth, shaking body) and a behavioral response of flight, withdrawal, or avoidance. In its extreme, fear can render a person paralyzed, feeling helpless and unable to cope (Ohman, 2008).

Link feelings of courage to feelings of self-esteem. One technique to contain or overcome fear is for the nurse to ask herself to think of a situation or an event in which she overcame a fear and stood up for herself or for someone whom she perceived to be vulnerable, or to think of a situation in which she took an unpopular position or resisted peer pressure. The nurse should describe the event, the events leading up to the incident, its context, what her thoughts and feelings were at the time, how she reacted, and her subsequent feelings and reactions after she took action. Once the nurse has described the incident, she needs to reread the description of the event and ask herself "What was the thing I feared most?", "In spite of others' reactions how did I feel about myself?", and "Did I feel that I did the right thing?" The nurse will discover that when she stood up and behaved in ways that were consistent with her beliefs and values, no matter how difficult, she felt good about herself. Nurses who answer these questions will recognize the link between showing courage and feeling good about themselves. Conversely, when nurses do not stand up for their patients, for themselves, or their profession, they undermine their sense of self.

Develop agency by using the "I" word. Courage grows out of voicing one's opinion, taking responsibility for one's own actions, and being heard. Remaining silent, suppressing one's thoughts, and subjugating one's own opinions contribute to feelings of helplessness, depression, shame, and thinking of oneself as being invisible and inconsequential. A graduate nursing student reported overhearing two physicians denigrate a nurse and the nursing profession. She listened and said nothing. Her silence made her feel ashamed that she was too fearful to stand up for what she believed. She felt she acted in a cowardly manner when she did not stand up for her fellow nurse and profession.

Courage begins by getting in touch with one's own thoughts and feelings and learning how to express them in appropriate ways. The nurse may begin this process by learning to speak in the first person—"I think," "I have observed," "I want." The nurse can also prepare some responses and rehearse using them, in order to respond when the situation calls for it without feeling flustered. With practice, the nurse will build his confidence.

Use the title "Nurse" and pay attention to how you present yourself. Bernice Buresh and Suzanne Gordon (2006) identified other techniques for helping nurses find their voice including using the title "Nurse" to introduce themselves when behaving professionally. The first technique relates to how a nurse introduces herself. There is much in a name. They suggest that nurses, when introducing themselves for the first time to a patient, colleague, and other team member, use the title "Nurse" along with their last surname, such as "Hello; my name is Nurse Jones, and I will be caring for you today." Nurses have a tendency to introduce themselves just by their first name, "Hello; my name is Norma, and I will be caring for you today." Nurses had always been referred to by their last name—Miss Nightingale, Miss Barrett, Mrs. Gilchrist—that is, until 30 years ago, when informality trumped formality. Buresh and Gordon suggested resurrecting "Nurse" as a title, to bring parity to the way health professionals introduce themselves. Doctors use their title and last name when first meeting a patient—"Hello; my name is Dr. Smith." Nurses should do the same. Alternatively, the nurse can introduce himself in such a way as, "I am Daniel Peters, a Registered Nurse. I will be your nurse today."

The importance of proper, formal introduction is to communicate to the patient the nurse's role on the health care team. It also restores and reasserts nurses' professional identity. Moreover, when nurses begin to use the title "Nurse" to introduce themselves and to greet staff and patients, and adopt a dress code that communicates professionalism, they begin to see themselves as professionals. When they see themselves as professionals, they act profesionally. These simple techniques may sound superficial, but they are important in building pride and instilling self-respect. When nurses are proud of who they are and the work they do, they will have greater self-respect and hold themselves in higher esteem. People with high self-esteem are more likely to be confident, find their own voice, and act with courage out of commitment for what they believe to be right. When nurses find their own voice, they are in a better position to give the patient voice.

Develop competency through acquiring knowledge and practice. Competence breeds confidence, and confidence builds courage. The more competent, skilled, and technically adept a nurse is, the more likely he will feel confident in his judgment. Competence takes time to develop. It is acquired through formal learning, experience, and reflecting on that experience. Competence develops through practice: practicing a skill, honing a talent, and developing a capability. Practice involves repeating an activity until one gets it right and feels comfortable performing it. However, there are different ways of practicing something. Daniel Coyle (2009), in his book *The Talent Code,* discovered the importance of "deep practice."

"Deep practice" holds the key to competence and excellence. It is practice that comes from mistakes and by stopping, focusing on, and analyzing what has gone wrong and then making adjustments, both small and large, until the person gets it right and then repeating, repeating, repeating, until a level of proficiency and competence has been achieved. It is by immersing oneself in the experience, and confronting the challenge, rather than giving up or avoiding it, that a person finally gets it right, and it is in getting it right that the person builds competence, which in turn boosts confidence. Consider a nurse who is skilled at drawing blood. She just "knows" how to locate the vein and knows which veins will not collapse. She is recognized for her skill by her peers and is valued for her competence. This skill was developed and honed with repeated experience by feeling the resistance of veins, sensing how to move the needle ever so slightly, and so forth. She has developed this skill over time. Consider too a nurse who "senses" her patient and can detect whether the patient is comfortable and needs to be repositioned, or a nurse who feels that her patient is depressed and makes time to sit and talk with her. Nurses need training to retrain their senses, attend and attune to their own and their patient's needs, and learn skills of professional social engagement. I return to these ideas in Chapters 6 through 8.

Perceived Self-efficacy

Self-efficacy is an important determinant of whether a person attains his desired goals. When a person believes he has the skills and the know-how to execute a course of action to achieve specific goals, he is then more likely to try and will eventually succeed. Self-efficacy, simply put, is the person's belief that he can perform a behavior that will produce a desired outcome. Self-efficacy is concerned not just with the belief that "I *will* do" but also with the belief that "I *can* do it" (Maddux, 2002). When the person thinks she can achieve something, this in itself is empowering. Often, these thoughts are sufficient to motivate the person to take action. Albert Bandura (1997), a psychologist and father of self-efficacy theory, defined *self-efficacy* as the "belief in one's capabilities to organize and execute the courses of action required to produce given attainments" (p. 3).

Self-efficacy theory is premised on people's need to gain control and have some influence over their own lives. Individuals who do not feel they have any control and do not believe they have the ability to exercise control over certain aspects of their environment are more likely to live in fear; to feel apprehensive, depressed, and helpless; and to experience high levels of stress (Maddux, 2002). On the other hand, individuals who believe that they have the ability to control at least some aspects of their lives are able to actively plan for the future, cope better, and find ways to make things happen (Bandura, 1997).

Relationship to Strengths-Based Care: Self-efficacy is about feeling empowered and being empowered. Recall that empowerment is one of the major cornerstones of SBC. Empowerment requires a degree of self-efficacy. Advocacy is about empowering oneself in order to empower others. Through self-efficacy, one empowers the self in an attempt to achieve one's goals and change one's own future (Hendricks, Hendricks, Webb, Bonner-Davis, & Spencer-Morgan, 2005). A person with high self-efficacy will be *agentic*; that is, he will have a can-do attitude and will know how to make things happen. Self-efficacy also affects how much effort a person is willing to expend to accomplish a goal and how long she will persevere and work to overcome obstacles. It also determines a person's openness to help and ability to tolerate frustration and cope with stress from environmental demands (Bandura, 1997). Remember that self-efficacy is tied to a specific situation. This means that one can have high self-efficacy in one situation but not necessarily in another.

Approaches to promote self-efficacy: Both nurses and patients need to develop self-efficacy. When the nurse develops a can-do attitude she will be in a better position to advocate for her patients. Moreover, it is important that the nurse helps patients promote their own sense of self-efficacy if they are to become empowered, learn how to advocate for themselves, assume greater responsibility for their own health and health care decisions, and help themselves heal and repair.

Nurses can use the techniques listed below to develop their own self-efficacy. They can also apply them to the development of self-efficacy in their patients and families.

Seek out environments that are innovative and support creativity. Self-efficacy beliefs are influenced by the responsiveness of an individual's environments (Maddux, 2002). Innovative environments encourage exploration that in turn enhances the development of the person's belief in himself. These environments subscribe to the philosophy "Nothing ventured, nothing gained." Not only do nurses need to hear this from others, but they also must begin saying this to themselves. In the course of trying out new things and achieving success, nurses will come to believe in themselves and their abilities. On the other hand, controlling environments paralyze and retard such development.

Try to do new things (performance experiences). Performance (i.e., the act of doing) and experience are the best and most effective ways to acquire efficacy beliefs (Bandura, 1997). The experience of how well the person succeeds or fails forms the basis about her belief in her ability to accomplish goals and control her environments. In other words, success gives rise to a belief that one can do. It is in the doing that the person comes to understand the limits and expansiveness of his own capacities and learns what knowledge and skills he needs to acquire so that he can achieve the desired results.

Observe and learn from others (vicarious experiences). Another source of information for developing self-efficacy is through *vicarious experience* (Bandura, 1997). This means observing how somebody else gets things done. Much of learning and acquiring skills is through watching and observing others.

Imagine and then rehearse different "what if" scenarios. Imagining what an experience is like before it has occurred is another way to develop self-efficacy. When nurses imagine themselves in a difficult situation, they can think of different scenarios on how to handle it. In other words, they can rehearse beforehand how they will respond by practicing different responses. In doing this, they will feel prepared and will likely handle the situation more effectively than if they had not anticipated, strategized, rehearsed, and practiced. Most important, if a particular situation does arise, they will be more likely to handle the situation appropriately and meet with success, which will in turn boost their confidence and show them that they indeed "can do it."

Seek out feedback and give feedback (verbal persuasion). Verbal persuasion is an important source of self-efficacy (Bandura, 1997). It involves being encouraged by others to try things and to take small risks. Verbal persuasion also comes through discussing alternatives, and being mentored and coached. Individuals are more likely to try new things when they trust others, have confidence in them as mentors, and feel they have people on whom they can rely to help them know how to better handle a situation.

Learn how to regulate emotions (physiological and emotional states). People feel more self-efficacious when they are calm than when they are distressed or anxious (Maddux, 2002). Thus, strategies to control anxiety will also improve a person's belief that they can do it. When individuals are anxious or upset they are less likely perform at their optimal level than when they have their nerves under control. Nurses need to consider how to control their emotions, such as by reducing, managing, or controlling anxiety and stress.

Now let us once again return to Nurse Catherine Gros and her nursing of Marie and her mother, Linda, and how she advocated for them. From getting to know this family and listening to Marie's and Linda's concerns, what they wanted, and what was important to them, Catherine knew that Marie wanted to keep the baby and that Linda wanted this for her daughter. Catherine also knew that the health care team thought it best for all concerned that, when born, the baby be placed in a foster home and be given up for adoption, even though Marie had told the health care team that *"this is my baby and I want to keep my baby and I want to raise my baby myself."*

Catherine described how she advocated on this family's behalf: *"I understood what their goals were, and I had to begin working with the system in order to really articulate and bring Marie's and Linda's voice into the meetings because decisions were being made on their behalf based on the clinical judgment and expertise of the teams. Their voices were absent. So that was a big part of my role, saying, 'You know, this woman is very attached to this child, and wants to have this child and the grandmother's very invested in this as well and is very fearful that if this doesn't work out that her daughter will take a turn for the worse.' In other words, this could be a very positive thing in the daughter's life and there is some research to support that a life event like that can really turn someone around. There are mothers who have been on drugs and the child is what helps them to turn their lives around. The baby can be an impetus for a very positive change, and I think that's what the grandmother was looking for. There was a lot of hope but a lot of fear; fear of not being in control of the decisions that might come down."*

Catherine spoke about how she brought a change in attitude. She had experience and knew that she needed to develop a working alliance with the team and help them see Marie and her mother in a new light. Catherine was able to acknowledge and recognize the team members' concerns. Catherine continues with the story:

"They began from the position that 'This is horrible, the mother's smoking and we know smoking is bad, and we want a healthy baby.' There was caring there, and they [the nurses, the team] were very invested and very upset. There was a lot of emotion around this case and a lot of debate. I reflected back to them [the nurses and team] that 'You really care about this person and this family and what's going to happen to them.' So, by starting where they were at and working with their strengths, I was able to learn from them what their goals were and what interventions they had tried and what their outcomes were. When we talked about it, it was very clear that they weren't getting where they wanted to go. They wanted Marie to quit smoking and they wanted Marie to detach from her child because they knew the plan was to remove the child to foster care at the time of birth. So it was a real dilemma for them that she was attached to the child."

After much soul searching that took courage and self-efficacy, the team decided to give this family a chance. As Catherine related, *"We said 'What's the goal here? It was to keep the baby safe.' If we put in structures that will keep this child safe that you can live with, why not?"* The team negotiated with the family that Linda, the grandmother, along with her partner, would play key roles and would assume responsibility for the care of Marie's newborn with the support and close monitoring of social services.

Key Summary Points

- SBC requires that nurses develop specific qualities to practice it
- There are 11 essential basic nurse qualities that are grouped within four categories of strengths: (a) strengths of mindset, (b) strengths of knowledge and knowing, (c) strengths of relationships, and (d) strengths of advocacy
- Strengths of mindset include qualities that are required to establish a set of attitudes, outlooks, philosophies, or values that affects one's way of behaving. Specific strengths include mindfulness, humility, open-mindedness, and nonjudgmental attitudes
- Strengths of knowledge and knowing are needed to acquire and use information from formal sources (books, monographs, articles, etc.) and from experience. The specific basic strengths for developing knowledge and for knowing include curiosity and self-reflection
- Strengths of relationships are qualities that are needed to connect with others and for creating and maintaining collaborative partnership. Specific strengths include respect and trust, empathy, and compassion and kindness.
- Strengths of advocacy are qualities that are needed to protect, stand up for, and defend another person. Specific strengths include courage and self-efficacy.
- There are many approaches and techniques to develop each of these strengths

Retraining the Eight Senses for Nursing Practice

6

LEARNING OBJECTIVES

After reading this chapter, you should be able to:

- Explain what is meant by *apprenticeship* and *formation* within the context of professional nursing education.
- Describe the three apprenticeships involved in becoming a nurse.
- Identify the five "outer" and three "inner" senses and how they are used in practice.
- Explain the role of the eight senses in clinical practice.
- Describe the requirements for training and retraining the senses.
- Relate the way the brain rewires itself to retrain the senses and describe some strategies to affect the retraining.

In the 1970s, Alvin Toffler, sociologist, author, and futurist, wrote the book *Future Shock* about how technology would transform our lives. He later expanded on these ideas about illiteracy and learning in the 21st century. Forty years later, Patricia Benner and her colleagues wrote about educating nurses for the future. These visionaries have much in common. The following quotations identify what learners need to be prepared for the 21st century.

> The illiterate of the 21st century will not be those who cannot read and write but those who cannot learn, unlearn, and relearn. (Alvin Toffler)

> Nursing educators must teach for a practice that works deliberately in the social spaces of mechanistic medical diagnoses and treatment and the patients' lived experience or illness or the prevention of illness in their particular life, family, and community... Helping students learn to use the knowledge effectively in their practice is one of nursing education's great challenges. It is best achieved through integrating all three professional apprenticeships, the knowledge base, skilled know-how, and clinical reasoning and ethical comportment,

in all teaching and learning settings. (Benner, Sutphen, Leonard, & Day, 2010, p. 80)

They have identified the issues and set forth the challenges that need to be addressed to be prepared to function in this new age of science, technology, and information. Toffler was writing about our lives in general, whereas Benner and colleagues specifically addressed educating nurses for the 21st century. Although Benner and colleagues directed their remarks to educators, it is students who need to take heed of what is going to be required of them in their role as professional nurses. Both Toffler and Benner et al. understand that in today's fast-paced world, characterized by rapid change and uncertainty, the only way to have some control over the future is by the choices we make that involve learning: what we choose to know, how we choose to think, and the way we want to be in our personal and professional lives.

PROFESSIONAL LEARNING

All individuals seeking a career as a health professional need specialized knowledge and skills that can be acquired only through formal education and clinical training. Although each profession has its own focus of practice based on its mission, historical roles, and mandate and contract with society, each requires its members to undergo specialized training to fulfill these roles and obligations. The practice of helping professions such as nursing, medicine, psychology, social work, and the like is one of practical and moral engagement embedded in the professional–person relationship and not primarily a matter of carrying out a set of tasks and performing techniques and procedures (Dahnke & Dreher, 2011).

To be a nurse requires being able to connect in a meaningful way with the person who seeks help. Becoming a professional requires having and using skills of social engagement in new ways that are different from how the nurse may use them in personal relationships and casual interactions (this is covered in Chapter 8). A major focus of nursing education is devoted to training and retraining the senses to enable nurses to develop a clinical grasp of a situation, arrive at sound clinical judgments on which to make decisions, and then take appropriate actions (see Chapter 7). To accomplish this requires the ability to connect with and develop therapeutic relationships with clients, patients, families, and communities.

Benner and her colleagues (2010) provided the road map to professional nursing practice. They recognized that, beginning with the nurse's initial education and continuing

> Learning to nurse requires training and retraining the senses to: see problems that would otherwise go unnoticed; attune to sounds and listen to patients so that they can be heard; discriminate and find salience in unexpected smells; touch and feel the body to detect subtle changes in skin quality; and sense a situation before understanding what is happening.

throughout a nurse's career, nurses must be engaged in learning. Because nursing demands technical expertise within the context of the nurse–patient relationship, nurses need to develop skills in the following three areas: (a) a broad knowledge base in nursing science that draws knowledge from the physical and biological sciences, the social sciences, the humanities, and nursing and medical science; (b) skilled know-how and expertise to deal with a broad range of clinical issues, concerns, and problems that affect a person and family's health, recovery, and healing; and (c) clinical reasoning and ethical comportment in every decision and action that a nurse takes. These three arms—knowledge, skills, and thinking—comprise the "new" apprenticeships whenever and wherever learning takes place beginning with initial training and continuing throughout the nurse's career.

APPRENTICESHIP AND FORMATION RECONSIDERED: NEW APPROACHES TO LEARNING

The "New" Apprenticeship

Benner et al. (2010) reintroduced the words *apprenticeship* and *formation* and imbued them with new meaning to signify a new approach to learning. For Benner, apprenticeship is *not* on-the-job training with minimal formal education and theoretical knowledge, as it had been in the hospital school training of the mid-19th through mid-20th centuries. It is not about observing and then imitating a "master," although the new apprenticeship retains this aspect; instead, the new, high-ended apprenticeship is used "to capture the experiential learning that requires interaction with a community of practice, situated coaching by teachers, and demonstration of aspects of complex practice that is not easily translated" (Benner et al., 2010, p. 24).

Experiential learning involves learning that is gained while nursing patients and their families. In contrast to formal, theoretical learning that is separated from actual practice, experiential learning marries theory and practice.

Situated learning, on the other hand, is situated in a specific context and with a specific patient. The opposite of situated learning is to ignore the context and treat everyone as if "one size fits all." Situated learning subscribes to the idea that it is knowledge of that particular person and his uniqueness that is required to nurse and provide patient-focused care.

Formation

Formation is a French word used as an umbrella term for education and training. Benner and colleagues (2010) purposefully elected to use the term *formation* to capture the nature, breadth, and extent of the learning and educational experiences involved in learning to nurse. A person does not just become a nurse by acquiring a set of skills, learning how to perform procedures, and becoming technically proficient. On the contrary, becoming a nurse involves a new way of being, adopting a stance of how to care for and be with another person to promote health, facilitate her recovery, and create the conditions for healing. Becoming a nurse involves being "formed" through meaningful experiences and transactions (Benner et al., 2010).

Formation also includes training and retraining the senses as well as reforming social engagement and social involvement skills (Benner et al., 2010). Senses need to be developed, honed, and refined through the acquisition of new knowledge and new skills. Similarly, social engagement skills need to be trained, and existing skills must be re-formed for use in a new context for different purposes.

Formation occurs over time as a nurse deals with new situations, learns about how to deal with different patient and family concerns, and acquires new knowledge and skills within a moral and ethical framework. In the process of becoming a nurse, one must learn new roles, assume new responsibilities, and revise one's own identity so that it includes "nurse" (Benner, 2011). Being a professional requires becoming a lifelong learner.

Much of nursing training focuses on retraining the senses, developing a professional gaze by becoming engaged as an astute observer (see Chapter 7), and re-forming social engagement skills to connect in different but meaningful ways with the person (see Chapter 8). (The term *professional gaze* is used here to mean a special connection that the nurse develops with the person to improve his professional systematic assessment of gathering salient information about the person to guide nursing action rather than as a way of objectifying and distancing from the person). In other words, people do not enter a profession and undergo professional training as "blank slates." They choose a career in their early to middle adult years. They come with strengths: capabilities, capacities, and life skills. A good deal of professional nursing training is in effect a form of retraining and re-forming that builds on the person's existing senses and strengths to be used in a new context (i.e., caring for people) and for a new purpose (i.e., working with patients and families to achieve new levels of health, recovery, and healing).

All humans are equipped with sensory systems. These systems are needed to enable a person to adapt to different situations, navigate different environments, get the most out of life and living, and to express one's own humanity and personhood. A person's senses develop as sensory systems that biologically mature and are shaped by experiences. For example, experiences cause the wiring and rewiring of a person's neuronal circuitry and a structuring and restructuring of the brain in unique ways that in turn affect how well the individual understands, knows, operates, and lives in her different environments, including how well she connects with others to form meaningful relationships. Experiences also affect how sensitive and attuned individuals are to external stimuli as well as how in tune they are with their own internal sensations that affect their thoughts, feelings, and behaviors. When an individual chooses a career in one of the health professions, she needs to undergo a retraining of her sensory systems and acquire a different set of knowledge and skills to meet the demands of her chosen profession and speciality area of practice.

DIFFERENCES BETWEEN HEALTH PROFESSIONALS AND "UNTRAINED" CAREGIVERS

Humans are biologically wired to care for and protect their more vulnerable members. Parents care for children, children care for ill and aging parents, siblings care for other siblings, neighbors help neighbors, communities mobilize their resources to care for those in need, and strangers care for strangers.

Caregiving involves both caring and giving. *Caring* is about being concerned for another and involves a degree of altruism, compassion, kindness, involvement, openness, honesty, authenticity, and commitment (Gordon, Benner, & Nodding, 1996: Mayeroff, 1971). Because caring occurs in the context of a relationship, caring for another is not just about doing *to* another person but also about how the receiver responds to being cared for (Gordon et al., 1996).

Giving, on the other hand, includes the qualities of caring just mentioned but goes beyond it. Giving requires having the knowledge and skills to identify, attune to, and meet another's physical, emotional, mental, and spiritual needs.

When dealing with health issues, caregiving involves understanding the underlying medical condition of the person's complaints to treat and find solutions. Caregiving involves a complex interplay among physical (doing), technical (medical), and interpersonal (talking and listening) knowledge and skills (Aranda & Brown, 2006). Caregiving involves judgment, decision making, and action. It requires knowledge, skilled know-how, and technical competence within a moral and ethical framework of caring (Gordon & Nelson, 2006). Effective caregiving requires that the caregiver understand the context in which care is being given and has developed a well-honed sense of timing. This requires perceptual acuity; skilled know-how; knowledge; and a way of being with the person that is mutually satisfying, promotes growth, and engenders feelings of empowerment (Benner, 2011).

Every situation has the potential of eliciting certain emotions, passions, and fears that shape responses (Demarais, & White, 2005). Part of becoming a professional involves changing the way the person feels, thinks, reacts, and responds. It short, caregivers must master the necessary moral, emotional, and intellectual practices as well as medical and technical skills (Gordon et al., 1996). The extent to which caregivers are able to master these practices distinguishes the untrained, lay caregiver from the professional health care practitioner.

In summary, professionals are individuals who have undergone specialized training and possess specialized knowledge to function with some degree of autonomy (Nodding, 1996). They are capable of understanding a situation, have sound and reasoned clinical judgment, are able to foresee difficulties and take actions that protect and safeguard the people whose care has been entrusted to them (Benner et al., 2011).

DEFINITION OF AND CONCEPTUAL USE OF THE TERM *SENSES*

For decades, when scientists and practitioners talked about the senses, they were referring to the five traditional senses, namely, sight, hearing, smell, taste, and/or touch. These senses are used to perceive stimuli originating from outside a person's own body (*Random House Dictionary*, 2010). In this context, the term *sense* is used as a noun.

Sense can also be used as a verb, to refer to perceiving something, become aware of something, and recognizing something for what it is. Sense can also refer to an act of understanding, that is, to grasp the meaning of something, as well as to refer to mechanical objects that sense or detect changes, such as in oxygen saturation levels (*Random House Dictionary*, 2010). Sense in this context is about knowing and understanding the environment and involves three additional, internal senses: being (a) aware of that which is happening inside oneself, (b) aware of one's feelings and thoughts, and (c) aware of that which is happening outside oneself in the surrounding environment and its impact on oneself.

Information gathered through the five senses and through sensing constitutes the backbone of clinical inquiry. Clinical inquiry requires *critical* inquiry, the intellectual processes of reasoning applied to making sense of the information on which to base clinical decisions. These two forms of inquiry form the foundations that underlie clinical practice.

Importance of the Five "Outer" Senses For Living

We experience our worlds through our five sensory systems, namely, eyes, ears, nose, mouth, and hands. It is through the sensory systems of the eyes (seeing), ears (hearing), nose (smelling), mouth and tongue (tasting), and skin-to-skin contact (touching) that sensory information is acquired. This information is needed for all aspects of living and functioning.

Sensory information does not exist just as a collection of images we see, or sounds that we make, or smells that we experience; instead, sensory information comes together as an integrated whole and is experienced holistically (Levitan, 2008). A person doesn't see without hearing, and doesn't hear without smelling, and doesn't smell without tasting, and doesn't touch without seeing. Sensory information is integrated and organized in such a way as to inform people about the dangers or safety of their environment, the sadness or joy of an experience, the beauty or ugliness of a situation, and so forth. It is in the encoding and decoding of the information from all of the sensory systems that people come to know and understand their environments and how to navigate in them.

Sensory information is the backbone of knowing, and knowing is the means by which we understand the world. It is little wonder that the human nervous system and sensory organs are the first to form in utero and that by the time an infant is born they are all functioning. By the end of the first trimester of pregnancy, all the structures of the sensory organs have been laid down, and by the second semester the sensory organs are functioning to varying degrees (Berk, 2010). For example, the fetus can feel by 10 weeks' gestation; taste by 14 weeks; smell by 15 weeks; hear by 16 weeks, with full hearing ability by 24 weeks; and see by 31 to 32 weeks (Smotherman & Robinson, 1995). By 22 weeks, the fetus is viable and can survive outside his mother's uterus because he is sufficiently equipped to interact and respond to the extrauterine environment.

At birth, a full-term newborn (40 weeks' gestation) has the capacity for human interaction and for connecting with those who care for him. Although the newborn's sight is the least developed of the sensory systems, the eyes are still equipped to see and prefer the shape of the human face. By age 1 to 2 months, a newborn can recognize and discriminate actual faces (Nelson, 2001). At birth, infants respond to touch. Some react positively and enjoy being cuddled, whereas others react adversely. Even preterm infants are highly sensitive to pain and can be readily calmed when they have skin-to-skin contact (known as *kangaroo care*) with another human being (Johnston et al., 2003). Newborns can distinguish several basic tastes, such a sweet, sour, and bitter, and prefer sweet, as in the taste of breast milk (Steiner, Glaser, Hawilo, & Berridge, 2001). Finally, smell and hearing are the most highly developed of the sensory systems. By 4 days of age, breast-fed and bottle-fed infants prefer the smell of breast milk to formula milk (Marlier & Schaal, 2005) and show preference for their own mother's milk over a stranger's milk. Infants are sensitive to mother's voices even in utero (Kisilevsky et al., 2009).

Thus, newborns come into this world primed for social interaction. Their very survival depends on it. They are well equipped to signal to their mothers when they need care. When they are wet, hungry, or in pain, infants are able to call on their mothers (or other caretaker) and get their attention by crying and fussing. They reward their mothers by cooing, cuddling, fixing their gaze on their mother's face, and throwing out the occasional smile. Very few people can resist an infant's smile, coo, or touch on the shoulder, all actions that invite further human interaction.

A child comes into the world with a certain genetic makeup that affects how she will react and interact within multiple environments (Rothbart, 2011). Every interaction, experience, situation, and circumstance, be it positive, negative, neutral, or a combination, will affect how an infant develops into childhood and then how that child develops into young adulthood, middle adulthood, and old age. Researchers have found optimal periods in which experiences affect the structure of the brain and shape its circuitry so that by the time a person enters young adulthood, her sensory systems have largely been developed (Casey, Tottenham, Liston, & Durston, 2005; Goleman, 2006). Having said this, it is important to note that the brain is remarkably plastic, and new experiences can modify the senses and retrain them for new or different purposes. Individuals can be taught to select sensory inputs that are salient in a particular context and interpret sensory information in light of new knowledge. I return to these ideas in the section of this chapter, Domains of Clinical Nursing Practice: *Requirements for Retraining the Senses*, which deals with training and retraining the senses for clinical practice and, more specifically, for Strengths-Based Care (SBC).

The Other Senses: The Importance of the Three "Inner" Senses

In mapping out the social brain, scientists—and more recently, therapists—have broadened their lens of study to include awareness and knowing. Rather than narrowly focusing on just the information that comes from the five sensory organs, scientists now have boosted the number of senses from five to eight (see Table 6.1). The first five senses are responsible for transmitting stimuli from the outside to the brain, hence the term *external* senses. In contrast, the sixth, seventh, and eighth senses are concerned with information about what's happening internally in one's own body, and sensing what's happening in another person (intuiting), before being able to articulate what is happening to oneself (Siegel, 2007). In this situation, these sensory systems function to help a person or clinician "sense" the situation and act accordingly (Benner et al., 2011; Siegel, 2010). Another way of thinking of the difference between these two groups of senses is that the five traditional senses are turned outward, whereas the sixth, seventh, and eighth senses are turned inward. A summary and description of the eight senses are provided in Table 6.1.

There is growing interest about how people "sense" their environment. Sensing is a way of knowing. All individuals sense their environments, and it is their sensing that subsequently directs their responses to specific situations. The accurate sensing of one's environment is a skill that must be learned. Individuals learn about their environments by dwelling in them, observing, noticing, and experiencing them, and by being told by more knowledgeable and informed individuals what is salient, and what things to attend to, that indicate safety or warn of danger. Consider people who have grown

TABLE 6.1

Summary of the eight sensory systems and their functions

Sensory System	Sensory Functions	Chapter in Which Primarily Discussed
1. Visual system: sight and images	Images are the stimuli; sight is that which has been seen based on interpretation. The visual system allows individuals to assimilate information from the external environment. Vision involves the ability to interpret stimuli from the outside gathered from the visible light reaching the eye. Vision is not simply the translation of retinal stimulation; it involves attending to and then interpreting the stimulation that results in a perception of that which has been seen.	6 & 7
2. Auditory system: hearing and sound	Sound is the mechanical wave that is transmitted and strong enough to be heard. Hearing is not simply the translation of auditory stimulation; it is a product of interpreting what has been heard. Sound is produced in many forms, such as voice, music, noise. Sound varies in intensity (soft to loud), pitch (high to low), and harmonic content. Hearing is used to detect danger, navigate one's environment, and communicate with oneself and with another being. Hearing sound is balanced with producing sound (listening and talking).	6 & 7
3. Olfactory and pheromonal systems: smells and odors	Smells are sensed by olfactory neurons that are geared toward detecting odor. Odors are chemicals that can be smelled. Odors are subject to interpretation and discrimination. Odors can range in quality from unpleasant/objectionable to pleasant and desirable and in intensity from strong to mild.	6 & 7
4. Gustatory system: taste and flavors	Ability to taste and detect flavors. Individuals receive stimulation through taste buds on tongue and in the oral cavity (mouth). Involves the recognition and discrimination among five flavors: sweet, sour, bitter, salty, and umami (savoriness). Flavor is linked to taste and smell. Taste is associated with quality (pleasant vs. aversive), temperature (hot vs. cold), and intensity (bold vs. subtle).	6 & 7
5. Somatosensory system: touch (somatic sense), temperature, proprioception	Involves a wide range of sensory neurons that, when triggered, affect many different sensory qualities and areas of functioning. System reacts to a wide range of stimuli that affects different receptors.	6 & 7

(continued)

TABLE 6.1

Summary of the eight sensory systems and their functions   (*Continued*)

Sensory System	Sensory Functions	Chapter in Which Primarily Discussed
(body position), nociception (pain)	Through the skin, the external world is perceived. Skin and use of touch have many uses: source of assessment; form of nonverbal communication; a therapy or therapeutic intervention; massage, healing touch, reflexology.	
6. Awareness of internal, bodily sensations	Awareness of specific bodily sensations, such as weakness in the limbs; tension or relaxation of muscles; and functioning of lungs, heart, and intestine. These sensations shape emotions and thoughts and direct responses to situations. A deep source of intuition.	6 & 8
7. Awareness of an awareness (i.e., meta-awareness) of thoughts, feelings, and intentions of oneself and of another person	A specific mindset that involves awareness of one's own and of another's thoughts feelings, intentions, concepts, attitudes, beliefs, hopes, and dreams. This mindset becomes the focus of attention. Enables one to gain deep insight and empathy.	6 & 8
8. Relational sensing	Awareness of relationships, things outside yourself, the I–thou connection. It is the sensing of relationship, connection with another being. Resonating with another being that involves an awareness of "feeling felt" and feeling understood. Enables a sense of connection, relating, and belonging to beings outside of ourselves (family, friends, community) and to a higher being, a greater cause.	8

Source: Information regarding sixth, seventh, and eighth senses are based on the writings of Siegel (2007), and Siegel (2010).

up or lived for some time in one area of a city. They understand the city's culture and way of operating. They know which areas are safe to walk in at night and which areas to avoid. Citizens of their own country behave very differently than tourists or new immigrants. Think of a person who is living in a country beset by conflict. Even its youngest members can detect subtle signs of danger. They can decode information more rapidly than an adult who is visiting the country. They know what to look for, what information to attend to, and what to ignore. They know what information is salient and what is not. Also, consider what happens when you walk down a street. Most people have learned to scan their environments. Have you ever walked down a street and seen another person approaching from the corner of your eye and, in a split second, you have crossed the street or increased your pace? Before you even understand why you reacted in the way that you did, something from your internal warning system sent you a message that this individual could be dangerous and that you need to take immediate action to protect yourself. This message may have registered as an uneasy feeling in your gut, a sudden increase in your heart rate, or more labored breathing. In effect, your gut sent the message "Beware." Consider a nurse who, while walking down the corridor of his unit, stops suddenly in his tracks, makes a U-turn and enters a patient's room, only to find that patient in distress. Something caught his eye as he passed the patient's room, a brief, split-second image that triggered his internal alarm bells that the patient needed help.

Some people have called this form of sensing or way of knowing *intuition*. We know that "intuitive" knowing plays a significant role in everyday functioning by informing us what is safe and what is dangerous, who can be trusted and who cannot, who needs help and who can manage on their own. All individuals, regardless of their work, possess these different senses, to varying degrees. An individual can be an expert in one area of her life but a novice in another. Consider an experienced baker who can judge whether to add more flour to a cookie recipe just by looking at the consistency of the batter but, when asked whether it is going to rain after looking at the cloud formation, is at a loss.

Thanks to advances in brain imaging, scientists have begun to map out the architecture of the sensory brain and how it functions. This is not new work. In the 1940s, Dr. Wilder Penfield, an American-born neurosurgeon working at the Montreal Neurological Hospital in Canada, began mapping out the functional areas of the brain and identified which regions in the outer cortex of the brain were responsible for different sensory and motor functions. He did this by using electrical probes that stimulated different areas of the cortical regions of the brain. The patient was awake and could report on what he experienced. The five external sensory systems were located in the upper regions or outer cortex of the brain (Penfield, 1975).

Until recently, few researchers could explain how experts *intuited*, or came to sense and anticipate something before it happened. In fact, experts could not articulate what made them respond the way they did, and scientists were at a loss to explain intuition from a neurobiological perspective. Now, scientists have uncovered that the brain processes information in the subcortical region of the brain, an area that some have referred to as the "low road" of the brain (Goleman, 2006; Siegel, 2010). A person takes in stimuli from the outer world, and this information is driven downward to the lower regions of the brain, beneath the cortex, where information is processed before registering in the "high road" or cortical levels of the brain. Thus, awareness is a function of the upper regions of the brain, the cortical regions. This explains why experts can sense a situation and act before they are able to articulate or explain their actions.

Use of the Senses in Clinical Practice

A major focus of nursing is the need to detect danger and to identify risk before danger occurs. That is why we focus on deficits. SBC goes beyond this and broadens the focus to look at the whole person and his "whole" situation. It involves retraining the senses to focus on and understand the whole and, in particular, what things are working that can be used to cope with deficits and minimize risk. Nurses use their senses to see things clearly, to select relevant information about the person and the environment. The goal is to see things clearly, to pick up salient information and interpret the information without distortion. When something is viewed as salient, the nurse is more likely to monitor it with intention and with precision, looking for specific features until the she sees the whole or most complete picture (Siegel, 2010).

Nurses come to understand and experience an event because of the way they experience the world. A person experiences the world in two ways: (a) physically and (b) experientially (Siegel, 2010). Although each can be described separately, in reality these two worlds are indivisible and irreducible and, in effect, are experienced holistically, as a seamless integration of the two.

The physical world is what is visible—what can be observed. When the nurse enters a patient's room, what does she see? She sees the physical arrangement of things in the material world: the size of the room, the number of beds, the chairs, an over-the-bed table, the type of lighting, the location of the window, the placement of the bathroom, the color of the walls, the pictures on the walls, the window treatments, its orderliness or messiness, cleanliness or lack thereof, and so forth. The nurse will also notice the type of equipment in use, both equipment that is expected to be there and that which is missing, and she will look to see that the machines are operating as they should be. She will note whether the patient's bed rails are up or down and whether the placement of furniture could compromise the patient's safety. At the same time, she will also make note of any unexpected and/or noxious odors. The nurse will listen for and be attuned to the expected as well as unexpected sounds coming from the patient, family, or anyone else in the room and will also make note of any unexpected sounds coming from the equipment.

While the nurse is scanning the environment and listening to what the patient is saying, she may reach over to touch the patient, noting his skin temperature (i.e., warm, cold, or hot), texture (moist, dry, firm or saggy), and intactness (smooth, clear, any bruises, markings, skin breakdown, redness, blotches, or tattoos). In addition, an SBC nurse will observe and listen for and note anything that provides any clues as to what makes the person unique. She may notice photos of the family, drawings from a grandchild, or the patient's overall demeanor. This scan may take just a matter of seconds and relies on the nurse's own visual, olfactory, auditory, and tactile sensory systems to provide her with preliminary information about the patient and the safety of the environment. The nurse begins to formulate a first impression of how her patient is doing, what he is like, and what, if anything, requires her immediate attention.

Equally important is the experiential world—the subjective feeling experienced from entering a patient's room and the images this evokes. By making eye contact with the patient, noticing her facial expression and body language, the nurse will make judgments about the person's mood, physical condition, and emotional well-being. From the nurse's own past professional and personal experiences, he will interpret the patient's body and behavioral cues, and will sense her pain or suffering, or detect an aura of peacefulness. All of these inputs will evoke feelings in the nurse and that call forth specific images and memories.

Consider Linda Evans, a nurse who recently lost her own father to chronic obstructive pulmonary disease. She returns to her duties as a pediatric nurse. She is in a heightened state of alertness and is particularly attuned to 4-year old Lisa who suffers from cystic fibrosis, who was admitted the night before in respiratory distress. Linda finds it almost unbearable to listen to Lisa's wheezing and struggles for breath. She notices the faint cyanosis on Lisa's lips and nailbeds that she might otherwise have missed if not for her recent experience in caring for her own father. Linda feels queasy; a knot forms in her stomach. In reflecting why she is having these feelings, Linda recognizes that listening to Lisa struggling to breathe reminds her of her own father's struggles.

In summary, Linda received inputs through her five senses. These inputs register and are interpreted in both the person's mind and body, causing both the body and mind to become "knowers," to signal what is happening on an emotional and intellectual level and to react accordingly.

The way sensing operates in everyday life is also the way it operates in clinical practice. What often distinguishes the novice from the expert nurse clinician is their instantaneous way of knowing and intuiting a situation before being able to explain "why" (Benner, 1984). This can even happen to more junior clinicians, when their own personal experiences have provided them with information they can use in making clinical decisions, as happened in the case of Dr. Daniel Siegel. Daniel recalls a decision he made when he was a pediatric trainee that went against the judgment of more seasoned, senior physicians. His decision saved the life of Maria, a 15-year-old girl. Maria had been suffering from headaches. In listening to Maria tell her story, something about what she told him captured his attention. Although he was unaware at the time of what he had heard or how he had put together the pieces of information that he had gathered to diagnose Maria's headaches the information that had registered in Dr. Siegel's subcortical region or "low road" of his brain nonetheless subsequently directed his actions and saved Maria's life. His story is told in Exhibit 6.1.

Re-forming and retraining the senses for clinical practice depends on what nurses need to know. Almost all senses need to be retrained to some degree. Consider, for example, the sense of smell. The vast majority of individuals can smell and differentiate odors. Some have more sensitive noses and are able to detect subtle differences among odors. Other people are oblivious to smell unless forced to deal with ones they find highly offensive, such as the smell from a skunk or odors from vomit or feces. Moreover, a sense of smell is very specific to an individual; what one individual finds pleasant, another may find offensive. That is one of the reasons there are so many fragrances and perfumes on the market. Certain professions require a highly developed sense of smell. Consider the work of sommeliers, who specialize in all aspects of wine services, including pairing wines with food. Sommeliers are knowledgeable and trained in wine pairing, and part of their training is learning to attend to and be attuned to the subtlest nuances in aromas that distinguish an ordinary wine from a fine wine that complements food.

The same is the case for individuals seeking a career in nursing or medicine. Doctors and nurses need to be trained to attend to and discriminate odors emanating from different orifices (e.g., skin–sweat, mouth–breath, urethra–urine, bowel–feces). Different specialty areas may require more training in a particular sensory system. For example, nurses who work with patients suffering from kidney disease need to be trained to detect subtle changes in the smell of a patient's breath, because early kidney failure is often accompanied by a distinct, offensive odor. This is a form of bad breath that differs from the other forms of bad breath that are caused by poor oral hygiene or a breakdown of bacteria. Also, the breath odor of patients suffering from kidney failure differs from the breath odor of a diabetic patient, the latter of which has a fruity quality when the patient is in keto-acidosis.

EXHIBIT 6.1

Personal experience *The sixth sense: Saving Maria*

Dr. Daniel Siegel related the following experience of using his sixth sense to be open to possibilities to solve the mystery of what was causing Maria, a 15-year-old, to suffer headaches. Maria had been complaining of headaches that some professionals attributed to stress and conflict with her friends. As a young physician, he listened to her story attentively. As he was writing, "Something grabs my attention in the way she points to her head and tells me that only when she sleeps on her right side does her head really hurts in the morning." It is her words "really hurts" that are red flags. He also believed that Maria's retina looked cloudy—a sign of increased cranial pressure—but his supervising physician, a neurologist, as well as an infectious disease expert, did not agree with his observations. They believed that the next step in Maria's evaluation was to do a spinal tap to examine her cerebrospinal fluid. As Dr. Siegel prepared to perform this procedure, his sixth sense kicked in: "A huge wave of 'No!' arose from my belly." He continued to explain the functioning of this sixth sense: "Then my subjective side of reality picks up a sensation and enters my awareness. I experience a sudden sense of panic." Having listened to his internal warnings, he told Maria, her mother, and the other staff members in the room that he would not proceed with the procedure. He insisted instead that Maria have a CT scan over the pleas from Maria's mother to go ahead with the tap. Dr. Siegel prevailed and was later exonerated when the scan revealed that Maria's massively elevated cranial pressure was due to parasites growing in her brain. The spinal tap would have caused her immediate death.

Source: Adapted from Siegel, (2010). Retold with permission from Dr. Siegel (personal communication, August, 2011).

In SBC, in addition to what is required of that clinical situation, nurses also need to retrain their senses to look for person and family strengths. This means they have to learn how to attend with the intention of observing what is happening, and to listen for the positives in order to connect to the person with awareness and understanding (see Chapter 9 for ways of uncovering and discovering strengths).

Domains of Clinical Nursing Practice: Requirements for Retraining the Senses

Even within the same profession, differences exist among its practitioners. Different senses need to be trained to meet the domains of nursing practice in different areas. Consider the nurse working in critical and acute care. He needs to retrain his senses to identify and manage life-sustaining physiological functioning in unstable patients (Benner et al., 2011). This means developing knowledge and observational skills to detect early signs of instability, such as a sudden change in cardiovascular functioning as evidenced by a change in the quality of a patient's pulse. Pulse is caused by pressure exerted on the arterial wall causing expansion of the vessel for a brief moment as the wave of pressure passes (Blows, 2001). All arteries demonstrate a pulse, but only a few are accessible to observation. The nurse may observe signs of cardiovascular distress by noticing the color of the patient's skin (sight) or detecting a faint sigh or murmur (sound); however, observation of the patient's pulse depends on touch. By gently asserting pressure on the arterial site, the nurse notes rate, strength, and quality. Consider a rapid pulse rate. It may be an indication of tachycardia, or a compensatory mechanism as a result of a systemic infection, or a sign that the patient is going into shock. Bradycardia, a slow pulse, may indicate a heart transmission block when the impulse from the sino-atrial node does not reach the ventricle and the ventricular contractions slow (Blows, 2001). The strength of the pulse also indicates different aspects of heart function: A weak pulse may indicate left heart failure due to the myocardium's inability to reach full stoke volume, or a loss of volume, such as that which happens with a bleed. In these cases, retraining the senses requires the nurse to learn how to locate a pulse; how to exert just enough pressure to feel the pulse so that its rate can be counted; and how to develop the proprioreceptors in his own fingertips to distinguish between a thready pulse, a pounding pulse, and so forth. The nurse also has to interpret the information in light of the information he has about cardiovascular physiology and to relate that information to knowledge of this particular patient (e.g., the patient's normal pulse, medical history, and current medical condition), in order to determine whether changes in pulse quality and rate are significant.

Some domains of clinical nursing practice apply to all areas of nursing. Some of these domains may have to be modified to meet the needs of a specific group of patients. On the other hand, there are specialized domains of practice relevant only to a specific population of patients. To illustrate this point, consider the domains of practice in acute and critical care nursing as outlined in Table 6.2 (Benner et al., 2011). All nurses need to be trained to provide comfort, safeguard and ensure patient safety, alleviate suffering, manage symptoms, and the like; however, comfort measures may have to be modified on the basis of whether the patient is a preterm infant, a postoperative patient, a patient who is comatose, and so on. Another example is that acute and clinical care nurses need to develop specialized knowledge and skills in managing crises and have the know-how to prevent hazards in high-tech environments such as an

TABLE 6.2

Domains of Practice in Acute and Critical Care Nursing.

- Diagnosing and managing life-sustaining physiologic functioning in acutely ill and unstable patients
- The skilled know-how of managing a crisis
- Providing comfort measures for the critically and acutely ill
- Caring for patients' families
- Preventing hazards in a technological environment
- Facing death: end-of-life care and decision-making
- Making a case: communicating clinical assessments and improving teamwork
- Patient safety: monitoring quality, preventing and managing breakdown
- The skilled know-how of clinical and moral leadership and the coaching and mentoring of others

Source: Adapted from Benner, Kyriakidis, & Stannard, (2011).

intensive care unit, whereas nurses in a rehabilitation or hospice setting, where there is little technical equipment, might not need this level of knowledge. Hospice nurses, on the other hand, may need to have specialized knowledge and skill in end-of-life care because active, life-saving treatment has shifted to palliative care.

Finally, the domains of practice can also include the nurse's orientation to practice. Nurses practicing SBC require skilled know-how in the following domains that reflect SBC values that were described in Chapter 3. These domains of practice include the following:

- Promoting health, facilitating recovery, and creating conditions for healing
- Understanding the person's individuality—what makes the person and her family unique by uncovering, discovering and working with strengths
- Caring for the whole, integrated person (i.e., holism and embodiment)
- Caring for patients' families
- Working with and negotiating multiple perspectives (i.e., subjective/objective realities) and different created meanings
- Supporting self-determination, an aspect of decision making
- Creating healthy, healing, and safe environments (i.e., in which the person and environment are integral)
- Working with patients' unique learning styles, respecting issues of readiness and timing
- Creating collaborative partnerships

Each domain of practice has its own knowledge and skills that require that the senses undergo retraining. Consider the story told by nurse Luisa Ciofani, who displayed how her formal knowledge and practical experience in neonatal, perinatal, and postpartum nursing, along with her strengths-based nursing orientation, direct the information she gathers to decide on the best course of action. Luisa was asked to intervene with a young couple, Mr. and Mrs. Gasper, by the couple's primary nurse, Danielle, who had cared for this couple during their pregnancy. Mrs. Gasper had just been told that her baby, an 8-month fetus, had died in utero. The death was very sudden and totally unexpected. Mr. Gasper was away at the time, and Mrs. Gasper was completely traumatized.

As Luisa related, "*She was being admitted for termination the next day. The patient had decided she wasn't going to see the baby. She didn't want to have anything to do with the baby and she was going to stay away from the baby as much as possible. Danielle, in her experience in caring for bereaved patients, knew that this wasn't necessarily the best decision.*"

Mr. Gasper had arrived by the time his wife was admitted to the unit for the pregnancy termination. Luisa continued: "*We talked about what the experience would likely be for them, the options that would be offered to them, and the reasons to choose a particular option or not. It was obvious that the couple was very loving together but both were completely traumatized by this sudden rush of events.*"

Luisa later reflected on her first impressions of this mother and this couple: "*I sensed they were open to different possibilities. When she first came, she had decided 'No, this is not for me—no seeing the baby, none of this, I want to deliver and go home, and if I can deliver without any pain that would be even better because I don't want to feel the contractions and feel I'm having the baby.' She was open to the possibility that maybe that wasn't the best approach. Mr. Gasper, who was with her at the point, also wanted to avoid whatever pain was possible for his wife. He was being very stoic in terms of 'No, we don't need that—no, no, no.' But I told them this: 'What we do is to open the doors and we don't close them until you tell us to close them. You can change your mind at the very last minute; you can change your mind after things are done.' They integrated what I was trying to tell her but, most of all, Mrs. Gasper was open to the possibility that her way might not be the best way even though that's what she thought. I told her that we would be respectful of whatever choice they made."*

Luisa sensed this couple's openness. Her impression of Mr. and Mrs. Gasper guided her decision to explore with them options that were different from their initial response of "just getting things over with as fast and as soon as possible."

Luisa continued with what happened to this couple: *"She delivered during the night and left very early the next day, and although I didn't see her I did learn from the nurse that she had seen and held the baby. I became quite involved. [It is our practice] that whenever a baby dies or a baby is stillborn, we offer the family baptism or blessing, or pastoral services 24 hours a day. Mrs. Gasper declined this service. However, the next day she called me in a panic and said 'I want my baby baptized. This is very important to me—I don't feel as though I've said goodbye.'"*

Luisa related that the baby's body had been transferred to another hospital for the autopsy. Although she had no idea when the autopsy was scheduled, she called Pastoral Services and was able to schedule a baptism for that morning. She asked Danielle to attend the baptism, and although Danielle was at first hesitant to go, as indicated by her response to Luisa: *"Oh, do you want me to go?"* Luisa answered, *" 'No, no, that's not the question. I believe that somebody needs to accompany this family through this experience, and I think you would be a good person to accompany them through this.' She debated about going or not but went. When Danielle came back, she thanked me for pushing her to go, and I said 'Well, you were really easy to push.'"*

Luisa later recalls why she asked Danielle to go: *"I understood that she would be good there. I wouldn't have done the same thing with everybody, with a less experienced nurse, or someone who hadn't worked with a family who had been bereaved, or who didn't have interest in that particular area. I wouldn't have been quite so open about sending them out there".*

It was Luisa's knowledge about Danielle, the situation, and what she now understands to be the parents' needs, which informed Luisa's actions.

Luisa continued to share her thoughts as to why she thought the baptism was so important for this couple: *"The baptism allowed Mrs. Gasper to parent her baby. She was very articulate about that in terms of being able to unwrap the baby on the altar, to have a sense of closeness with the baby, and to experience with her husband what made them both feel they were a community and that this baby had been born into a community. One of the volunteers from the hospital had knitted a blanket for the baby that the baby was wrapped up in. So, even people who didn't know this family were touched by the baby's life."*

Luisa also made the arrangements for the infant to be photographed. *"It was interesting, because the next day, Mrs. Gasper wanted to come to see her infant's photograph. Often families do not want to look at them right away. When I was with her, I said 'Do you want to look at the pictures?' and she said, 'Of course; that's my baby'—just like a woman whose baby hadn't died; the exact same response."*

In this story, Luisa displayed skilled know-how in several domains of practice of neonatal and postpartum nursing with a strengths-based nursing orientation, including skilled know-how in facilitating the parents' healing by creating conditions that allowed them to feel like parents and to give them experiences to ease their bereavement and grief. She also showed that she knew how to manage a crisis, care for the couple, and help them make choices. Finally, in making the case for the need for a baptism, Luisa showed clinical and moral leadership and the ability to coach and mentor others. It was her formal knowledge of fetal and neonatal loss, previous experience in nursing parents who had delivered a stillborn child, along with her belief in the parents' right to make choices that came together to direct her nursing. These considerations were at work when she reviewed with the Gaspers their options. Although this couple's initial decision was not to see their dead son, they later changed their minds after discussing their options with Luisa. Luisa also showed clinical and moral leadership and was able to make a case, communicate her clinical assessment to other members of the team when she made the arrangements for the infant's baptism, which required her to coordinate activities between two hospitals. She also showed clinical and moral leadership when she coached Danielle to attend the baptism ceremony that benefited both the nurse and this couple.

Luisa's clinical grasp of the situation, wise judgments, and quick, decisive actions contributed significantly to this couple's healing. Luisa continues with the story: *"We felt that they still needed help. So we referred this couple to a support group. Mrs. Gasper came back and told us that she felt she had progressed in her grief beyond the other people in the support group. She told us that some were mourning the fact that they hadn't seen the baby; they hadn't spent time with the baby, or had never held their baby. The baptism had put her in a good place because we had facilitated that whole experience for her."*

Luisa had been trained to observe the couple's reactions to devastating news and in how to listen to patients' pain and suffering without becoming overwhelmed. Luisa was aware that her own thoughts and feelings may differ from those of her patients'. She also was trained to identify strengths, how to ask questions that uncovered the meaning that a situation had for this couple, listen to the patient's needs, observe the couple's responses, and react accordingly in a situation-responsive manner. Her experience and instinct had taught her the importance of timing and "sensing" a situation—deciding when to move in a situation and when to hold back, how to plant seeds and wait until the person is ready to act. She has spent years retraining her eight senses and is now in her role as an expert clinical nurse specialist in perinatal and postpartum nursing.

HOW THE BRAIN RETRAINS ITSELF

As mentioned earlier in this chapter, recent discoveries have revealed that the brain is remarkably plastic. The most substantial evidence of neuroplasticity has come from examining the brain's response to various neurological insults. In persons who have suffered strokes, motor neuron recovery begins after several weeks, and growth-related processes evolve over time (Ward & Cohen, 2004). One study indicated that individuals diagnosed with early-onset schizophrenia and who had two years of social therapy displayed a substantial increase in hippocampal nerve genesis (growth) at the frontal subcortical level (Lewis & Lieberman, 2000). Similarly, in cases of patients with epilepsy, on whom a hemispherectomy was performed and the language center removed, new subcortical growth was observed after the patients' recovery of language (Devlin et al., 2003).

Three basic neurological processes are involved in retraining the brain: (a) creating and strengthening synaptic connections, (b) stimulating new neurons to grow, and (c) increasing the sheathing along the axonal lengths to enhance conduction speed of neuronal electrical impulses (Siegel, 2011). These processes result in alteration of the neuronal tissues that make up the brain when new synapses are formed or existing ones eliminated as a result of axons and dendrites being remodeled or reorganized. In other words, the connections between neurons are altered to form different connections. The remodeling of the axons and dendrites can occur in two ways. One method is by creating new and different neuronal connections, and the second is by increasing the strength of the connections. Both are considered to induce neuroplasticity; however, only the first process can strictly be considered a rewiring of the brain. Scientists have hypothesized that although rewiring the brain increases plasticity, increasing the number and density of connection among neurons provides a substantial boost in the storage capacity of the brain (i.e., memory). Learning may be slowed, however, because the neural network has become more indirect. In other words, messages have to pass through different parts of the brain and travel along additional pathways instead of taking a more direct route (Chklovskii, Mel, & Svoboda, 2004). This process is akin to taking a detour: The route is less direct, but it gets one to the destination.

The adult brain is different from the child's brain. Up until recently, it was assumed that children learn more easily than adults because their brains are developing. As part of growth and development, new neuronal pathways are being created, the brain circuitry is being laid down, and the neural connections are being strengthened. It is now accepted that development is not limited to childhood but instead is an integral part of the human condition. Development and learning continue throughout the life span, from conception until death. Adults, like children, are always learning, growing, and transforming.

Science has begun to explain differences between children and adults in regard to brain plasticity and how adults learn. What has been found may surprise you. Adults' newly minted neurons appear to be just as active as the neurons in a developing child but, interestingly, for about a month after they are formed (Ge et al., 2007). Further, it would appear that newly formed adult brain cells can "listen" (receive nerve stimulation) before they can "talk" (send messages to other nerves). A study of new nerves that were formed in the olfactory bulb of the brain found that such nerves can receive input from the higher parts of the brain only for the first 10 days after they are formed, and new synaptic connections do not form until after 21 days to allow the new nerves to send signals to other nerves (Whitman & Greer, 2007). This could indicate that new nerves need to be integrated into the existing brain structure before they introduce changes to the wiring of the brain. In other words, the brain doesn't just change automatically—it doesn't just rewire itself. The brain must determine the "added value" and efficacy of such rewiring before it alters its current neuronal structure.

Training and Retraining the Senses

Training and retraining derive from the need to develop new ways of seeing, hearing, smelling, tasting, and touching, as well as new ways of knowing what is going on inside a person in order to understand the nature of that person's concerns and then to plan care that is responsive and appropriate.

Training and retraining the senses involve rewiring the brain. The brain is neuroplastic (flexible) and, after repeated exposure to specific experiences, can change both its structure as well as the way the different areas of the brain function (Doidge, 2007). According to Siegel (2010), training "involves the purposeful harnessing of the power of experience to change the function and structure of the human brain" (pp. 217–218). The implications of this definition for training is that, for teachers, mentors, preceptors, and anyone involved in teaching students, regardless of who is the learner (i.e., entry-level students, seasoned nurse clinicians, patients/clients/families), considerable thought needs to go into selecting and creating learning experiences. These experiences will affect how the brain becomes rewired, that is, the direction and flow of energy and information. In turn, these changes will determine how a situation is perceived and, subsequently, the way the person functions.

Training refers to the acquisition of knowledge, skills, and competencies through formal education and practical experience. On the other hand, *retraining* refers to building on existing knowledge and skills, using the nurse's sensory systems in new ways to achieve different purposes. It involves transforming everyday experiences so that they are experienced differently through formal retraining of the nurses' sensory systems to attune to the clinical situation.

Every sense needs to be used for two purposes. The first is *assessment*, that is, how to use sensory systems to gather salient information. This involves deciding on what information to gather, what stimuli to attend to; how to distinguish the important from the unimportant; how to determine whether the information that the nurse has is sufficient to understand the problem, and how to grasp what is going on so that the nurse can arrive at an understanding as to the nature of the situation. The second purpose is *therapeutic intervention or approaches*: how to use the sensory systems in a different way so as to bring about or stabilize a person's health status, promote their health, address their concerns, meet their needs, and/or minimize harmful effects of a medical condition or treatment, and facilitate healing.

- *Retraining the senses involves* attending to and becoming attuned to things that may have gone unnoticed or taken for granted but now are salient.
- *Retraining the senses involves* acquiring knowledge and theory and then putting this knowledge and theory to a new use, such as by helping one refocus attention or reframe a situation so that it is understood and experienced differently. For example, a nurse who, as a student, was taught about attachment theory will look at how nurses can become secure bases for patients when patients are distressed and their loved ones are not available to calm them and reduce their anxiety and fears. Knowledge and theory redefine the boundaries of what the nurse should attend to and helps to refocus the senses.
- *Retraining the senses involves* learning how to shift attention and attend with intention to different stimuli in the outer world as well as to the nurse's internal

world. It involves learning to observe the environment for signs and listen to signals that suddenly take on different meanings and significance; to discriminate and distinguish that which is relevant and salient to better understand the patient's situation; and to organize this information in order to arrive at a clinical judgment, make clinical decisions, and take actions.

- *Retraining the senses involves* learning to interpret information by altering how the nurse perceives the situation through a new lens: a professional lens. In this case, nurses filter sensory stimuli and arrive at an understanding of the situation through the lens of strengths-based nursing. What the nurse "sees"—that is, his visual perception—is often affected by his own desires and preferences (Balcetus & Dunning, 2006). Part of retraining the senses is a need to focus on changing perceptions by altering perspectives and changing desires and preferences.

The major features of retraining the senses are summarized in Table 6.3.

Retraining the Senses for Strengths-Based Care in Different Settings, Specialties, and with Different Populations

Nurses require different training for different areas of practice. Nurses will be attuned and attentive to different stimuli and look for different signs and signals when practicing in different settings and caring for patients at different points in their illness–recovery–healing trajectory. Consider two nurses taking care of a patient who has suffered a head injury. The nurse caring for a patient immediately following a head injury, in the intensive care unit, is concerned with assessing the patient's mental and physical status. The patient's survival and the prevention of further deterioration are foremost in her mind. The nurse needs to retrain her senses to detect obvious and subtle changes in neurological status. In this situation, the nurse's immediate concern and the focus of her attention is looking for any signs of change in the patient's states of consciousness. The spectrum of alertness ranges from consciousness, confusion, delirium, stupor, to coma (Blows, 2001). In addition to assessing for what is not working (i.e., deficits), SBC nurses also attend to and evaluate what is working (i.e., strengths) and how what is working helps compensate for what is not working. The nurse understands the

TABLE 6.3
The nature of retraining

Retraining involves:
- **Building on existing knowledge** and learning to use the sensory systems in new ways to achieve different purposes
- **Attending to and becoming attuned** to things that may have gone unnoticed or things that are taken for granted
- **Learning to distinguish and discriminate**, sort out the important from the unimportant
- **Learning how to shift attention and attend with intention** to different stimuli in the outer world as well as to the practitioner's inner world
- **Learning to interpret information** by altering how one perceives the situation through a new lens—a professional lens
- **Rewiring the brain**/building new neuronal circuitry

importance of careful observation: to direct management and to gauge whether the patient is showing signs of improving or signs consistent with deterioration. The SBC nurse knows it is important to work with strengths to prevent further deterioration and support the body's innate healing mechanisms. This is what happens when the nurse assesses that the patient is sufficiently hydrated and that his pain is well managed and under control. The nurse also alters the environment and makes it more conducive to healing by attending to the decibel levels of the machinery, keeping noise levels at a minimum by lowering beeper volume, dimming the lights, and so forth. The nurse also ensures that the patient's sheets are clean and pulled taut for the patient's comfort. The nurse checks the patient's skin temperature by touch and thermometer, if needed, makes sure that the patient is covered with a warm, heated blanket. These measures are taken to promote sleep. It is during sleep that the body heals.

Contrast these concerns with those of a nurse in a rehabilitation setting, who is assigned to care for a patient who has suffered a head injury. One of the top priorities for the rehabilitation team is to understand how the brain was affected by the injury by assessing areas of function that have the potential to be restored and, if the damage cannot be reversed to pre-injury levels, then to consider ways to help the patient learn how to do things differently. Brain injury rehabilitation is designed to take into account that which is working (strengths) as well as assessing those areas that have been affected by the injury. Those areas that are working need to be strengthened, while at the same time the team must help the patient regain function in the affected areas (National Institutes of Health, 1998).

Rehabilitation is about restoring wholeness and creating a new level of health. As part of developing perceptual acuity, the nurse must retrain his senses to assess the patient's psychosocial and functional health patterns. He needs to know what to attend to when assessing the patient's patterns of mobility, sexuality, sleep and rest, sensory acuity and pain, communication, cognitive impairment, nutrition, elimination, skin impairment, and social relationships (Canadian Nurses Association, 2005). He also needs to understand how the patient and her family carry on with their lives and accommodate the patient's disabilities. This happens when the occupational therapist evaluates the person's physical home environment and alters it to help optimize the patient's level of autonomy when he returns home. The nurse and the team members seek to understand how the person copes with everyday challenges. Essential to healing is uncovering and discovering the person's strengths and working with them to manage that which is not working. The nurse needs to learn what to listen for, such as how the patient conserves and expends energy, participates in her own care, deals with anxiety and depression, and the like. The nurse also needs to be sensitive to the person's and caregiver's age, gender, and cultural variations and to be attuned to their strengths. Finally, the nurse needs to retrain his senses to attend to the patient's and family's behaviors that indicate that they are ready to direct their own care.

Maria Boggia, a rehabilitation nurse, shared what she attuned to when working on a neurological unit to care for Mr. Schmitt, a 62-year-old engineer and project manager. Mr. Schmitt was used to being in charge. When Maria met him, he had undergone a repair of a leaking aortic aneurysm. During the postoperative period Mr. Schmitt had suffered several severe complications that left him partially paralyzed.

Maria shared her first observation of Mr. Schmitt: "*I saw a man who was totally devastated by what had happened to him. There was a body, but there was nothing else—there was just a body in that bed. He made very little contact with me, barely answering questions; he had really turned inside. You could see that he was closed and turned toward the interior, this gentleman. His wife did most of the answering. He just lay in bed. He had a lot of difficulty because he was totally dependent for basic needs like washing, dressing, and toileting. He was incontinent of urine and stool: He had a lot of needs—his skin had broken down all over his back. It was a total mess. I knew we had a lot of work to do and we started the next day, me and the [restorative nursing assistant]—we took charge of the case.*"

Maria describes Mr. Schmitt's attitude as one of "*'Do whatever you want with me' type of attitude, 'Throw me wherever you want, I don't really care.' This was the attitude, and I thought, 'Okay, this man has lost all hope and he doesn't know what will happen to him.' I had nursed other paraplegic patients and I had the experience. I saw this gentleman with a lot of potential and I needed to communicate this to him now...that he still had the possibility of a good life.*"

Where to begin? Maria began working with Mr. Schmitt's on his basic needs, as Maria recalls: "*I had to explain what we were going to do in terms of his routine, his bowels, his urine, how we were going to work, to explain to him what the objectives were, and what I was aiming for—again he was looking at me, not really understanding and just going along with me...No matter what I was going to say to him, at that point, I don't think that was the right strategy. I had to show him. I had to do for him so that he could realize, and if he's going to see it, he's going to believe it because he's going to experience it and he's going to embark on it with me. So just by talking to him, I didn't feel—physically he was not ready because of his body—he had pressure sores and we were so focused on him getting better with that and not deteriorating. His body was not ready, and mentally he was not ready.*"

Maria assessed that Mr. Schmitt was not ready, both physically and mentally, to became a partner in care. She saw her role as beginning with tending to his body and his physical needs, as a way to restore and bring a new level of wholeness to Mr. Schmitt, the person, by beginning where he was at mentally and physically.

Maria described the context of her care, which involved not just attending to Mr. Schmitt's basic needs, but also helping him and his wife gain a glimpse into a life that could be. As Maria described, "*I don't think he knew what to expect. Of course, he wanted to be like he was before, but he didn't know what to ask for. So I was telling him that we could do intermittent catheterization. We could remove the catheter and he could learn how to do this eventually for himself. He didn't understand that, so he just let me do whatever I needed to do for him at the beginning. But I knew I was dealing with a very intelligent man, someone who had been in control of his life; someone who was able to decide for himself. He had a lot of support from his wife. I knew that eventually I could get him to participate with me. He did eventually join us. He started saying what he wanted and, in fact, he even suggested different things that I was doing—'Maybe we could do it differently, maybe we could do it this way.' It was nice because I started seeing him engaging, seeing him participating, and deciding for himself and taking control. I just needed to help him, at the beginning, to see that there was some hope and there were some things that were possible. My role, at the beginning, was to make him believe that there was a future to have, to have a quality of life.*"

As Maria observed and assessed for strengths, she gained insights into Mr. Schmitt, the person, and he helped her to see what was possible. She looked for strengths, found them, and used them to alter the course of Mr. Schmitt's recovery and rehabilitation.

The Mindset Required For Retraining the Senses

The essential qualities nurses need to practice SBC were described in Chapter 5. Before proceeding, you may want to review them.

Daniel Siegel (2010) identified three mental processes—*inner openness, objectivity,* and *observation*—that can help practitioners focus and then get in touch with their own inner feelings and thoughts. These mental processes enable them to develop their sixth, seventh, and eighth senses. Developing awareness and getting in touch with one's own thoughts and feelings are critical in becoming a nurse and practicing SBC; however, it is not easy to do. Part of the difficulty is that the mind wanders. Siegel illustrated the three mental processes as a tripod, because tripods provide stability to the camera that allows it to form its internal image (see Figure 6.1).

The first leg of the tripod, *inner openness*. Siegel (2010) defined inner openness as "cultivating the receptive states within ourselves that rest beneath the surface layers of judgment and expectation" (p. 102). Inner openness allows the clinician to embrace uncertainty, to let events to unfold before acting, to understand that anything can happen, and to be open to all eventualities and recognize opportunities. Unlike the discussion of openness in Chapter 5, which referred to being open to the patient, openness as used here refers to a nurse being open to her own thoughts and feelings. In other words, the nurse needs to be aware of and in tune of what is going on inside of herself so she can hear her patients and be more receptive to them.

FIGURE 6.1

The tripod: Openness, observation, objectivity.

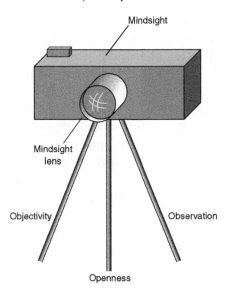

Source: Reprinted with permission from Siegel, (2010).

To be in tune with their inner selves, nurses need to begin by attending to what they are thinking and feeling and how they are responding to their patients at the time that an incident happens. Openness means that the nurse is fully present when he is with his patient. He is able to experience the situation as it actually is, rather than as he would hope or like it to be.

The second leg of the tripod is *objectivity.* Objectivity enables a nurse to identify with patients, understand their concerns, and bear witness to their suffering without becoming overwhelmed. Objectivity is important because it allows the nurse to be responsive to her patients. When nurses overidentify with their patients, they may not be able to see the situation clearly. In retaining a degree of objectivity, the nurse is in a better position to select and sort information, separate the relevant from the irrelevant, and the important from the less important, while at the same time empathizing with the person by acting out of compassion and with genuine concern. Objectivity also prevents nurses from becoming burned out.

The third leg of the tripod is *observation.* Observation involves witnessing, noticing, and recording what is happening to the patient. When a nurse is receptive to what is going on inside herself (*inner openness*), he is able to set some boundaries to prevent himself from becoming overwhelmed by what the patient is experiencing (*objectivity*). This allows him to witness his patients' experiences and suffering. He is then in a better position to help patients understand and work through what they are experiencing and make meaning of their situations.

The nurse helps the patient weave together the events as they unfold. She does so against the backdrop of what she already knows about the patient as a person. The nurse can supply the commentary because she has spent time reflecting on what she has witnessed. She can comment on what she knows from her own personal experiences and also from her professional experiences of what she has learned from other patients. In short, the nurse plays an important role in helping the patient rewrite his narrative and construct a new script about his experiences with illness or other insults (Liehr & Smith, 2008).

Unlike storytelling, which is often told in a linear, chronological order of events, a narrative is about integrating memory (what one already knows) to make sense of events. In the process of helping patients narrate their experiences by helping them label their emotions and thoughts, nurses help patients discover who they are, what is meaningful to them, and make sense of all that they have been through. Equally important is that the nurse comes to learn more about his patients, the people—who they are and what is important to them (Charon, 2001; Munhall. 2009). The narrative is now recognized as an important tool not only to get to know a patient but also as a therapeutic approach in helping a person heal (Frank, 1998; Skott, 2001).

Nurse Joann Creager brought this very mindset to her work with Mrs. Chan, a 72-year-old Chinese woman who was transferred to a long-term care unit following a stroke. Up until the stroke, Mrs. Chan had been a very active member of the Chinese community. She was a widow and had lived for many years on her own. She had enjoyed success in many careers: as a teacher; a musician; and, in her last career, in managing real estate properties. The stroke had left her paralyzed on her right side. Although she could manage somewhat on her own, she was not well enough to return home. She found this decision difficult to accept. Other than the stroke, she was in good physical condition, despite having diabetes and hypertension. Both were well controlled. Mrs. Chan spoke Mandarin and little English, and Joann spoke only English and no Mandarin. Despite these differences, they found a way to communicate. They formed a bond. Joann served as Mrs. Chan's trusted advocate during her year-long stay on the unit.

Very soon after Mrs. Chan's arrival on the long-term care unit, she began having difficulties with some of the staff. Joann described the situation: *"I knew it was going to be a rough road over the long haul because she had very specific needs. She was having trouble expressing them because of the language barrier. But it went beyond that. I think, because of the difficulties with language, the assumption among some of the staff was not that there were language problems but that she had dementia, and because many of the things she was asking were not things patients usually ask for, the staff considered her requests to be unreasonable. Therefore, they couldn't meet them."*

Joann learned that Mrs. Chan had concerns around her bathing: *"Mrs. Chan had a very specific ritual around bathing. When she went to the shower, it wasn't enough to be washed and rinsed once. She wanted to be rinsed at least twice, which some staff members found completely unacceptable."*

Although Joann didn't understand why rinsing Mrs. Chan twice during her shower was such an issue for the staff and yet so important to Mrs. Chan, she slowly pieced the puzzle together: *"What happened in the shower room was so unacceptable on both sides, and the two stories were presented very differently. Some of the staff labeled this woman as difficult—'Oh my God, this woman, she just never stops and you can't make her happy— she just wants to shower and shower and shower and shower.' However, for me that just didn't make sense. Most of our elderly patients get cold easily, their skin is thin and they don't want to spend hours and hours under the shower. So right away it didn't make logical sense to me. So I asked myself, 'What is going on here?' And then you have Mrs. Chan trying to tell you, it was hard for me to grasp at first, she has a fear of soap residue being left on her skin. She wants to be thoroughly rinsed twice."*

Joann, in piecing together Mrs. Chan's narrative, came to understand that Mrs. Chan believed that her diabetes and hypertension were responsible for her stroke and that the soap residue left on her skin contributed to her having a stroke: *"She believed that her diabetes and her hypertension had been the cause of her stroke. She was absolutely, extraordinarily afraid that there would be another [stroke], and she was going to make sure that there wasn't. To the best of her ability, she was going to make sure her blood pressure and her blood glucose were under good control."*

Part of that control was making sure that the soap residue on her body was completely rinsed away—hence the need to be rinsed twice. How did Joann make this connection? Even though Mrs. Chan spoke a little English but mostly Mandarin, and Joann spoke no Mandarin, nonetheless Joann was able to find a way to communicate with Mrs. Chan: *"I learned that—although it was very hard to understand her in English, if you listen to [people] for awhile then you pick up a lot from their body language and you start hearing what they are trying to say. Just stopping and letting your ear get tuned to how they are speaking, what it is that is bothering them…And I think that's what I did with her…Not only that, she was very articulate and very literate. She wrote. She kept journals of her care every day."*

Joann was successful in communicating with Mrs. Chan: "*I know from speaking to her son, he said 'My mother tells me she talks to you all the time. You understand what she's saying.' I was flattered, but it also reflected my sense that we understood each other.*"

Joann credits her own background and childhood experiences in developing the skills needed to connect with others from a different culture or who are labeled "difficult." Joann's inner openness, objectivity, and observation led her to this understanding: "*I spent my entire childhood and adolescence being the outsider. Being a military brat and going from school to school, neighborhood to neighborhood, I wouldn't have been able to articulate what was going on when I was a kid, but looking back I now know what I did... When you have this sense of being alone and not acceptable or not accepted, it can be stultifying and soul destroying. So, you find a ways to get around that. And oddly enough, the way of getting around that is often making alliances with others who feel equally marginalized. For different reasons... I learned early on to listen to people that everyone else thinks are weird or not worth listening to.*"

This story illustrates the three legs of the tripod (see Figure 6.1) that contributed to Joann's ability to connect and care for Mrs. Chan. Joann showed an openness to try to understand the staff's and Mrs. Chan's narratives. In her desire to understand the situation, her own inner openness led her to understand that there existed not only the differences in their belief systems but also what Joann came to understand was a "clash of cultures." Some of the staff too readily labeled Mrs. Chan as "difficult" because of what they interpreted as her unreasonable demands. They also labeled her as suffering from "dementia" because of her inability to speak English. Joann found just the opposite. By training her senses to listen, see, and hear what was going on inside herself as well as Mrs. Chan, Joann got to know Mrs. Chan, not just the patient but Mrs. Chan, the person. Joann developed a deep and abiding respect for Mrs. Chan because of Mrs. Chan's persistence to take back control over aspects of her life.

Joann explained how her own *inner openness* helped her overcome initial responses and respond in new ways: "*My own alarm buttons can be set off by what people say to me or by what I read and think... Nonetheless, I go into a room to speak to someone thinking 'All right, I'll leave this wide open and see what it is even if it really seems like it's going to be complicated, difficult, or painful. Maybe it won't be to the same degree. Maybe if I can leave this open enough I'll still be dealing with the not-so-nice aspects of a person but maybe not at the same level of intensity.'*"

Joann was in touch with her own bodily sensations and used her sixth and seventh senses (awareness of internal, bodily sensations and awareness of thoughts and feelings) to guide her actions.

Joann also showed *objectivity* in her work with Mrs. Chan. She identified with Mrs. Chan just enough to want to learn more about her, but not enough to be overwhelmed by Mrs. Chan's own distress that she could not see what was transpiring between Mrs. Chan and the staff. She also wanted to understand why the staff was distressed by Mrs. Chan's bathing ritual. She did not take sides until she had a chance to explore all perspectives and to explain why the staff and Mrs. Chan behaved as they did.

Finally, Joann mastered the art of *observation*. Her specific role, among her many roles, was to serve as a witness, observing and weaving together the many threads of Mrs. Chan's narrative. Over the course of the year, she observed Mrs. Chan's determination to recover some of her lost functions. At night, Mrs. Chan went on the stairwell, located just outside the unit, to practice going up and down the stairs to retrain her paralyzed leg to walk. Mrs. Chan showed the same gutsiness in dealing with this health challenge as she had during her lifetime.

Joann learned from Mrs. Chan that, as a young girl, she had fled China during the cultural revolution of the 1960s and come to Canada, where she rebuilt her life by taking advantage of opportunities. She was a woman of many talents, a highly respected teacher, businesswoman, artist, who had become a stalwart, trusted, and revered member of the local Chinese community. Joann had retrained her senses by developing a mindset guided by SBC. This was Joann's lens from which she viewed the world. It was in getting to know Mrs. Chan that she came to admire and respect her and forge a very special connection between them.

TOOLBOX: TOOLS FOR RETRAINING THE SENSES

In becoming a health professional, a significant amount of time is spent on training and retraining the senses through the acquisition of theoretical and formal knowledge concurrently with knowledge gained in practice. Every experience, each interaction, directly and indirectly influences the development of how senses are used to form observations; how observations become the basis for ideas; how ideas are reformulated to become concepts; and how concepts direct sensations and observations that, together, contribute to nurses' learning and subsequent ways of knowing. It is knowing that is at the heart of clinical practice, which in turn directs actions.

> Every experience and each interaction is an opportunity to develop the senses to form observations, to note how observations become the basis for ideas that evolve into concepts, and how concepts direct sensations and contribute to nurses' learning a way of knowing and a specific approach to practicing nursing.

There are many strategies and techniques that make up the nurse's toolbox to facilitate the retraining of the senses. In today's fast-paced, constantly changing world in which individuals are bombarded with choices and a vast array of learning opportunities, it is important to learn how to learn. In other words, it is important to understand the training process and to take charge and manage one's own learning activities (Bjork, 2011). In this section, I discuss some of these basic tools, which are based on the knowledge of how the brain rewires itself to "learn" and how we come to "know" ourselves and learn about the world. The former draws on ideas from the new cognitivism and the latter from phenomenology. Many people separate these two approaches as distinctly different and opposing, but I find there is overlap and draw inspiration from both.

Recall that the way the brain retrains itself is through three basic neurological processes (Siegel, 2010) as described earlier: (a) creating and strengthening synaptic connections, (b) stimulating new neurons to grow, and (c) increasing the sheathing along the axonal lengths to enhance the conduction speed of neuronal electrical impulses. Each of these processes affects the state of neuronal firings. With enough firings targeted at specific areas, the neuronal architecture of the brain and how it works can be altered or created. Thus, there are certain experiences that affect these neuronal processes, resulting in a retraining of the senses. In other words, it is having knowledge of these processes and using them to plan learning experiences that promote the retraining of the senses in learning to nurse and develop expertise in practice. The following three major forms of experiences develop and strengthen these neurological processes:

- Exposure to novelty
- Benefiting from mistakes and obstacles
- Practice and experience

A summary of these three major experiences, along with specific strategies for retraining the senses is found in Table 6.4.

Exposure to Novelty and New Situations

Novelty is important to learning. Many people believe that the human brain is attracted to new information and novel situations. Moreover, individuals often remember something new and are more likely to remember it if the context is somewhat familiar (Fenker & Schutze, 2009). When nursing students rotate between different clinical settings and nurse different patients, they are called on to use their senses in different ways. Some aspects of the situation may be familiar, whereas others may be novel, a surprise. The familiar, even that which occurred at some distant past and has been forgotten, can be recalled and relearned with greater efficiency if it becomes relevant again (Bjork, 2011). Paradoxically, the same applies to the unknown and the unfamiliar. Although novel information does not exist in memory, once it is encountered, it

TABLE 6.4

Summary of experiences for retraining the senses with suggested strategies to maximize learning

Experiences For Retraining the Senses	Suggested Strategies for Maximizing Learning
1. Exposure to novel experiences	• Taking time to reflect on what is new and novel • Taking time to write observations • Sharing observations with others
2. Benefitting from mistakes and obstacles	• Facing mistakes, not avoiding them • Seeking feedback • Overcoming obstacles by looking for opportunities and creating possibilities
3. Practice and experience	• Seeking out experiences just beyond one's comfort zone • Dialoguing about one's practice and experiences with peers • Observing, modeling, and imitating • Learning by teaching others • Mental imagery, rehearsing, considering hypothetical "what-if" situations • Developing a portfolio to assess progress and plan learning

is more likely to be encoded into memory. In fact, novel information often facilitates memory of the familiar. It is by attuning to the familiar and distinguishing what is novel in the situation that helps direct and focus the learner's attention. Consider the case of a student nurse working in a neonatal unit. In caring for a newborn, the nurse is expected to monitor the newborn to ensure that her systems are functioning; to detect subtle changes in her condition; and to distinguish the normal from the abnormal, the expected from the unexpected. Part of this assessment involves examining feces, not a normal activity in which the average person normally routinely engages unless one happens to be a parent. The nurse needs to retrain her senses as to what a 2-day-old infant's feces looks like, including its color, consistency, and odor. Moreover, the student nurse needs to learn to distinguish between the feces of a bottle-fed and a breastfed newborn to assess the baby's health and to pick up abnormalities that may signal that something may be wrong with the digestive system.

Take time to reflect on what is familiar, what is new and novel about the person, the health issues, and the nursing experience. It is important that a nurse takes the time to reflect on what he has just learned. Even with repeated exposure to the same experiences, learning is always new because the context always changes. Patients are unique, their situations and circumstances change, and their environments are never the same. It is important for a nurse to then become aware of what is new—what makes this experience different. In noticing, detecting, discriminating, and distinguishing specific features of the situation, a nurse can then identify important indicators that might be missed by an untrained eye. Nurses need to take time to think about what they have observed, place that observation in its new context, and ask themselves the following questions:

- What did I already know?
- What was new?
- What surprised me?
- Had I ever seen, heard, smelled, or felt anything like this before?

By answering these questions, nurses will focus on the novel, and, recall, it is the novel that is more likely to be remembered. Retraining involves novel information, including being in unfamiliar situations and dealing with problems and issues as a professional for the first time.

A nurse can also note whether the situation has a somewhat familiar "feel." Even first-time experiences may have elements that have been experienced before. In fact, the nurse may experience a feeling of déjà vu, a sense that she has been here before, that something about the person or the situation "feels" familiar. Tapping into the familiar, the slightly familiar, and even the novel, will help a nurse call forth and build on what he already knows. When an individual has to work to retrieve information and to encode it into memory, the likelihood that he will learn increases (Bjork, 2011).

Take time to record experiences in field notes or a journal. It is even better when a nurse records his experiences. In the process of recording an incident, writing about an event, describing what is known about a patient, and reconstructing their dialogue together, the nurse may become aware of a new detail or details that he hadn't considered previously. The act of writing causes the learner to slow down, process and review the information, and reflect on what has been learned. Memories may surface about things that were noticed or were heard but had not been registered into consciousness at the time. The nurse can then revisit the situation and, perhaps, see things in greater detail.

Detailed field notes or journaling should include a description of the event and its context, as well as the circumstances surrounding the event. This allows the nurse to re-create what happened. When observations are placed in context, it helps the person to encode the experience in memory, thereby making recall and retrieval easier (Siegel, 1999). After the nurse has described the event, she could add a reflective section to her notes, such as "what I learned" and "future questions to pursue." The nurse can follow up on her questions by consulting the literature or discussing the questions with her instructors, peers, expert nurses, and the like. It is also important that after writing field notes or entries in a journal to set aside time to re-read what was written. Rereading, remembering, rethinking, and reflecting are powerful tools that reinforce and strengthen neuronal connections, thereby enhancing learning and retraining the senses.

Share observations with teachers, preceptors, and peers. Another tool to retrain the senses is participating in clinical conferences, journal clubs, class discussions, or grand rounds. These forums afford nurses an opportunity to develop insights and to get in touch with their own thinking. These experiences contribute to learning in three ways. First, listening to oneself helps raise awareness about one's own ideas. Second, when others make comments or raise questions, this can stimulate new ideas, cause one to reinterpret the information from a different perspective, and consider new possibilities. Third, a skilled practitioner develops the ability to explain the salience of an observation by linking the observation to a specific action and a specific action to an observable outcome.

These strategies have one thing in common: They are important sources of feedback. Feedback is the fuel of reflection, and reflection is the mechanism that promotes new learning and is the means by which one comes to know. Exposure to novel situations that are then reflected on, and about which feedback is received, serve to reinforce and strengthen new neuronal connections. In continuing the example of retraining the senses to observe a newborn's feces, once the nurse has learned what to expect to see and smell in a newborn's feces, he will inten-

> Feedback is the fuel of reflection. Reflection is a habit of the mind that promotes new learning and is an important tool to retrain the senses.

tionally look at the quality of the stool and smell its odor in order to detect, discriminate, and distinguish subtle differences in the digestive processes of breastfed and bottle-fed newborns.

Benefiting from Mistakes and Obstacles

Another way to help retrain the senses is learning from obstacles and mistakes. Until recently, mistakes were viewed as negative. However, there is now growing evidence that making mistakes is an important experience that is required to learn. Taking this one step further, without making mistakes, learning is thwarted. Making mistakes—and, more to the point, learning from them—is involved in change. Apparently, overcoming obstacles and learning from mistakes help maintain myelin sheaths and create a well-integrated neuronal circuitry (Coyle, 2009). In fact, in a recent study, scientists discovered a protein that is responsible for correcting errors of neuronal connections within the cerebellum and that it often takes several attempts by this protein to make the correct connections. The cerebellum has very precise connectivity that allows the brain to use sensory information (input) and convert it into an exact motor response (output). It would appear that the incorrect connections last for only a relatively short period of time and are then removed once the correct connections have been made (Kalanovsky et al. 2011).

Face mistakes, don't avoid them. The most common way people deal with a mistake, error, obstacle, or perceived problem has been to avoid it by trying to either forget it happened, deny what happened, keep others from knowing how bad things are, refuse to think about it, wish for a miracle, drink and eat to excess, and the like (Edgar, 2010). The reason for these ways of coping with making mistakes is that mistakes often threaten an individual's sense of self, undermine self-esteem, and spark feelings of inadequacy and vulnerability. Mistakes are routinely met with criticism and accompanied by feelings of shame. Blame and shame go hand in hand.

For a long time, developmental psychologists and educators have known that learning from mistakes is a very effective way to learn something new. Now we have some insight into why this is the case. Coyle (2009) discovered that struggling or operating at the edges, trying something new or venturing into the unknown or unfamiliar territory, increases the likelihood of making errors and mistakes. Yet it is these very experiences that make a person smarter and help with memory retention. This is because the person is forced to slow down, think about what he has done wrong, refocus his attention, and correct the error. *Thinking, focusing,* and then *correcting* help to generate neuronal impulses, and the more impulses that are generated, the faster a person learns. Moreover, repetition adds layers to the myelin that sheaths axons and strengthens neuronal connections and conductivity. Thus, mistakes often result in the development of new skills and insights.

However, to learn from mistakes and be changed by them requires that one expend some time and effort. Think of a situation in which you made a mistake or something that you regretted doing. Take the time to reflect on what happened. Review the events leading up to the mistake, your own state of mind at the time (e.g., tired, preoccupied), personal factors (e.g., lack of knowledge, inadequate information, stress, or lack of sleep), and other factors within the system (e.g., miscommunication or poor communication) that may have contributed to the error, in order to understand and explain why things happened the way they did. Consider how different actions could have resulted in different outcomes. Now complete the "Reflect and Connect" exercise found in Exhibit 6.2.

Ask for feedback. Feedback is important in learning about both positive and negative aspects of mistakes. The nature, quality, and timing of the feedback are important factors that can influence how much one benefits from a mistake.

Feedback comes in many forms. One is formal feedback provided by others in the form of criticism, constructive suggestions, and compliments. When feedback is given in the form of criticism or in a negative, angry tone of voice, the person receiving the feedback often responds by shutting off her critics or shutting down her information-retrieval systems. She cannot hear the message and, if she does hear the

EXHIBIT 6.2

Reflect and connect *Critical incident report of an error or mistake*

Think of a situation in which you made a mistake or an error or something that you regretted doing. Take the time to reflect on what happened. Review the events leading up to the mistake, your own state of mind at the time (e.g., tired, preoccupied), personal factors (e.g., lack of knowledge, inadequate information), and other factors within the system (e.g., miscommunications, poor communication) that may have contributed to the error in order to understand and explain why things happened the way they did. Consider how different actions could have resulted in different outcomes and its impact on you and others.

1. **Details of the incident.**
   Describe the incident in as much detail as possible. Describe the events leading up to the incident. Describe what else was happening at the time. Who else was involved? What were their roles?

2. **Thoughts, feelings and concerns.**
   Describe your thoughts, feelings, and concerns just before the incident, at the time of the incident, and after the incident. How long did these thoughts and feelings last? What actions did you take to deal with these thoughts feelings and concern?

3. **Factors that you think contributed directly or indirectly.**
   List personal, family, and situational factors that played a direct or an indirect role in the incident. Explain why you think they played a role. Rate each factor as to its significance on a scale of 0 to 10, with 0 indicating *not at all significant* and 10 indicating *extremely significant*. Try to justify your rating.

4. **Impact on yourself, my family, others.**
   Describe how this incident affected you personally and professionally. Has it affected any one else in your family circle, social circle, or work circle? If yes, describe whom it has affected and how they have been affected.

5. **What you have learned.**
   Describe any changes in your mood, attitude, ways of behaving and any other emotional or behavioral responses since the incident. What actions have you taken to deal with this experience? How helpful have these actions? Explain. How are you feeling now?

feedback, its message can be distorted or misinterpreted. The way to handle this type of feedback is not to respond immediately. It is important to take some time to let one's emotions and tempers subside before discussing the matter. Another technique to defuse a negative, potentially volatile situation is to say, "I know I have made a mistake and I want to learn from it. Can I make an appointment to see you at another time after I have had a chance to think about it?" In handling the situation in these ways, both parties have a chance to cool down and cool off. It allows the person to focus on the content of the feedback and not on the negative emotions arising from the feedback. The person can then take the time to review and reflect on what happened, why it happened, what he learned from the incident, and consider how best not to repeat the mistake.

Positive feedback, which reinforces what one has done well, is just as important for learning. Often, a nurse may not be aware of the how her nursing has affected others. Increasing the level of awareness of what she has done well increases the chances of intentionally repeating an action or behavior. Positive feedback helps one develop strengths.

The most useful feedback is that which gives examples of specific behaviors rather than feedback that deals in generalities. Corrective feedback points out what was right or wrong. The person provides specific examples from the incident to illustrate his points. This form of feedback enhances future performance.

The timing of feedback can have an important effect on behavior. Researchers found that, when people were learning a technique or how to perform a new procedure, they profited the most from a simulated practice session when feedback was given immediately afterward (Boyle et al., 2011). Students' learning curves were smoother and faster, and they subsequently made fewer errors. However, there are situations when delaying feedback is more beneficial than when feedback is given immediately. In situations where students need time and space to process the experience, delayed feedback may be more informative and effective (Metcalfe, 2011).

Attend to the sixth and seventh senses and develop these senses. Few journeys are ever smooth. Everyone faces obstacles, bumps, and hitches while working toward a goal. Some people are easily deterred and give up, while others find alternative routes. The latter group tends to remove obstacles, create detours, and continuously seek opportunities. They train their senses to see possibilities. They do so by relying on their sixth and seventh senses (viz., awareness of bodily sensations and awareness of their own thoughts and feelings) to guide them. They have come to listen and trust their 'inner voice' and are in tune with their 'gut' reactions. Experienced clinicians have a well-honed intuitive sense (Benner et al., 2011). Intuition develops through reflecting on action, trying out different things to see what works, and analyzing why certain solutions worked or didn't work. Expert nurses, who rely on their intuition to guide them in practice, treat every experience as a learning opportunity. They learn from every experience: trial and error, successes, mistakes, and failures. They also use what they have learned in their personal lives to benefit and guide decisions in their professional lives.

Intuitive learning is a form of implicit learning. The reason that an individual often cannot articulate the basis for his decisions is because information is being processed in the deeper regions of the brain, namely, the subcortex, which is not immediately connected to the higher regions of the cortex, where rational thinking takes place (Siegel, 2010). More specifically, brain imaging data have revealed that the caudate and putamen, in the basal ganglia of the brain, are central components of both intuition and implicit learning, supporting the relationship between the two concepts of learning (Lieberman, 2000). Intuition develops with experience. Intuitive learners are not impulsive because they know the importance of waiting for the right moment to act. They welcome obstacles, for they know that often an alternative route turns out to be a better route.

Practice and Experience

Few ideas can be learned from a book alone. Proper training of the senses can come about only from understanding the theoretical while learning from experience.

For a long time, it was well known that practice and experience were essential for developing new competences and acquiring new skills, as summed up in the well-known adage that "practice makes perfect." What has been unclear is the number of hours required to achieve expert status in a given craft or field—that is, until now.

There is growing evidence that a specific number of hours are required to develop a competency, refine a skill, and retrain a sense. In the bestselling book *Outliers*, Malcolm Gladwell (2008) popularized the idea of the "10,000-hour rule." In a nutshell, if a person wants to shine in her chosen field, she needs to put in 10,000 hours acquiring knowledge, perfecting that skill, and honing that talent through practice.

The apprenticeship model of training is based on diverse experiences of many hours of practice. Almost all craftsmen learn their trade through apprenticeship. They spend the better part of each day mastering their chosen field by acquiring formal knowledge; observing a master; having experiences in different areas; and practicing, practicing, practicing basic skills of their trade until they have mastered them. Consider that it takes 10 years to become a master sushi chef and head chef, and 8 years to become a master carpenter or master gardener. Professionals agree that, regardless of training, the most important route to becoming a master is by having the "right" experiences and then being given opportunities to practice and deepen one's knowledge and perfect one's skills.

Benner, inspired by the Dreyfus Model of Skill Acquisition, identified the five levels of skill proficiency in becoming a nurse—(a) novice, (b) advanced beginner, (c) competent, (d) proficient, and (e) expert (Benner, 1984; Dreyfus & Dreyfus, 1996)—and found that it took 7 years to progress from novice to expert. Not everyone will achieve expert status even with 7 or more years of experience; however, they will develop expertise in a given area. Nonetheless, achieving some level of competency requires practice, and with more practice, there is an increased likelihood of developing expertise in a chosen clinical specialty.

With repeated practice, neuronal connections are strengthened until they become so well established that they are an integral part of a person's neurological circuitry. With repeated practice, a nurse becomes more perceptually aware. She develops and hones her perceptual acuity by becoming more aware of and attuned to subtleties, pays attention and notices the smallest detail, discriminates among differences, and sees similarities and patterns that would otherwise be missed by the untrained eye or by an inexperienced clinician. When previously unrelated neurons begin to work together, they learn how to fire more effectively together and with greater dependability.

> With repeated practice, the nurse becomes more aware of subtleties, notices the smallest detail, detects distinctions between seemingly unrelated data, and identifies similarities and patterns that would otherwise be missed by the untrained eye or by the inexperienced clinician

Practice through simulated learning. Until the relatively recent advent of simulation learning, health care professionals acquired knowledge and skills in the classroom and then applied what they had learned in the clinical area with patients without the benefit of prior practice. Patients were placed at risk and treated as "guinea pigs", and learners did not have the benefit of practicing a skill, of being able to make mistakes and correct them before trying things out on a "real" patient.

Advancements in simulated learning equipment technology, such as the medium- to high-fidelity patient simulators, have made simulated learning an integral aspect of most nursing curricula. Case studies and role play, using trained actors, are also used to help nurses learn skills and acquire the necessary competence and confidence before meeting and caring for actual patients in the hospital or clients at home.

Simulation has become an increasingly important teaching strategy in most nursing programs. The two theoretical orientations of simulation learning are (a) experiential learning and (b) situated learning. *Experiential learning* occurs when the student is fully engaged in an experience, particularly when the experience is relevant and related to the theoretical idea being learned. *Situated learning,* on the other hand, is premised on the idea that most learning has some element that is specific to a given situation and that learning is enhanced when that which is being learned is placed in its rightful context (Anderson, Reder, & Simon, 1996).

In a concept analysis of simulation learning, Bland, Topping, and Wood (2011) identified four critical attributes of what constitutes simulation learning: (a) creating a hypothetical opportunity that was (b) an authentic representation of real life practice; (c) active engagement of students in learning; and (d) repetition, evaluation, and reflection. For example, for simulation to be effective, it had to be warranted because the actual experience was not available. However, the simulation has to be based on real cases, not constructed ones that exist only in the imagination of those making them up. The learning environment has to encourage interaction. Finally, the simulation has to be of such quality as to be able to motivate students to want to be involved in learning.

High-fidelity simulation learning has been shown to be an effective substitute for traditional clinical learning experiences. However, what is the evidence that students learn clinical skills? Does this form of learning experience translate into effective performance? Gates and his colleagues asked these very questions. The findings of their study are found in Exhibit 6.3.

Seek out experiences that are difficult—just beyond the learner's competency. One of the most effective ways to retrain the senses is to seek out learning experiences that are moderately challenging. Experiences that have a desirable degree of difficulty have been found to enhance memory (Metcalfe, 2011; McDaniel & Butler, 2011). In other words, individuals should not seek the easy route but one that challenges and pushes them slightly beyond what they have already mastered (Metcalfe, 2011). A complementary theory that enhances learning was proposed by the Russian developmental psychologist Lev Vygotsky (1978), who proposed that optimal learning is exposing children to learning opportunities in the *zone of proximal development.* If an experience or learning activity is found to be too easy or is too familiar, the individual often responds by becoming bored, and the activity becomes too routine. In these situations, the individual—in this case, the nurse—goes on automatic pilot and zones out. On the other hand, if the challenge is beyond the individual's capabilities and competencies,

EXHIBIT 6.3

Empirical study *Enhancing nursing knowledge using high-fidelity simulation*

The Problem

The use of high-fidelity simulation as an accepted substitute for traditional clinical learning experiences in nursing education has gained acceptance over the past decade. The California Board of Registered Nursing now allows up to 25% of student clinical learning to occur in simulation laboratories, the hypotheses being that the students who participate in a simulation experience will have a higher score on an examination of course content covered in the simulation than students who did not participate in that simulation.

The Issues

Little research evidence has documented the efficacy of simulated learning experiences, particularly on objective outcomes such as examination performance.

The Study

This study examined the effects of high-fidelity simulation participation on knowledge acquisition in 104 undergraduate nursing students. All 104 nursing students enrolled in the course agreed to participate in the study. The students were part of 12 clinical groups, each of which were randomly assigned to either the gastrointestinal (GI) bleed or pulmonary embolism (PE) simulation scenario. A total of 53 students took part in the PE simulation, whereas 51 students participated in the GI bleed simulation.

The Findings

The results from both the PE and GI bleed models indicate there is more than an 8% increase in examination performance for students who participated in high-fidelity simulation compared with those who did not. Further, as all students had equal access to the information tested on the examinations, meaning that the simulation experience did not include any additional new information that was not already covered in course material. The 8% increase is equivalent to an increase of almost one full letter grade when viewed on a traditional grading scale.

The Bottom Line

The findings provide beginning evidence that high-fidelity simulation can be an effective substitute for traditional clinical experience.

Source: Adapted from Gates, Parr, & Hughen, (2011).

when left alone, without support and scaffolding (i.e., assisting another person and giving him the competencies and skills that he is missing or has yet to develop), the individual may become frustrated and give up. This is what happens when a person becomes overwhelmed and decides to quit rather than to persevere.

Both frameworks (i.e., desirable level of difficulty and zone of proximal development) stimulate, contribute, and enhance learning, particularly when the learner is actively involved. The person needs to select learning opportunities that have a desired level of difficulty and to be in a zone just beyond her comfort level. In selecting an experience or learning activity, the nurse must first be aware of her own capabilities, competencies, and level of mastery. Then, she needs to seek out activities that she considers to be desirable that will contribute to her own development as a nurse. Finally, she needs to ask for corrective feedback and to select experiences that are familiar yet different enough to intrigue, to stretch her abilities to acquire new knowledge and skills.

Dialogue about your practice and experiences with supervisors, peers, and colleagues. Nurses advance their knowledge when they dialogue with others about their own experiences. There are many forums in which to share experiences, including clinical conferences, case presentations, grand rounds, and the like. Sharing experiences can occur one on one, during small group discussion, and in more formal presentations. In preparing for a presentation, discussing an issue with peers, the nurse has an opportunity to organize her thoughts and to reflect on what she already knows as well as what she doesn't know. She also has time to think about the meaning of an experience by asking herself: "What was it about the situation or the patient that is interesting, problematic, or challenging?" In the process of preparing for a presentation, the nurse has an opportunity to get in touch with her own thoughts and feelings. This activity brings the experience to a higher level of awareness. In other words, the experience had been processed in the "low road" or subcortical region of the brain and, by reflecting on it at the cortex level, the nurse is conscious of what made the experience significant. Engaging in this process of reflection and thinking helps the nurse to develop her seventh sense.

Observe, model, and imitate. An important human learning mechanism is to observe somebody you admire and wish to be like. This observation and imitation of a role model is known as *social learning*. In wanting to be like the role model, and adopting some of the role model's attitudes and behaviors, a person will attend more carefully to details of the role model's behavior. The first step in the process is to identify a person who can serve as a role model and then to pay careful attention to what the role model is doing and why he is doing it. When the role model explains why he looked for what he did, and explains how he did something, the observer will be more likely to reproduce or 'imitate' that behavior and try out what has been observed. Both good and bad practices are acquired through modeling another's behavior.

Learn by teaching others. One of the most effective ways to retrain the senses is to teach others. The famous Chinese teacher and philosopher of the 5th century BC, Confucius, wrote: "I hear and I forget. I see and I remember. I do and I understand." Mel Silberman (1996), a proponent of active learning, elaborates on this:

> What I hear, I forget.
> What I hear and see, I begin to understand.
> What I hear, see, discuss, and do, I acquire knowledge and skill.
> *What I teach to another, I master.*

In teaching others, nurses must first get in touch with what they did and the reasons for their choices and actions. To teach another person, the teacher must first become a student, a learner.

Mental imagery, rehearsing, and considering hypothetical "what-if" situations. Perceptual learning is, as the name implies, learning to perceive differently (Tartaglia, Barmert, Mast, & Herzog, 2009). Extended training and repeated practice improve one's performance. This is thought to occur because of changes in neural synapses brought about by repetitive and repeated stimulation. Moreover, one can bring about such changes in the synapses just by using mentally generated signals. In other words, imagining a practice situation in the absence of actually engaging in it can improve perceptual learning.

Rehearsing, a form of imagery training, is commonly used in nursing education to prepare for clinical practice. Rehearsing involves reviewing what could happen and thinking about different ways of responding before the nurse is in the actual clinical situation (Benner et al., 2010). Pilots rehearse flight paths before embarking on a mission. Surgeons practice and review in their mind a complicated surgery before actually performing it.

All of simulation learning is about practicing and rehearsing, both in real life and in one's mind, before engaging in the actual event, including interacting with a person and family or performing a procedure. Not only does rehearsing prime nurses to anticipate what could happen but it also helps prepare them to respond in different situations should they happen. When nurses think in terms of "what-if"s, they are imagining and thinking through different eventualities so that if a particular situation does occur, they will be better prepared to respond (Benner et al., 2010). Imagining and rehearsing strengthen neural synapses in the brain that result in improved performance. This means that rehearsing before entering the clinical field, thinking about it, and considering "what-if" hypothetical situations are important strategies for retraining the senses.

Develop a portfolio to assess progress and plan learning. Many professionals have used a portfolio to document and keep track of their progress. Think of architects, designers, and artists who carry around large black cases that contain materials as proof of their accomplishments. A portfolio usually contains papers, drawings, projects, comments of others, and so forth. Health care professionals are now beginning to use portfolios in their work.

A portfolio is simply a collection of materials used for many purposes: to facilitate professional development by encouraging self-assessment and self-reflective skills, document professional achievements, show how course content can be used to further develop expertise in practice, and keep track of progress made to attain learning outcomes. A portfolio also can be used as proof of one's competence. In short, a portfolio encourages and promotes responsibility in directing one's own learning, and serves as a tool to guide lifelong learning and chart professional growth (Pearce, 2003).

What types of materials would nurses collect for their portfolio? The contents should reflect what and how the portfolio is being used at various points in a nurse's professional career. As an educational tool to encourage professional training, it could contain the student's own learning objectives listing the knowledge, values, attitude, competency skills, and behaviors one would like to achieve at different stages of a program of study; plans for meeting the objectives; and, finally, the evidence to illustrate how those objectives were met. It could contain course materials, course plans, field notes with supervisors' comments, papers, exams, clinical evaluations and the like.

A portfolio should also contain narrative accounts of specific clinical encounters and incidents, narratives and case studies of patients' illness experiences, and reflective notes on what made these particular experiences seminal and memorable, in short, turning points in becoming a nurse and expert practitioner. In fact, using narratives and case studies of real patient situations is a critical learning strategy to help the learner integrate content and weave together the many themes and threads of a person's story (Ironside, 2006). Analyzing, discussing, interpreting, questioning, and reflecting are involved in clinical reasoning and thinking (Benner et al., 2010; 2011). These strategies help one develop habits of the mind. Furthermore, narrative pedagogy relies on analyses and interpretations, and is an important tool that helps one see possibilities and unfolding realities, learn how to deal with ambiguity and uncertainty, and consider situations from multiple perspectives (Ironside, 2003; 2006)

If the nurse is using a portfolio to track professional development, then it is important to set aside time at regular intervals to review the material in it. If the purpose is to advance and track one's learning progress and set direction for future learning, the portfolio can be beneficial at the end of a unit of study to examine and reflect on where one began at the start of a new course; what one has learned; and what experiences, both positive and negative, advanced or contributed to learning. If the portfolio is being used to develop skills and demonstrate competence, it should contain evidence of skills achieved. If the goal is to further one's own learning and develop specific competencies, then it is important to identify one's own learning needs and develop a learning plan, outlining a program of study and the strengths and resources that will be needed to make this happen. These learning needs should be realistic, specific, and achievable (Pearce, 2003)

Key Summary Points

- The ideas of retraining the senses for clinical practice have been inspired by the work of Patricia Benner (2010; 2011) and Daniel Siegel (2004; 2008; 2010), even though each represents different schools of thought: Benner belongs to the school of interpretative phenomenology and Siegel to the new cognitivism.
- The formation of a person's sensory system is determined by the interaction of that individual's sensory organs with sensory stimuli and the interpretation of those stimuli in specific areas of the brain. Sensory systems respond to the person, family, physical surroundings, and other environmental stimuli that, together with information from internal sensations of the body, create *representations*, or new ways of understanding and knowing.
- The sensory system consists of five "outer" senses: (a) sight, (b) sound, (c) taste, (d) smell, and (e) touch, which are responsible for transmitting stimuli from the outside to the brain. In addition, the person's whole being, including brain and body, responds to two "inner" senses as well: awareness of (a) internal bodily sensations and (b) the thoughts, feelings, and intentions of every person involved in one's relationships, which allow a person to be aware of his own self as well as of another person (intuition).

- Becoming a nurse requires a retraining of the sensory systems to focus on information that is clinically relevant, such as new sights, sounds, smells, taste, and touch, and increasing self-awareness of sensations arising from one's own body. Nurses need to be attuned to, discern, and then train their senses to meet practice demands of their professional roles in order to be responsive to their patients.
- Retraining requires a nurse to have a mindset of openness, objectivity, and observation.
- Different domains of clinical nursing practice require senses to be retrained for different purposes, to work in specific settings, deal with different medical conditions and clinical issues, and work with specific groups of persons and family.
- Retraining the senses for SBC requires that a nurse be retrained to assess for what is working, what is functioning, and what the patient/client/family does best, in addition to what is not working while taking into account different settings, specialties, and populations.
- Nurses need to develop a toolbox for retraining the senses. These tools can greatly help in retraining the nurse's neurological processes. There are specific tools and strategies under the three major forms of experience: (a) exposure to novelty and new situations, (b) being able to benefit from mistakes and obstacles, and (c) exposure to repeated practice and experiences. There are specific tools or strategies involved in rewiring the brain and consequently in retraining the senses.

Nursing's Professional Gaze: Observations for Clinical Judgment and Decision Making

7

LEARNING OBJECTIVES

After reading this chapter, you should be able to:

- Explain clinical and critical inquiry and the role each plays in developing the nurse's professional gaze, clinical reasoning, and decision making
- Identify the different meanings associated with the term *observation*
- List the essential elements of the observation process, including what, why, who, when and where to observe
- Identify the components of observation and how each relates to perception, memory, and interpretation
- Describe the five external senses and their role in observational acuity
- Describe how salience, relevance, and relatedness contribute to judging the effectiveness of an observation and the tools for improving each

Leaning across the bed behind him, the doctor placed her stethoscope at precise points on Phil's back, and began to listen. As she listened she created around herself a screen of privacy. Her eyes disengaged. She folded herself into the stethoscope, in toward Phil's back, attending to the sound as a musician might. Then she began concentrating on an area midway down his right side. She was tracking something within his body, moving the stethoscope an inch to the left, and inch to the right, as if comparing two notes. Suddenly she was satisfied, and leaned back, tugging the stethoscope out of her ears. Kathleen Jamie, poet (cited in Atkinson, Macnaughton, Saunders, & Evans, 2010, p. 1733)

Using Jeannie as an intermediary to relay the words that were too painful for her to tell her family herself, she apologizes because she no longer has the strength to continue fighting. That isn't living, she tells them. "I am ready to die," she whispers weakly.

But they interrupt, try to contradict her, and promise that there is still hope.

Jeannie Chaisson [primary nurse] stands silently during this exchange and then intervenes, asking them to try to take in what their loved one is telling them. Then she repeats the basic facts about the disease and its course. "At this point we have no treatment for the disease," she explains. "But we do have treatment for the pain, and we can make her comfortable and ease the suffering." Jeannie spends another hour simply sitting with them, answering their questions and allowing them to feel supported. The family is finally able to heed the wishes of the patient—to leave in the catheter, not to resuscitate her if she suffers a cardiac arrest. Give her enough morphine to stop her feeling pain. Let her go.

The woman visibly relaxes, lies back, and closes her eyes. Jeannie approaches the husband and daughter with whom she has worked for so long and, with a look of great sympathy and affection, hugs them both in turn. Then she goes out to talk to the medical team.

Before leaving to go home, Jeannie again visits her patient. The husband and daughter have gone for a cup of coffee. The woman is quiet. Jeannie sits down at the side of her bed and takes her hand. The woman opens her eyes. Too exhausted to say a word, she merely squeezes Jeannie's hand in gratitude. For the past three years, Jeannie has helped her fight the disease and live as long as possible. Now she is here to help her with her most difficult work. She is helping her to die. (Suzanne Gordon, 1997, p. 11)

Part of being human is having the ability to gaze. A *gaze* is the way in which one person looks on another and how the other person looks back. A professional's gaze can be both literal and metaphorical (Shapiro, 2002). The literal gaze is about how the health care professional observes, looks at, inspects, assesses, analyzes, and interprets an issue or a situation. At a metaphorical level, a gaze symbolizes the broader, more intangible dimension of the relationship. It is about how two people come to gaze on one another, the connections that they make, and the meanings that are created. This view is in stark contrast to that of philosopher Michel Foucault (1973), the philosopher, who coined the term *medical gaze* to refer to the detached, objectifying gaze of medicine that precludes meeting and acknowledging the patient (P. Benner, personal communication, December 13, 2011).

The medical gaze focuses on understanding the medical condition for the purpose of arriving at an accurate diagnosis and prescribing an effective course of treatment. The gaze tends to dissect, segment, and disassemble. The first passage presented at the beginning of this chapter eloquently captures the physician's clinical gaze. As Atkinson and colleagues (2010) wrote:

> Poet Kathleen Jamie's account of the clinical examination of her husband, the physician's stethoscope makes a connection to the patient that enables a cool intimacy that is both intensely caring in the attentiveness to the specific body and impersonal and abstract in the application of generic knowledge. (p. 1733)

On the other hand, nursing's professional gaze is about understanding uniqueness, wholeness, and strengths. Nursing involves knowing: knowing the person, family, and community, their strengths and what defines their uniqueness. This involves knowing the person and family, their history, circumstances, and situation. It is about knowing their hopes, goals, and dreams, as well as knowing the person's physical and emotional responses to his medical condition and treatment. It also involves knowing the person and family's health and illness experiences and narratives. It is this knowledge and knowing that their nurse needs to have in order to help the patient, client, and family cope with their challenges.

The second passage at the chapter's beginning sensitively captures the work of one nurse's clinical gaze. Journalist Suzanne Gordon's account of Nurse Jeannie Chaisson, who served as the intermediary between her patient and the patient's family, encompasses life and death; despair, anguish, and peaceful acceptance; letting go and connecting; suffering and healing. Jeannie's very presence is the instrument of comfort, skilled know-how, and advocacy. Jeannie has the capacity to be fully present, attentive, and authentic; to know when to listen and when to explain; when to mediate and when to comfort; when to act and when to step back; and when to lead and when to follow. Nursing's professional gaze is a tapestry that comprises many threads of knowledge and technical skills woven together and applied with compassion and a commitment to caring and moral being.

Thus, nursing requires technical expertise and skill in engaging, forming, and developing helping relationships, as well as skilled know-how in practical, ethical, and clinical reasoning (Dreyfus, Dreyfus, & Benner, 2009). Each of these aspects of nursing is dependent on nurses' development of their own professional gaze, which is shaped by their nursing orientation and clinical experiences. Nurses need to develop their gaze—both the literal and metaphorical gazes—to be able to systematically assess the person and family by becoming involved and connected with them while at the same time learning to be objective in their observations. This is the delicate balance that nurses must strike if they are to provide exquisite nursing care.

INTERRELATED THINKING PROCESSES

Nursing practice could be described as "a set of nursing actions to achieve specific clinical outcomes." If we limit the description of nursing practice to this conception, we would be doing nursing a disservice, because it is a rather simplistic description. Nursing is a far more intricate and complex enterprise (Ellefson, Kim, & Han, 2007). Nursing actions, activities, and interactions are an outgrowth of complex thinking processes. What determines the nature of the way a particular nurse engages with a particular patient in a particular situation and in a particular way is shaped by many factors. Ellefson and her colleagues (2007) identified three interrelated processes involved in the "thinking" work of clinical nursing practice: (a) professional gaze; (b) clinical construction, and (c) clinical engagement.

Clinical work begins with nursing's professional gaze. The term *professional gaze* indicates the clinician's "ways of knowing and perceiving, a particular stance towards the world" (Lawlor, 2003, p. 30). A nurse's gaze is affected by many things, but foremost her gaze is shaped by her values and beliefs, which are reflected in her nursing orientation and frames of references (see Chapter 2). These determine what the nurse selects to attend to and where she then directs her energy, efforts, and actions.

Clinical work also involves *clinical construction*, which includes all the "thinking" work of figuring out the problem that has yet to be identified and, then, putting together the puzzle in need of solving. It includes a number of thinking processes, including clinical grasp, clinical reasoning and clinical decision making (Benner et al., 2011).

Clinical reasoning begins with having a clinical grasp of the situation. The nurse's clinical grasp directs clinical judgments, which then serve as the basis for clinical decision making and subsequent actions. Together, these tasks direct clinical engagement, that is, how the nurse relates to and enters into a relationship with the person and family.

Nurse Sarah Shea described a brief encounter with Mr. and Mrs. Mustafa, a young couple from Syria, whose newborn son, Ishmael, was taken to the children's hospital for emergency cardiac surgery. Sarah met the Mustafas on the unit as she was preparing Ishmael for open-heart surgery. She accompanied this couple through the ups and downs of their son's illness journey—from diagnosis, to surgery, to recovery. The diagnosis came as a surprise, as did their son's need for surgery. The surgery was long and difficult, as was the post-op course. Ishmael had several cardiac arrest episodes and other complications.

Sarah described why she became involved with the Mustafas prior to, during, and immediately following their son's surgery: *"One could be blind or one could see the distress in this family both physically and emotionally. I chose to become involved with them. I think it sounds silly to say, but this is what we do as nurses—it is just who we are and we make conscious decisions in our interventions. In terms of launching into that process, it comes to the point where it's not a choice. You launch into that process of gathering data the moment you see them; you start speculating, hypothesizing, identifying risks, strengths, and deficits. You start putting that together almost subconsciously."*

In gathering information, observing, listening, and attending to what is happening, Sarah began to construct a picture of this couple: *"This was a family that needed a nurse and they needed nursing. And it was very easy as they were so engaging, just to launch in and realize very quickly that they were under enormous stress, had few resources, were fairly isolated, but did have some strengths—so let's work with these."*

Sarah identified a number of the Mustafas' strengths as individuals and as a couple that proved critical to her success in connecting with them and subsequently affected how she worked with them: *"[They were] intelligent, articulate, and with unity as a couple. I think they were able to prioritize within themselves what their own needs were. They were able to recognize that bringing in other family members was not going to help. They were able to put into place that support in advance. In terms of friends, I think they were kind of isolated. They felt that they would have to care for friends instead of having their friends care for them."*

Sarah also described why she was able to engage them as a couple: *"This was a family that was fairly open to my being there in the first place. This was not a closed family; they were fairly open to approach, so it was fairly easy to build rapport with them. We didn't have to struggle with that at all. I basically had to say hello and they were receptive. I think they were also looking for any lifeline that they could get, because this was hours before their child went into the operatingroom."*

Sarah's clinical construction varies with the events that unfold as she senses the situation and responds sensitively to changing circumstances. In preparing Ishmael and Mr. and Mrs. Mustafa for surgery, Sarah stayed with them, ensured that they had access to their son, answered their questions, and helped them navigate the system. During the operation, Sarah's role was one of comforter. She carried out this role by being available, being fully and attentively present when she was with them, and by giving them instrumental support.

"I was able to sit with the family and hold hands, pass tissues, and bring glasses of water. At this point, this is what they really needed. My goal was instrumental support—just to keep them literally conscious. They were so overwhelmed—even hyperventilating. I was concerned for them and for their physical well-being. I gave them time to be alone as a couple. I also made myself available to answer any questions as they came along. I also focused on pulling in strengths from the family, as they preferred to stay isolated as a couple. They had family here in the city, and when I offered to call people in they preferred not to. They didn't want grandparents coming in. They said that that would actually increase their anxiety. And with time they were able to digest what was happening with the support we were able to provide with teaching and drawing on past experience. The couple, whenever they had tough times before, preferred just to be together and remain quiet. That's how they always had done things in the past. They would walk and walk and walk and I would bring in whatever updates I could get."

Sarah began her clinical work by identifying with and bearing witness to this young couple's stress and distress. She found herself unable to ignore or turn a blind eye to their suffering because her own professional gaze did not allow her to act otherwise. In reflecting back over this experience, Sarah felt that she was successful in meeting this couple's needs in a way that they had wanted her to. Sarah attributed her success to her ability to connect with this couple, to shift her focus as the situation changed, work with this couple from a position based on what she already knew about them and what she subsequently learned, and to capitalize and work with their strengths. She had gathered this information over the course of several shifts because she had taken the time to observe and to spend time talking with them, getting to know them and what they wanted for their son and their family.

"I spent a total of five or six shifts with them over six weeks. It was a family in definite distress. There was no denying that. On two separate events, I just felt that without the benefit and support of nursing, their stress wouldn't have been mitigated at all. If we had just been there to push drugs on this child or if I'd let them stay in the parents' room (on the unit) and hadn't spoken to them at all or spent any time with them their stress levels would have been astronomical. I do feel that what we were able to do (referring to herself and her colleagues) was because we were all on the same page. Whenever we would sign off, we would say 'Oh, I was able to do this for the family, I was able to do that.' By the end of their stay in hospital, their son was doing better than what we had expected. . . . We were able to get them through the rough patches until they were able to see him, and we were able to get them to relax a little bit. They were able to say that they were feeling a little less stressed, that their stress was more manageable, and they could get through this crisis. They were able to talk about their

feelings a bit more and to formulate their thoughts to a greater extent. We, as nurses, were able to have an impact."

Thus, clinical engagement begins with nursing's unique, professional gaze. It is the nurse's values and beliefs about nursing that direct observations. Nurses need to train and retrain their senses to become astute observers. Accurate and detailed observations are required for clinical reasoning and clinical decision making. More specifically, it is the thinking work of nursing that directs nurses' actions to achieve specific outcomes.

However, we have seen only the surface of some of the thinking work of nursing: The processes involved are far more complex and involve reasoning, emotion, being in touch with one's own internal bodily sensations, analyzing and synthesizing various pieces of information, and the like. Having said this, a question still needs to be asked and addressed at a very basic level: What is the thinking work of nursing and what does it involve?

THE ART OF CLINICAL THINKING

Clinical judgment and clinical decision making are endpoints of the clinical reasoning process in which nurses take action based on their understanding and assessment of the presenting problem, issue, or concern. Some researchers have said that clinical judgment is considered the "assessment of alternative actions," whereas clinical decision making is considered "choosing between alternatives" (Dowie, 1993). Benner, Tanner, and Chesla (1996) defined clinical judgment as "the ways in which nurses come to understand the problems, issues, or concerns of client/patients, to attend to salient information and to respond in concerned and involved ways" (p. 2). Clinical judgment and decisions often follow from an understanding or clinical grasp of the situation.

Clinical Grasp

Clinical grasp is the orienting activity in which the nurse situates the information that he has gathered about the patient and the patient's situation. To arrive at a clinical grasp of a situation, the nurse needs to know what information to attend to and then evaluate the aspects of that information that are clinically salient, that is, important. It also involves honing one's skills of perceptual acuity so that one's observations are accurate (Benner et al., 2011). In deciding what information is salient (i.e., important), the nurse needs to develop skill in making qualitative distinctions among different pieces of information and then prioritizing those pieces of information in terms of their degree of importance.

An essential aspect of nurses' education involves developing their sense of salience. A sense of salience is acquired in the classroom and, in the clinical setting, through nursing patients, clients, and families. There are many pedagogical approaches to develop salience, such as when an instructor or teacher selects an experience to teach a specific concept, draws the students' attention to specific information, points out the significance of an observation, focuses on and reinforces certain concepts, draws relationships between disparate behaviors, or directs the students to pay attention to some information while explaining why other information is of less significance (Benner et al., 2011).

Learning to nurse also requires developing *habits of the mind,* a term that refers to a set of thinking skills that are needed to analyze a situation in order to learn and to arrive at some new understandings. These skills include asking questions (see Chapter 8 and 9), self-reflection and mindfulness (see Chapter 5), listening to patients' stories and ongoing narratives (see Chapter 8), and benefitting from one's own personal and professional experiences and the experiences of others by reflecting, relating, and connecting.

Learning from experience is an ongoing process. It involves understanding how context shapes a person's behavior and illness experience. It also requires that nurses gather considerable information about the patient and family about their concerns. It also involves trying to understand the nature of their issues by integrating new information into what is already known, identifying patterns of responses, and shaping and reshaping what has been learned and understood in a different light (insight; Rashotte & Carnevale, 2004).

Dr. Daniel Siegel (2010) identified four streams of awareness that are involved in clinical work (as introduced in Chapter 5). These four streams are referred to as SOCK—*S*ensations, *O*bservation, *C*oncepts, and *K*nowing:

1. *Sensations* are the most direct input of data into one's field of awareness. They emanate from reactions to external events and feelings that are registered within own body
2. *Observation* is the capacity to sense one's self and witness unfolding experiences
3. *Concepts* are constructed ideas and models of a person's inner and outer worlds. The inner world is how you personally experience an event or see yourself, whereas the outer world is the ways others view you
4. *Knowing* is a nonconceptual, nonlanguage–based way of understanding that is commonly thought of as intuition

These streams of awareness operate at all times and in all clinical situations. Consider the nurse who is getting a patient out of bed for the first time postoperatively. The patient is in pain and moves gingerly. The nurse knows from studying post-op recovery that patients are at risk for fainting when they first get out of bed. Consider the following scenario: As the nurse prepares to get the patient out of bed for the first time since surgery, he is aware that his heart is beating faster and that his abdominal muscles are more taut than usual (a sensation). He notices that, as the patient sits at the edge of the bed, the patient turns ashen and complains of feeling lightheaded and dizzy (an observation). The nurse believes that the patient is going to faint (based on the concept of the physiology of the autonomic nervous system's response to a sudden change in position that results in a dramatic drop of blood pressure accompanied by peripheral vasoconstriction). He senses that she is going to faint (an example of knowing something intuitively before having a chance to analyze what is about to happen). The nurse has a clinical grasp of the situation and therefore moves closer to the patient to prevent her from falling (using his clinical judgment and clinical decision-making skills). The nurse rings the call bell for additional help and, with his arm firmly planted on the patient's neck and back, gets the patient to lie back onto the pillows before she actually faints.

The nurse then applies a cool compress to the back of the patient's neck. With the assistance of an aide, the nurse places the patient in a Trendelenberg position (i.e., lying the patient flat on her back in a supine position and elevating the foot of the bed so that the patient's legs and feet are higher than her head) all the while carefully watching and noting how the patient is responding to his nursing interventions (and thus completing SOCK, i.e., using sensations, observations, concepts, and knowing). This type of sequence of events usually takes place within a matter of seconds, at an intuitive level.

Learning from experience involves developing the systematic and methodical skills that lie at the heart of the art and science of clinical and critical inquiry.

CLINICAL INQUIRY-CRITICAL INQUIRY PROCESS

Clinical inquiry is about gathering information from many sources, first to identify and clarify the issues and then to define the problem. Methodical inquiry requires astute observation and excellent communication skills for the purpose of collecting information in a systematic and deliberate way.

Critical inquiry also involves skills of analysis, synthesis, and interpretation so that the nurse can develop an understanding or a clinical grasp of the situation. Clinical grasp begins with clinical inquiry and is dependent on critical inquiry. Nurses identify problems through a complex set of thinking and reasoning processes, including learning how to do the following:

- Make qualitative distinctions between observations
- Sort information into degrees of importance in light of what is known in the scientific and empirical literature and from previous clinical experiences
- Explore the role of context as it affects the patient and family's responses (Benner et al., 2010; Benner et al., 2011)

First, the nurse gathers information and then, analyzes and interprets that information. In light of these interpretations, the nurse then decides what information is missing and what further information is needed. The clinical inquiry–critical inquiry process continues until the nurse arrives at a clinical judgment and makes clinical decisions or decides on a course of action. Expressed another way, clinical decision making is based on the quality of information gathered through clinical inquiry and analyzed through critical inquiry.

What is Clinical Inquiry?

Nurses' work has been likened to detective work (Benner et al., 2011). It begins with the nurse's desire to know and the need to understand the issues before deciding on what actions to take. All too often, nurses begin to work on the solution before they have a clear understanding of the issue. Nurses cannot work with patients to deal with a problem or resolve an issue until they know what they are dealing with (Benner et al, 2011). Having a clinical grasp begins with investigation. As good detectives, nurses are continuously asking questions, generating hypotheses, following up, consulting with others, verifying information, brainstorming possibilities, pursuing more leads, and so forth.

Detective work begins with the investigation, which often commences by situating the concern within its proper context, that is, finding out more about why the concern is an issue and getting a detailed history of the concern: when it began, how long it has lasted, how disruptive it has been to the person and family's level of functioning, how the person has tried to deal with it, and the like.

The nurse begins the inquiry from a position of not knowing and is motivated to know (Munhall, 2009). The nurse also assumes that situations are complex, and it is only with methodical detective work through which the pieces of the puzzle are identified and then pieced and fitted together that a clear picture might begin to emerge.

Thus, sound detective work begins with good clinical inquiry, and good clinical inquiry requires that one be trained in the art of sensing, observing, listening, dialoguing, and questioning. This chapter focuses on training to become an astute observer, and Chapter 8 focuses on training in the skills of becoming an attentive listener and engaging in clinical conversation, including dialoguing and questioning.

Consider the story told by Nurse Luisa Ciofani, who was asked by the community nurse to see Josie, a three-month-old and her parents, the Argyles. Josie had not only failed to gain weight but had lost a significant amount of weight since her birth despite the best efforts of her mother to feed her. Mrs. Argyle was breastfeeding Josie on demand. Josie seemed to spend hours at the breast, so the situation was puzzling. The nurses and doctors alike could not figure out why Josie continued to lose weight let alone gain weight.

Luisa recounted her first visit to the Argyles and little Josie: *"I went in (to their home) and what I saw was that the baby had two states: either really sleepy or frantic, nothing really in between.... I tried to watch Josie breastfeed but she fell asleep on the breast, so we took her off. The mom had lots of milk. We pumped her and then I tried to bottle feed Josie. Josie would suck, suck, suck and then open her mouth and the milk would all pour out. Suck, suck, suck then open her mouth... So she wasn't swallowing—this little two-, maybe three-pound baby just wasn't swallowing. The parents were saying that she was better at the breast than what I saw but I thought, 'Well, I don't know if I believe you because she's losing weight—she's not swallowing, so how can I imagine that she's swallowing at the breast?'"*

Luisa continued to relate the events as they unfolded. She noticed that the Argyles *"were very caring about this infant. They were completely restructuring their lives to take care of Josie. They had both taken time off."* She also noticed that Mr. Argyle had developed an ingenious strategy to get his baby to feed.

"Josie had gained, I think, forty grams in one day. What Mr. Argyle would do was put the bottle in the baby's mouth. Because the baby wasn't swallowing, and the baby would suck, suck, suck, then he'd pull the bottle out, dab the baby's face with a cold facecloth and the baby would go 'gulp' and then swallow. And I thought, 'Wow,' he has developed this technique all on his own! I'm not sure it was the best technique but Mr. Argyle recognized that his baby wasn't gaining weight. He knew that he didn't want to come to the hospital because he doesn't like hospitals, so he thought 'I have to get milk into this baby' so he had developed this strategy to get milk into his daughter."

Luisa also observed how committed Mrs. Argyle was to breastfeeding: *"She had a breast pump and good milk production. She would pump while her husband was working on getting milk into the baby, so that together they could nourish this baby. I followed them a couple of times over the phone. This is the first baby I've ever sent to occupational therapy because I thought, 'This baby isn't swallowing.'"*

Luisa explained this couple's style of interacting also characterized how they interacted with her. It was one of constant negotiation: *"Josie is at the breast full time. They were constantly negotiating; she didn't want to give the baby bottles and [Mr. Argyle] thought 'Well, intake is important,' so recognizing that, 'If I'm giving breast milk in a bottle, that's okay.' He just consumed all that knowledge and became this expert relating to his baby's care. . . . They, as a couple, were constantly negotiating—'The baby's weight is fine today, you can weigh her on Saturday.'"*

Then, one day, Luisa recounted how the Argyles wanted to skip their appointment with the occupational therapist: *"'The baby's doing better; do you really think we should go?' And I didn't share everything I was thinking with them, but in my mind I was thinking: 'A baby that doesn't swallow, full term, good weight, I don't understand it' . . . So I told them 'Yes, I want a baseline.'*

Luisa described her thinking and what she explained the Argyles: *"They were able to recognize I have concerns about their baby—this is not how full-term babies act. So I said, 'She seems to be getting better, but at least if something happens later on we will have had a baseline visit, assessment by an expert in swallowing who can guide you and who can recommend different bottle nipples that might be easier to use than you're using right now.' And they agreed, they said 'Okay, we'll go, because you're telling us to go.' They were open to doing the best thing, but only with negotiation, as it had to be done on their terms."*

Luisa's knowledge of how infants feed, combined with her astute investigative work of how this infant, Josie, was feeding, led her to conclude that the problem was swallowing, not sucking or other failure-to-thrive reasons. Luisa had a good clinical grasp of the situation because of her clinical and critical inquiry skills.

What is Critical Inquiry?

Critical inquiry is the act of analyzing the information. This involves a complex process of sorting information, selecting what is important, looking for links between separate pieces of information to find patterns, interpreting information, validating information from different sources, gathering additional information, and then beginning the cycle anew. The process continues until the nurse is confident that she understands the issues: what is at stake, and what is in need of immediate attention, and what can wait (i.e., prioritizing). The reward of methodical critical inquiry is having a clinical grasp of the situation.

Let's continue with the example of Nurse Luisa Ciofani's detective work. She had discovered that Josie's failure to thrive was related to a problem with her swallowing mechanism. She discovered this when she looked for a pattern of behavior by connecting seemingly unrelated pieces of information. She reflected on the information that she had gathered and what she had been told. She looked inward to understand her own reactions and was guided by her own feelings, thoughts, and bodily sensations. She engaged in all these activities until she believed she had a solid grasp of the issue. Nurses appreciate that their ability to develop a clinical grasp depends on the quality of information gathered, and that information quality is affected by the nurse's skills of observation and a trusting relationship with the person and family.

THE HEART OF PROFESSIONAL GAZE: THE OBSERVATION

Observations begin when the nurse is fully present while interacting with a patient and when his eight senses are primed to get to know the patient as a person and find ways to deal effectively with that person's concerns and complaints. Because nurses have the most contact with patients, they are in the best position to learn about the person and family and to make important observations about how they respond to their health challenges under a variety of conditions and when dealing with many situations. Nurses are also the "eyes and ears" of doctors and other team members, providing them with salient information that enables them to carry out their work.

Every encounter is an opportunity to get to know the person and the family and to learn something more about them and from them. For example, nurses, in particular those who work in hospitals, are among the few select groups of the health care professionals who can observe the person's body with impunity (Short, 1997). Moreover, patients and families often entrust nurses with the most sensitive and intimate information about themselves and their lives. Patients, clients, and families tend to be more open and divulge more information when they are in periods of transition; when they experience uncertainty and feel vulnerable. Thus, nurses can come to know the person and family as a whole in ways that few other health care professionals can.

Historical Roots: The Critical Role of Observation

Medicine and nursing have historically placed great importance on the skills of observation because they know that sound clinical decisions begin with astute observation. For medicine, the importance of astute observation is primary. It helps a physician to arrive at an accurate diagnosis. As early as the 4th century BC, Hippocrates, the father of medicine, wrote about the importance of observation:

> It is the business of the physician to know in the first place, things…which are to be perceived by the sight, touch, hearing, the nose, the tongue, and the understanding. (Henderson, 2011)

Hippocrates also wrote on the importance of knowing the patient as a person to understand the disease: "It is far more important to know what person the disease has than what disease the person has" (Henderson, 2011).

The famed physician Dr. William Osler—a founder of modern medicine and one of the four founders of Johns Hopkins School of Medicine (the first modern school of medicine)—wrote in the late 1800s on the importance of observation. Osler echoed the sentiments of Hippocrates: "There is no more difficult art to acquire than the art of observation, and for some men it is quite as difficult to record an observation in brief and plain language" (William Osler, n.d.). In a similar vein, he wrote, "Medicine is learned by the bedside and not in the classroom. Let not your conceptions of disease come from words heard in the lecture room or read from the book. See, and then reason and compare and control. But see first" (William Osler, n.d.).

In the field of nursing, Florence Nightingale (1860) wrote of the centrality of observation in nursing: "It may safely be said, not that the habit of ready and correct observation will by itself make us useful nurses, but that without it we will be useless, with all our devotion" (p. 112).

Nightingale understood that a patient's first and last line of protection was dependent on being cared for by a nurse who is a skilled, astute observer. At the time she was writing, nurses were the first line of defense, serving as doctors' eyes and the ears and informing them about what they saw, which in turn influenced the physicians' judgment and decisions. Nurses also served as patients' last line of protection insofar as they had within their power the skill to detect subtle changes in a patient's conditions and to "rescue" a patient from further deterioration and even prevent death. As Nightingale (1860) wrote,

> Nurses are the first line of a patient's defense when they serve as the "eyes and ears" of doctors. They are also the last line of protection when they detect subtle changes in a patient's conditions and act to "rescue" patients from further deterioration or even death.

> Let people who have to observe sickness and death look back and try to register in their observation the appearances which have preceded relapse, attack, or death, and not assert that there were none, or that there were not the right ones. A want (i.e., missing) of the habit of observing conditions and an inveterate habit of taking averages are each of them often equally misleading. (p. 120).

Nightingale recognized that patients' safety was at stake and that nothing could replace a patient's need for constant vigilant and careful monitoring. Almost 150 years later, a landmark study that examined the effects of the nursing shortage on patients found that patients' safety was severely compromised when there were not enough skilled nurses (Clarke & Aiken, 2003) to care for them. In other words, there were not enough nurses who were continuously observing changes in patients' conditions. The term *failure to rescue* entered the nursing lexicon to describe what happens when nurses or other caregivers fail to notice and intervene in a timely manner to prevent a condition from deteriorating, a potential untoward reaction, a complication, or even mortality. Joanna Streppa, an expert nurse, knows that when she notices "fish-smelling breath" on a patient she needs to act quickly. From experience, she has learned that foul fish breath indicates that the patient is about to "crash" and is an early sign of pending respiratory distress.

Finally, Nightingale (1860) understood that observation was key to health promotion, illness prevention, and healing. Nurses worked with the "laws of nature" governing health and healing. Nightingale believed that these laws were all around us, just waiting to be discovered. It is by working with the laws of nature—such as providing fresh air, clean water, healthy nutrition, and the like—that nurses could help patients self-heal and support their innate human mechanisms of healing.

Thus, it is hardly surprising that, for both medicine and nursing, observation became an important focus of students' education and training. In medicine, conducting the physical examination and taking a detailed medical history is how doctors have traditionally understood the patient's complaints. Nurses were taught skills to detect abnormalities or changes in patients' conditions. To do so, however, both doctors and nurses needed to retrain their sensory systems and learn how to do the following:

- *Auscultate* (hear) to listen for normal and abnormal sounds of the heart, chest, and intestine
- *Palpate* (touch) to feel the internal organs of the abdomen for the expected and unexpected in order to assess its internal workings, as well as feel the quality of the skin and integrity of muscles and tendons through skin-to-skin contact
- *Inspect* (look at) the surfaces of the body, namely, the skin, eyes, nose, ears, and the external orifices (i.e., mouth, anus, sexual organs) and the lining or mucosa of the orifices
- *Taste* bodily fluids such as perspiration and urine (in times past, doctors used to taste these fluids to diagnose such conditions as diabetes, with its characteristically sweet-tasting urine)
- *Smell* for unusual breath and bodily odors emanating from the body's orifices (e.g., pores, mouth, rectum, vagina)

In addition, physicians and nurses learned how to take an accurate and detailed history. They knew that, if they gained the trust of their patients; asked open-ended, exploratory questions; and attentively listened to the patient's story, they would be able to either diagnose the problem or at least begin to generate a list of possible diagnosis to rule out.

Until the late 1980s, the physical examination was a routine part of any visit to the doctor. Patients expected it. Today, the physical examination has become a rarity as doctors have increasingly turned to technology to help them arrive at a diagnosis. They have come to rely more and more on the results of clinical laboratory tests and radiographic images from X-rays, magnetic resonance imaging, and positron emission tomography scans as the sources of their clinical information. Moreover, detailed medical histories have been cut short, and brief encounters are replacing the more established, long-term physician/nurse–patient relationship. The physical examination is becoming a lost art in medical practice. A quick romp through the history of the medical physical examination is outlined in Table 7.1.

PHYSICAL EXAMINATION AND STRENGTHS-BASED CARE

In contrast to medical practice, the physical examination has recently become a routine part of advanced nurses' practices. Nurses are being trained in physical and mental assessments to detect problems before they occur and to diagnose some medical conditions. Nurses who practice Strengths-Based Care (SBC) integrate physical and mental assessments as part of their practice, but with a difference. In the course of observing for abnormalities and noting problems, nurses who practice SBC also are attuned to

TABLE 7.1

The history of the role of the physical examination in medicine's clinical inquiry

Era	Role of the physical examination in diagnosis
5th to 3rd Century BC: Hippocrates, Galen, and the humoral theory of disease	Disease is caused by an imbalance of the four humors: (a) blood, (b) yellow bile, (c) black bile, and (d) phlegm. *Hippocrates*: Dismiss supernatural causes and concentrate on empirical evidence gathered by an examination of the body, that is, inspection of the tongue, palpation of the abdomen, and so on. To diagnose, the nurse needs to learn about the patient's habits, way of life, work, diet, and so on. *Galen*: Greater emphasis on anatomy, physiology, pathology, and logic. Palpated abdomen to locate spleen and liver. Examined stools for consistency and composition. Spent many hours conversing with the patient to arrive at a diagnosis.
Late Middle Ages:13th to14th centuries: Medical school reform and separation of practitioners into physicians and surgeons	Physicians were educated in the university; surgeons were craftsmen. Physicians stopped practicing hands-on physical examination. Scholarship was valued over sensory experience; reason was more valued than clinical observation; mental activity was more important than manual procedures. High reliance on patients' accounts of their signs and symptoms to make a diagnosis because these took precedence over what the physician could observe. Use of thermometers was shunned because the information given by the thermometer often contradicted patients' reports—patients reported chills that contradicted registration of elevated temperature.
17th century: Social standing of physicians and surgeons	Humoral theory of disease was replaced by the scientific-based medicine of today. Doctors wanted to know as much as possible about the internal state of the body. The hands-on physical exam made a comeback, accompanied by new technology, such as the stethoscope.
19th to 20th centuries: Rise of scientific medicine	Rapid advancements in pharmacology and high-tech imaging emphasized biochemistry and radiology. Attentive listening to patients' stories was time consuming and deemed unnecessary as a clinical inquiry tool to arrive at a diagnosis and provide treatment. Physician–patient relationships have been replaced by the "medical encounter."

Source: Adapted from Henderson (2011).

looking for strengths—uncovering and discovering what is working and what is functioning well. Nurses generally rely less on technology to gather information and more on their senses for gathering relevant data. They use data from laboratory findings, but they treat them not as data that replace listening to the patient's and family's history but rather as information that supplements, validates, and confirms what they have learned from talking to the patient and family.

The pioneers of medicine and nursing attributed great importance to observation. Learning how to observe and what to observe differentiated the professional from the layperson. They also understood what was at stake when practitioners failed in their duty to acquire the skills of observation and to learn how and when to artfully use these skills. The antonym, or opposite, of *observing* is *missing*. When nurses miss what is happening to and with their patients, or fail to understand the salience or significance of a behavior or sign, symptom, or event, they place their patients and families at risk that something untoward could happen to them. In other words, they fail to protect their patients, and in so doing place them in harm's way. They are unable to provide safe care, let alone quality care.

> Quality care begins with astute, accurate, detailed, and clearly communicated observations. The person and family's safety and well-being are dependent on the nurses' power of observation.

Quality care begins with accurate and detailed observations. Nurses need to be trained in the art and science of observing by retraining their senses. Patients' safety and well-being depend on nurses' power of observation. Astute observations make the difference between safe and effective patient care as opposed to inappropriate and unsafe care (Peden-McAlpine & Clark, 2002).

CONCEPTUALIZATION OF OBSERVATION

The word *observation* involves noting, paying attention to, being conscious of, having knowledge of, and being aware of something. It encompasses paying attention or attentively caring for somebody. Observation is often followed by *documentation*—recording and describing what one has seen (see http://www.merriam-webster.com/dictionary/observe).

The word *observation* is associated with the sensory system of sight. To observe means to see, detect, and perceive by the eye. However, seeing encompasses more than just vision and sight. The term *seeing* has multiple usages in the English language (see http://www.merriam-webster.com/dictionary/see).

- Seeing is about *knowing, experiencing, discovering, judging, and grasping*, as in "Oh, I see!"
- Seeing involves forming a mental picture by being able to *visualize* or *imagine how something is*, as in "I can still see her as she was 30 years ago"
- Seeing is about *understanding and perceiving the meaning or importance of*, as in "I see what you mean"
- Seeing is about *being aware or recognizing*, as in "I see his strengths"
- Seeing is about *imagining possibilities*, as in "I now see what else can be done"
- Seeing is about *examining* and *watching*, as in "I want to see what will happen if we wait"
- Seeing is about being a *spectator, attending an event as an observer*, as in —"I went to see that DVD on how to insert an IV"
- Seeing is also about *accompanying somebody on his journey*, as in "I went to see them to be with them"
- Seeing is about *investigating* and *inquiring*, as in "I will see what is possible" or "I will see to that"

Observation includes looking, watching, and seeing (Dahnke & Dreher, 2011). It involves monitoring and scrutinizing for the purpose of attending to something with intention. In short, observation is how a practitioner senses and is witness to unfolding experiences (Siegel, 2010).

Nurses retrain their senses and hone their skills of observation to attend to relevant details in a situation that are considered salient; however, to decide what is salient, clinicians require knowledge—knowledge gained in the classroom and in the clinical setting. Nurses' training needs to focus on developing perceptual acuity through intentional attention, attunement, and discernment. To develop their professional gaze of making astute observations, nurses also need to increase self-awareness (sixth, and seventh sense), develop imagination, learn to witness how patients and families navigate life, and cope with illness and any transitional events and life experiences (eighth sense). Even when the nurse has had a long-term relationship with the person, there is always something new to learn, investigate, and inquire about.

- *Observing* involves the use of all the senses, not just sight. Input is received via the five sensory systems—visual, auditory, olfactory, gustatory, and somatosensory—and is then interpreted and integrated to create an impression of that which has been observed or experienced. In today's health care environment, observations are extended to include observing images generated by technology, such as ultrasound, and consulting laboratory test results (Barnard, 2009).
- *Observing* is about receiving stimuli or inputs. It begins with selecting, attending to, perceiving, and interpreting. Seeing often comes before one can formulate impressions and express them in words. The observer needs to "sense" the situation (Berger, 1972).
- *Observing* is about sensing the world. The act of seeing involves attending to many things simultaneously rather than just one thing at a time. Observation involves putting together all the separate pieces of information to create the whole, and it is this whole on which the nurse acts. Consider what happens when a person observes a flower. She immediately forms an image of a rose or a tulip or a lilac on the basis of what they have observed about the flower's form, shape, color, and scent as a whole. This image is then compared with previous images and matched. The person can then conclude that what she is holding in her hand is indeed a flower and, more precisely, a rose.
- *Observing* involves more than one person; it includes both the person who is being observed and the person who is observing. In a nurse—person relationship it is important to keep in mind that the nurse is observing the person and the person is observing the nurse. Observation is a reciprocal process during which the information that each person gathers will affect and define how they will interact and relate to each other.
- *Observing* requires clinical imagination which is required for clinical forethought. *Clinical forethought* refers to the nurse's thinking activities that help him anticipate potential problems (Benner et al., 2011). This requires on-the-spot thinking in action. Thinking-in-action involves perceptual awareness of the situation so that one can make a rational decision. Clinical forethought involves the following:
  - *Future thinking*, which is envisioning all eventualities and preparing for them by organizing the environment, putting things into place. An example of future

thinking is when people put bars in bathrooms to aid stability or remove throw rugs to prevent falls.

- *Intimate knowledge* of a specific individual and familiarity of specific conditions, the usual ways of responding, and the usual responses to treatment.
- *Anticipation of risks* and *crises*, as when a nurse takes specific actions so as not to contaminate a sterile field. This also involves
  - Seeing the unexpected,
  - Looking for what is missing, and
  - Thinking about what one expects to see and then comparing what is with what one had expected to see.

Many of these features are described in Rashotte, King, Thomas, and Cragg's (2011) descriptive study of what is involved in nurses making a decision about when to administer *pro re nata* (PRN) antiseizure medication to children in hospice and palliative care settings. Their study is summarized in Exhibit 7.1.

THE ART OF OBSERVATION

Nurses retraining of their senses can be guided by interrogatives:

- WHAT to observe
- WHY to observe
- WHOM to observe
- WHEN to observe
- WHERE to observe
- HOW to observe

What the nurse observes is related to the reason or purpose for the observation. The nurse needs to ask the question, "Why?" For example, "Why am I observing?" Answering the "why" question will help the nurse know what information she needs to gather. For example, a nurse observes for many reasons: She may want to get to know the patient, understand the patient's medical condition, detect early signs of deterioration, be interested in how the patient is responding to treatment, make sense of the person's lived experience with illness or trauma, and so forth. She may also hope to arrive at a clearer understanding of the problem (i.e., clinical grasp) or find an answer to a specific question. Once the nurse has asked the question—"Why am I observing?"— then she will have a clearer understanding of *what* to focus her attention on.

What to observe is also guided by a nurse's orientation of practice with its underlying value system (see Chapters 2 and 3). For example, when a nurse practices SBC, he will observe for health and healing; look to uncover the patient's uniqueness; seek to understand how the body and mind function as a whole; observe the effects on the patient of her physical and social environments, including her dynamics in different relationships and during various interactions; watch and listen for indicators of self-determination and readiness, listen to the patient's perceptions as well as her understanding of her situation (meaning), be sensitive to how the patient wants to collaborate with the nurse and other health care providers in her own care, and so forth. The nurse is primed to attend and attune to the person's strengths: what is working

EXHIBIT 7.1

Empirical study *The importance of observation in the moral experience of nurses'
administration of PRN anti-seizure medication to children receiving palliative care*

The Problem

How are nurses' moral experiences affected by the factors behind their decision making related to the administration of PRN antiseizure medications to children with long-term seizure disorders in palliative care?

The Issues

To understand the nature of nurses' decision making related to the administration of PRN antiseizure medications to children living with a long-term seizure disorder in a palliative care program and the importance of observation as it relates to the nurses' moral experience.

The Study

A qualitative design that used both interpretive (hermeneutic) and descriptive (phenomenological) elements to address the study question. Six nurses who had had at least three individual experiences in deciding on the administration of PRN antiseizure medication were interviewed.

The Findings

Nurses underscored the importance of observing the child and being constantly alert to a seizure. They attended to any visual and auditory signals they thought indicated an impending seizure, such as a change in the child's usual way of behaving. Nurses identified the importance of "knowing" to guide decision making: knowing this child, who she was, what she was like; knowing the history, nature, and pattern of this child's seizure; knowing in general about the medical entity of seizures; knowing how to monitor a seizure, the types and dosages of seizure medications, and the management of adverse effects of seizures and medications; and knowing the parents and their preference for treatment.

Nurses used multiple sources to gather information about the child and family. They believed that getting to know the child and his family was the best guide in making decisions about when to administer antiseizure medication that respected the parents' wishes while being consistent with their own assessment.

The Bottom Line

This study revealed the moral dilemmas and resulting moral distress that nurses may experience when deciding on when and when not to administer antiseizure medication. The process of decision making required skilled know-how in gathering relevant and salient information as well as having both in-depth general and specific knowledge of that particular child and family.

Source: Adapted from Rashotte, King, Thomas, and Cragg (2011).

at all levels—including at the biological/physiological, cognitive, emotional, social, and spiritual levels—in what situation, and under which conditions. The nurse is further primed to attend and attune to family strengths: how families create health-promoting environments, manage and support day-to-day living and function, provide emotional and instrumental support during health and illness, have available resources to access and use appropriately (e.g., financial), protect and ensure the survival of its members, facilitate coping, and the like. Finally, the nurse is also primed to attend and attune to community strengths: how communities develop resources to support families and patients; how policy and decisions occur; and the availability of basic necessities, such as quality housing, food, safe communities, green spaces, and the like.

In addition, what nurses choose to observe is guided by goals. To illustrate this idea, let's return to the study conducted by Rashotte et al. (2011), which is described in Exhibit 7.1. As they stated in the article, nurses expressed a number of goals for their nursing care that included stopping the seizure, reducing the number and length of seizures, making the child comfortable, preventing over-sedation, reducing bodily stress, preventing harm, especially to "not have the seizure kill the child," and meeting parental goals for seizure care. Each of these goals requires general knowledge about seizures; that is, the nature of seizures, seizure care, comfort, stress and so forth, and specific knowledge about the person.

All "what" questions begin with acquiring general and then specific knowledge about a particular patient and family and their responses to the medical condition and its treatment. General knowledge may include that regarding the medical condition and the treatment, as well as the biological, psychological, emotional, and behavioral responses. Particular or specific knowledge relates to how general knowledge is expressed by a specific patient.

Let's return again to Rashotte et al.'s (2011) study. If the goal of the study had been to determine when to administer a PRN antiseizure medication, what general information would nurses need to know? They would need to know the causes of seizures, have knowledge of the anatomy and physiology of seizures and its progression, risk factors, triggers, morbidity and mortality rates, and so forth. They also would need to know about treatment options, including knowledge of pharmacology, such as the various drug classifications, actions, dosages, side-effects, modes of administration, and so forth. They would have to have some understanding about physical growth and development as well as the developmental challenges of each age group, including knowledge of children's capabilities and competencies at a given age.

Given that pediatric nurses want to make decisions that respect parents' directives and that would be consistent with parental practices, they would have to have specific knowledge of that child's family, the family's dynamics, family communication patterns, family beliefs, family organization, and family decision-making styles (Walsh, 2006). This knowledge would be used to guide their observations. In addition, general knowledge would not only help direct nurses in terms of what to attend to but also would help them to interpret their observations. Nurses also need to gather information about the patient and his experiences by observing him, being attuned to what he is saying, and how he is behaving.

Whom to observe refers to the unit of the nurse's concern. The unit can be an individual (i.e., person, patient, client), family, groups, a community, or a population. Nurses' focus of care is on both individuals and families: individuals within the context of the family and the family as it is affected by its individual members (Gottlieb & Gottlieb, 2007). Nurses, even if they are not nursing at the family level (Wright & Leahey, 2009), should at the very least be family-minded, that is, observe the person through a family-oriented lens (Gottlieb & Carnaghan-Sherrard, 2004). *Family-minded* means that nurses are aware that individual family members are part of a web of relationships and that all are affected by those around them. People are linked to their families genetically, biologically, emotionally, socially, culturally, and historically (Gottlieb & Gottlieb, 2007). This principle is referred to as *linked lives*. Families are always present, and they often play a significant role in each of its member's lives even when they are not physically present to appreciate their influence on shaping values and making decisions. What determines "whom" to observe or ask about depends on what the nurse is trying to understand, her own theoretical orientation, and her level of knowledge and skill of nursing at the family level.

In Rashotte et al.'s (2011) study, the "whom" includes the child and his or her parents. Nurses needed to get to know that particular child and his history of seizures. They needed training to observe and decipher what was normal behavior for that child and what was expected behavior for children in that age group. They watched carefully for any changes in the child's normal pattern or way of behaving and were attuned to the most subtle cues or changes that could signal an impending seizure. Nurses also had to learn about each child's parents: what was important to them, how they made decisions, their health/illness beliefs, and their goals for their child. This required training in how to gain parents' trust and engage them as well as a knowledge of family dynamics.

When to observe involves both time and timing. Nurses need to have sufficient knowledge of the phenomenon of interest to know how frequently they should observe a particular patient (Gottlieb & Feeley, 1999). A significant part of any nurse's day is deciding when to observe patients. Nurses operate at heightened levels of alertness, watching out for the unexpected and unusual. When practicing from an SBC orientation, nurses note strengths while remaining vigilant for sudden and subtle changes in a patient's condition. The level at which the nurse is expected to observe depends on the patient's condition as well as the routines, rituals, policies, and procedures of a specific unit.

When a patient's medical condition is unstable, nurses increase their level of observation to continuous one-to-one monitoring (Moore, Berman, Knight, & Devine, 1995). Think of nurses in intensive care units, critical-care units, and recovery rooms and the amount of time they spend observing patients; monitoring vital signs; and watching for subtle, imperceptible changes in their patients' conditions, which can include reading the output from monitors that may indicate that the patient is going "sour." The level of vigilance required of a nurse decreases as the patient's condition stabilizes or when the crisis abates or is averted.

The facility's unit policy also affects a nurse's observation schedule. On most clinical units nurses spend a significant portion of their day undertaking routine clinical observations, that is, those that are considered necessary because they are warranted by the diagnosis, treatment, and existing ward policy or directives. In some institutions, nurses spend a significant portion of their day taking vital signs (i.e., TPR: temperature, pulse, respirations, and measuring blood pressure). A survey of the effects of such routine observations revealed that almost forty percent of nurses felt they were a waste of time, and over half the nurses said they believed that such routine observations heightened patients' anxiety (Burroughs & Hoffbrand, 1990). Often, unit and hospital policies are based on a fear of missing something that might result in a legal suit rather than on research evidence or on the assessment of that person's condition.

Timing plays a role in deciding when to observe. Rashotte and her colleagues (2011) identified two aspects of timing that affected the decision of when to observe, namely, the importance of (a) marking time and (b) waiting.

- *Marking time* required that the nurses become more aware of the passage of time. Time takes on different qualities depending on the event. For example, Rashotte et al. (2011) found that when children were having a seizure, nurses became acutely aware of time, feeling that the seizure seemed to "take forever"
- *Waiting.* The length of time spent observing depended on what the nurses knew about the condition, the progression of an illness, or the expected length of time for a symptom to resolve. Again, in the case of observing a seizure, the researchers found that waiting was involved in observing the beginning and end of a seizure, and this information informed treatment decisions

Nurses also need to be attuned to the patient's and family's need for space, which will influence the times when it is best to observe. *Space* in this case refers to emotional space: when to speak and when to be silent. Silence is often called for, and happens when families are overwhelmed and need "time out." It also happens when trust has been violated. Recall Nurse Lyne Charbonneau from Chapter 3, who described such an event, when a nurse had caused an error that jeopardized the health and recovery of a young couple's preterm son. The Alonzos' infant son had been born twenty-four weeks preterm. The year before, they had lost an infant, born twenty-one weeks preterm. This son was quite sick, having had suffered an intracranial hemorrhage the first week of birth, and he was transferred to the neonatal intensive care unit of a university children's hospital. A few weeks after arriving, the baby's condition stabilized. Then an incident occurred: a nurse made an error that destabilized the infant's condition once again. Before this incident, Lyne had developed a trusting relationship with the parents.

After the error, and the team had met with Mr. and Mrs. Alonzo to disclose what had happened, it was hardly surprising that Lyne felt them withdraw and distance themselves from her. She described their change in attitude: *"They didn't have questions. They didn't make eye contact, so they really wanted to close off the discussion. They were not able to say that but they were showing that is what they wanted.... And what I did is I just gave them some time. I adapted to going at their pace. I didn't impose myself. They saw me near the baby. They knew I was there and if they had questions they could come to me, but I kind of respected this distance."*

Lyne made herself available but did not impose herself on them.

Every clinical encounter is an opportunity to gather information and learn something more about the patient and his issues. The answer of *where* to observe is simple in all situations. Nurses need to function in "observation mode" during every encounter and every interaction, while providing bodily care, administering treatments, and engaging in clinical conversation. The concept of "where" also applies to any forum in which the nurse's patient and family are discussed: in a unit report, during informal talks with colleagues, or during rounds. These situations afford nurses the opportunity to look and listen for and to attend to different types of information. In SBC, nurses use their listening and observation skills to note the aspects of the person and her situation that will help them understand that person and how best to care for her, all the while being guided by SBC values.

PRECONDITIONS REQUIRED FOR DEVELOPING A PROFESSIONAL OBSERVATION GAZE

To become an astute observer requires that the nurse adopt a specific mindset and acquire skills of social engagement and relationship building.

Mindset. Becoming an astute observer begins with the nurse herself. Observation begins with a curiosity to know more about the person and his family and situation. The nurse needs to be curious about who this person that presents as a patient is, what brings the person to seek help, and what the person expects from the health care system and different health care professionals. The nurse also needs to be open to looking for and listening to different ways of thinking, be willing to pursue unchartered paths, and be alert to the unexpected. The nurse navigates between two worlds—being fully present in the moment while at the same time thinking about what else needs to be explored. (This strength is more fully described in Chapter 5 in the section titled "I. Strengths of Mindset.")

Skills of engagement and relationship building. Nurses need to be fully present when they are with a patient if they are to see clearly what is happening, hear what the patient is saying, listen for unexpected sounds, and be attuned to unexpected smells. Being fully present requires that the nurse be fully alert. This enables him to watch, attend, attune to,

> Becoming an astute observer begins with being fully present. It requires training in how to focus, be alert and vigilant, be attuned to and in tune with what is going on, reflect prior to, during, and after an encounter, and seek feedback from different sources at different times.

and listen with intention. It is when the nurse is engaged with patients that he can listen to subtexts and attend to subtle and overt bodily cues. These ideas are more fully elaborated in the Chapter 8.

CAVEAT

There are many other preconditions for good professional observation, such as those that have to do with the person and one's work environment. However, I have elected to discuss two of the most essential nurse preconditions because observation is the primary responsibility of the nurse, and only the nurse can decide how much time and energy she will spend observing.

Components of Observation

The above two preconditions influence observation, but they are not actually involved in the complex act of observing. The act of observing actually involves three elements:

- Perception
- Memory
- Interpretation

Perception

A person sees only what he looks at, and what the person decides to look at is a matter of choice (Berger, 1972). As Berger reminded us, the photographer's way of seeing is reflected in what he chooses as his subject. Consider how a nurse, when first entering a person's room, quickly scans the environment. He may choose to attend to the patient's appearance and take a mental snapshot of how the patient is doing. He may also choose to scan the physical environment, to note that everything is as expected. Then, just as the nurse is about to leave the room, something may capture his attention. The "something" may be an item in the room that catches his attention, or it may be a feature of the patient's appearance. The nurse may then elect to investigate what has caught his attention. The "something" that has captured his attention may be unexpected, out of place, missing, or a signal from within the nurse's body (i.e., an uneasy, queasy feeling) that something is amiss. As part of the nurse's investigation, he situates his observations in context by taking into account other things in the patient's immediate environment or circumstance to help interpret what that "something" means. The nurse forms an image, a way of seeing—in short, a perception. This perception is not based on what was actually seen but rather on the person's *own way* of seeing it (Berger, 1972).

Observations consist of two forms of representations: (a) sensory and (b) perceptual. *Sensory representations* comprise information, in the form of sensory signals, that is transmitted to their respective areas of the brain. They include information from the eight sensory systems: the five external signals transmitted via the five traditional sensory systems (e.g., visual, auditory, tactile, etc.) and the three internal signals transmitted as a result of internal bodily sensations (i.e., awareness of that which is happening inside oneself, awareness of one's feelings and thoughts, and awareness of that which is

> Sensory information is the "raw material" that informs the nurse about the person and family state of health, recovery, and healing asnd is the basis for clinical judgment and decision making.

happening outside oneself in the surrounding environment and its impact on oneself). Both forms of sensory information are registered in the brain but are thought to have minimal categorization (Siegel, 1999); in other words, they are registered in the brain but are not interpreted. Thus, a person may sense something, but what she or he senses still needs to be interpreted before the significance of the information is understood. Another way of thinking about sensory information is to think of it as raw material before being processed and transformed into a product.

Perceptual representation, on the other hand, is a more complex form of processed information than its sensory cousin (Siegel, 1999). A perceptual representation results when one constructs pieces of information received through the senses, compares them with what has been experienced in the past, remembers what has previously happened, and creates expectancies of what that information should be and how it should function. In other words, perceptions are subjective. They comprise information filtered through memories of things that are known, that which "feels" familiar, has already been experienced, or approximates to something close enough to predict its meaning by guessing what it might be. This involves filling in and completing missing information. Thus, the mind "constructs" perceptual reality from bits of selected data received through the senses and then combines it with what is already known or familiar. This explains why two individuals observing the same situation may see the same thing very differently. Prior experience will affect what the nurse selects to attend to and how she attunes herself to what is important. This helps to explain the difference between an experienced nurse and a novice nurse. An experienced nurse knows what is salient and already knows what information is important, what is less important, and what is nonessential and unimportant. If the situation is totally new, then the information received as a stimuli remains a sensation or sensory input in need of interpretation.

What factors affect perception? The most influential factor involves memory and its modifiers.

Memory

Memory is the means by which past events affect future functioning. Siegel (1999) defined *memory* as "the way the brain is affected by a past event or experience which then alters or affects future responses" (p. 24). Memory involves the recalling of past events to make sense of current experiences. It plays a critical role in processing information and is key to interpreting the information gleaned from sensory input.

Although there have been major advances in our understanding of memory and how it works, in general terms the consensus is that memory involves an unknown number of processes that helps a person deal with the sensory information that comes from events and experiences. The first act involved in memory is *perception*, followed by *encoding*, and the final act is *retrieval* of the stored information (Insel, 2011; Siegel, 1999).

Encoding involves receiving information from sensory systems, processing inputs, and then relating and combining the information with what has been previously experienced. Retrieval involves recall and recollection, that is, being able to call forth a stored response to some new cue, signal, event, or experience in order to help interpret the information in a new situation. Between encoding and retrieving are processes of storing information—deciding where information is to be stored, the form in which it is to be stored, and the length of time it is to be stored.

The mind works as a whole and recalls things as wholes (Siegel, 1999). Memories are about experiences, not about individual signals, specific stimuli, discrete sensations, or one element of a whole. When the mind retrieves information, memory often brings forth the event, and one recalls the context in which the event previously occurred. Memory is always situated; in other words, the person recalls what other things were happening at the time, how he was physically feeling (somatic state), how he was feeling at an emotional level (emotions and mood states), what he was thinking (cognitive state), and what he was doing at the time (behavioral state). For example, recall what you were doing when you first heard of the attacks on the World Trade Center and the Pentagon on September 11, 2001. What do you remember about that event? You will probably first begin to call forth images of the planes hurtling into the Twin Towers or the towers imploding. In recalling this event, your memory will be able to tell you where you were when you first heard the news, what you were doing, your first thoughts, your emotional response, and so forth. As another example, think of the first patient you nursed who died while in your care, or the first error you made or "near miss" you had. What do you recall about that event?

Memory is not a conscious process; most of the time, people are unaware that they are processing sensory inputs. They process sensory information almost automatically. However, a person can be trained to attend to specific stimuli. Consider the story told by Raphael, a physiotherapist. He can recall the first time he was observing an operation, the activity in the operating room at the time, his own behavior, and his feelings of embarrassment. Raphael had been working in rehabilitation with patients who had had hip replacements. One day, a surgeon, with whom he had worked with for a number of years, invited him to observe an actual hip replacement operation. During the surgery, the nurse asked Raphael to hand her the sponge on a tray across from where he was standing. Raphael automatically leaned over the patient and the sterile field to retrieve the sponge on the tray. Today, many years later, Raphael can vividly recall the events of that incident in the most minute detail. It is as if he was still there and time has been suspended. Never having been in an operating room before, Raphael had no understanding of asepsis or knowledge of a "sterile field." Raphael responded automatically. He had no mental model of the operating room and therefore could not anticipate what could happen or what would happen next. Raphael recalls "the horror" on the nurse's face as she observed him contaminating the entire surgical field. He can conjure up images of the nurses' facial expressions and his feelings of embarrassment. Every time he evokes this memory, he can even "feel" the temperature of the room.

Prior experiences shape our anticipatory models. The way this works is that, moment to moment, the brain is trying to figure out what is going on. It does so by matching what is happening to what it already has stored in memory. A person's prior experience biases her current perceptions and allows for more rapid processing (Siegel, 1999). If a situation is familiar, a person will know how to respond. Raphael now knows the "rules" and how to behave in the operating room during a surgery.

Modifiers of memory: Familiarity, stress, emotional state, and thoughts
Until recently, researchers thought that the brain registers that which the sensory system encodes without modification. It is now understood that the brain does modify observations before storing the information in memory.

Familiarity. Some encounters are more easily remembered than others. Humans tend to remember incidents, events, and encounters that are familiar. Nurses will become more efficient observers, know what is salient in a situation and what needs to be attended to with repeated exposure to the situation and practice in dealing with it.

These experiences will indelibly be encoded into their memory. When certain signals are received through sensory systems, ones that are familiar will be the most readily matched and accurately interpreted.

If a person has never encountered a particular situation, then there can be no match in that person's memory; however, if some elements of the situation that are familiar, although not exactly the same, the information gained from the observation could be modified and then stored in this new form. This is what happens when a nurse says to herself, "What I am seeing feels familiar," or "I feel that I have been here before," or "I know that person and what he is going through. I had a similar case last month."

Stress. Observations are filtered through memory. Stress affects memory. Low levels of stress have little to no effect on memory, but high levels of stress can impair memory over the long term (Siegel, 1999). The release of glucocorticoids, such as cortisol, tends to block hippocampal functioning. The hippocampus region of the brain plays a critical role in the encoding and storing of information in memory. Stress can facilitate recall when emotional memory is involved; in other words, when an event or thought arouses emotion, memory can be improved. To explain this observation, scientists have found that when cortisol levels are higher (an indicator of stress), the amygdala (the area in the brain where emotion is situated) response is stronger (Wolf, 2009). Individuals are more attentive to details when they have to be alert and they are aware that something can go wrong. Nurses can more easily recall an event or an experience in situations where there was some tension (emotion) and that thus called for them to be more vigilant. They will be more likely to recall the experience and describe it in more precise detail. High-stress situations will heighten memory because of high arousal levels. The autonomic nervous system is called into play, but only for a short period of time. Individuals will eventually crash. Think of soldiers in Afghanistan who remember every rock, every bend in the road, because their life and the lives of their fellow soldiers depend on it, but they can recall this for only short periods of time.

Emotion and thought. Memory is affected by the observer's emotional state, her state of mind. *State of mind* refers to the emotions a person is experiencing during important or significant events. The person can experience a wide range of emotions, such as joy, happiness, guilt, anger, depression, anxiety, and fear. Each type of emotion is accompanied by a physiological reaction that might alter their thinking. That's why almost anybody can recall in minute detail and be able to reexperience the events when they first learned about, for example, 9/11 and Michael Jackson's death, many years later. It is as if the details of the event have been branded into one's memory.

Consider an incident told by Jody, a nursing student in her senior year of her undergraduate program. Jody was assigned to care for Mike, a member of a biker gang. Mike was a good-looking man, but his tattoos, shaved head, leather jacket, and studs were all that Jody could see. Mike was never alone; one of his gang members was always with him. Mike had been admitted to the hospital in critical condition following a serious gunshot wound from an altercation with a rival gang. Mike made a good recovery and was transferred to a step-down unit when Jody was assigned to be his nurse. Every time Jody entered the room, she experienced fear. As she recalled, *"I would go in, do what I had to do, and leave as quickly as I could."* She told her fellow students to keep an eye on the room and, if she was not out within a few minutes, to call for help. Jody was on high alert: She anticipated trouble because her appraisal of this patient was that he was dangerous and could cause her harm. Even before Jody entered Mike's room to administer care, she found herself aware that her heart was racing and her breathing was more rapid and shallow. When asked by her teacher about Mike, the person, Jody could tell her very little. She just attended to what she had to, and even then she failed to remember very many details about Mike's condition, let alone Mike as a person. Thus, Jody's emotional state affected the information she selected to attend to and how it was appraised. As Siegel (1999) summarized, "The person's emotional processing prepares the brain and the rest of the body for action" (p. 124). Thus, people's emotions will affect what they are thinking and their physiological responses and ways of experiencing a situation (Siegel, 1999). Jody, coming from a different culture and social class than Mike, had had very little experiences with gangs. Her knowledge of gangs had been constructed from bits of information she had seen on television and in movies or read about in magazines and newspapers, but not from any personal experience. Her fear of Mike, the gang member, affected how she interacted with Mike, the person.

Appraisal. Often, a person's emotions and emotional state are the first things of which that person is aware as he appraises the situation (Aldwin, 2007). Appraisal helps the individual evaluate the situation and decide whether and how to act. The appraisal system is directed by past experiences that have been stored in memory. It is also affects a person's current emotional reactions, the social environment, and her expectations of what could happen. Let's return to Mike and Student Nurse Jody. Jody's knowledge of Mike came from preconceived ideas influenced by her own past; her lack of experience with street gangs; and what she had read in Mike's chart, overheard from other nurses, and observed about Mike during their brief encounters. Jody may also have attended to and selected different cues in Mike's demeanor, such as a certain look in his eyes, his tattoos, and the way he dressed. Then one day, an incident occurred that altered Jody's perception of Mike. Mike had been experiencing severe pain, and Jody decided to administer his analgesia intramuscularly. When she entered the room with the needle, Mike began to whimper. He was terrified of needles. All of sudden, Jody saw Mike, not Mike the *frightening* patient but Mike the *frightened* patient. This experience transformed Jody's perception of Mike. No longer terrified of Mike, Jody reached out to calm him. She stayed with Mike for a few minutes after administering the analgesic until he had calmed down enough and was able to doze. Jody observed Mike's vulnerability and could thus be better attuned to Mike and attend to his needs.

Nurses are also affected by their patients' emotions and emotional states. Think of how a nurse's mood is affected when a patient is happy after hearing good news or when a patient is depressed or sad when the news is bad. Emotions and emotional states are contagious, and the patient's mood often affects the nurse's mood, even if only temporarily. Conversely, a nurse's mood and attitude can have an effect on the patient's behavior. Patients have mentioned how much they are affected by a nurse's smile, a gentle touch on the arm, and small acts of kindness. Mood—that is, the general tone of emotions—shapes the interpretation of perceptions and biases a person's thinking and memory (Siegel, 1999).

People are more likely to retain an event in memory and reexperience it anew if there were strong emotions accompanying the event. Let us again return to Nurse

Lyne Charbonneau and her relationship with the Alonzos. Recall that a nursing error had seriously compromised the recovery of their son and may have further caused damage to his already-fragile brain, making his long-term prognosis uncertain. Lyne remembers all too well feeling "devastated" for this family and ashamed because it was a nursing error that had put this newborn at further risk.

Lyne remembers exactly how she felt at the time. Her memory of the details surrounding the event was affected by her strong emotions at the time: *"I really felt powerless as a nurse, as a human being…I had this relationship with this family and that made it worse. It was not only having to tell them (terrible) information like this, but also the timing of it. The fact that the baby was more stable for maybe a week or two so the parents thought that maybe the baby was out of the woods…. I just thought that it was so unfair for these parents."*

Interpretation

The third component of an observation involves the interpretative system. Sensory information is interpreted through a complex system of assigning meaning to what has been observed and then creating a narrative to describe and explain the observations.

Information from the sensory organs may or may not register with a person, depending on the significance assigned and the interpretation given. Information is filtered through the person's beliefs, assumptions, knowledge, past experience, and the meaning or significance she attributes to the event. The meaning or interpretation assigned to the information directs subsequent actions. This in turn creates a new set of beliefs and assumptions, which in turn determines what new information to gather next.

Beliefs. What an individual observes is not just what he sees but also what he knows and believes to be true (Berger, 1972). Consider how knowledge and beliefs alter what a person selects to attend to and then affects how that information is subsequently interpreted.

During the mid-19th century, the medical community, including Florence Nightingale, subscribed to the *miasma theory* of disease. This theory explained that diseases such as cholera and the Black Death were caused by miasma, the Greek word for *pollution*, a noxious form of toxic air caused by decomposing matter that was believed to be poisonous (Dossey, 2000). The medical community at the time focused on removing the foul smells associated with disease. They did not know about germ theory. If they had, they would have shifted their observations and actions from contaminated air to contaminated water, the actual source of cholera. Thus, the nurse will see only what she believes to be true. In other words, she will select and attend to stimuli that fit with her current belief systems.

Beliefs often affect assumptions, and assumptions in turn affect beliefs. *Assumptions* are ideas that are taken for granted or automatically accepted as truth because they are thought to derive from evidence and experience, even when the evidence is questionable. Ideas and theories that are taken as truths are transmitted from one generation to the next among members belonging to a specific cultural, ethnic, or religious group. A particular assumption may have come from one person's experience and is told and retold until the group takes the idea as truth even though they may not have experienced the situation firsthand. There are many "facts" in older textbooks that are still accepted even though empirical research has since proven them incorrect or inaccurate.

Research has revealed that a significant number of nurses rely on information taught to them during their nursing training to make practice decisions (Estabrooks, 1998; Estabrooks et al., 2005). In other words, they are basing practice decisions on outdated, and oftentimes incorrect, information.

In everyday practice, nurses choose to attend to only specific aspects of an experience. That which draws a nurse to attend to one aspect of a person's experience or to listen to one thing and ignore another is guided by the nurse's knowledge, practical experience, beliefs, and assumptions. Nurses then explain or interpret the selected data by adding meanings (i.e., cultural and personal meaning) to interpret the information that could explain why something is the way that it is. The nurse then derives an assumption that is based on these meanings. It is these interpretations that then lead him to draw new conclusions, and it is these conclusions that direct his further actions. This sequence of events leads to certain actions, and within this sequence of events there is a reflexive loop that directs and selects specific information. This process is known as the *Ladder of Inference*, and it is shown in Figure 7.1

FIGURE 7.1

Ladder of inference.

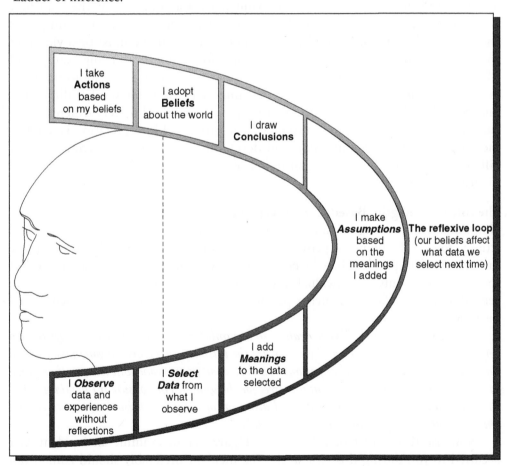

Source: Based on the work of Chris Argyris and developed by Peter M. Senge (2006).

(Argyris as cited and developed by Senge, 2006). As Nurse Sharyn Andrews explained, "*Miscommunication, misunderstanding, and mistrust can occur when a nurse 'goes up the ladder' too quickly.*"

Consider different individuals' reactions to the following scenario: A homeless person approaches a man and asks him if he has any change to spare. The man has to decide whether or not to give the homeless person money. If he believes that the person is a drug addict and will use the money to buy drugs (an example of added meaning), then he will most likely refuse the homeless person's request (his "logical" conclusion). On the other hand, if the man believes that this homeless person reflects a social injustice and inequity in the distribution of society's wealth (another example of added meaning) and that, as a more fortunate individual, he has a responsibility for the well-being of his fellow citizen (his belief and assumption), he is more likely to give the person money (his "logical" conclusion). What happens when the homeless person asking for money of the man is a young, strapping man or is a mother with a young baby? Does the man select different information and respond differently because of a different set of beliefs and meanings that he uses to understand the situation? If the person is a young man, he might assume that that person is lazy and should be working rather than asking for a handout. On the other hand, for the woman with a young baby, the man may believe that a woman's natural instinct is to protect her children (an assumption) and the fact that she has resorted to begging means that she must be a victim of an abusive partner or a single mother who can't find work (both being examples of added meaning). He might then ask the mother to tell him more about her partner or, in the other example of added meaning, may ask her about her difficulties finding work. Therefore, the interpretative process can lead to very different conclusions and result in different responses. The process of interpretation is in effect the process of creating a meaning and developing a narrative—putting together different pieces of information that have been selected to make sense of them and to create a coherent story.

The role of Strengths-Based Care interpretation

Now think of how strengths-based thinking would alter a nurse's interpretation of and attitude toward the homeless person, in contrast to those who view homeless people through a deficit, problem-based lens. Nurse Maryse Godin made this point, not just about the judgments of individual nurses but also about the health care system in general. On the surface, a homeless person is judged negatively by most members of the health care system.

As Maryse explained, "*We've dealt with a number of homeless people who get treated very negatively by the system, and yet they are the ultimate survivors. Anyone who lives on the street for fifteen years . . . that person should be dead as everyone will tell you that 'you'll catch pneumonia.' If you put me on the street for the winter, I'm not sure if I would survive. But there's an awful lot of negativity and dismissal of what is a person's ability to control one's own care when you don't quite fit the mold.*"

Now use the Ladder of Inference in Figure 7.1 to examine an incident that occurred to you during this past week. The incident preferably should come from your clinical work. If you have not yet worked in the clinical area, think of an upsetting experience in your personal life that happened this past week. It could be an incident, an event, or interaction that made you feel uncomfortable or that upset you. Write about what happened. Try to re-create the event in as much detail as possible using the questions in the figure. You should now answer the questions found in Exhibit 7.2.

Once observations have been interpreted, they need to be translated from what one has seen, transformed into images, and then put into words so that others can also imagine, share, and understand them. Thus, the observer needs to find words to articulate, describe, and explain her experiences to another person. The problem is that words can never quite capture the experience (Berger, 1972).

OBSERVATION: INTEGRATION OF ALL FIVE SENSES

Nurses rely heavily on what they see, hear, smell, and feel and, to a lesser extent, taste, to learn about the patient and her environment so they can understand the clinical significance of her concerns. The flow of information from the different sensory organs (vision, hearing, smell, taste, touch) is integrated to create a whole. An observation is experienced as a whole and not as sum of stimuli or bits of information transmitted from each sensory system. Returning to the example of a flower, its smell might suggest a flower, as does the information gained from touching it. But smell and touch alone are insufficient to determine what the object is. It is only when all the information is put together that a person not only identifies the object before him as a flower but also can identify its type and can distinguish it from others—whether it is a rose and not a tulip or an iris. This of course assumes that the observer has stored in his memory different categories of flowers. The observer also needs to be aware what thoughts and feelings are evoked when he sees a rose, hears the word *rose*, or smells a rose. For some people, a rose evokes negative emotion, especially for the person who has been pricked by a rose's thorns. However, for most people a rose evokes positive feelings and thoughts because they associate a rose with beauty, elegance, romance, and love.

> **CAVEAT**
>
> A good practitioner relies on information from all sensory systems, although information from one sensory system may be given more weight depending on the context and situation and its believed significance.

Consider the nurse who is assessing a patient's level of respiratory distress. He may give more weight to what he sees (e.g., rate of respiration, hyperventilation, shallowness or depth of respiration, dyspnea, changes in breathing rhythm accompanying any change in body positioning, cyanosis, edema in extremities, or increased anxiety) and hears (e.g., labored, gasping, wheezing respiration) than to what he smells (e.g., sweet breath odor) or to the information he gathers through touch (e.g., cold, clammy skin) (Blows, 2001).

EXHIBIT 7.2

Reflect and connect *The Ladder of Inference: Linking beliefs to assumptions to meaning to actions*

1. Choose an incident with a patient from your clinical experience that happened this past week that upset you or made you uncomfortable.
2. Write down what happened in general terms. What upset you?
3. Now take a small part of the conversation and try to re-create it.

   Take a piece of paper and divide it in half. On the right-hand side, write down what you and others actually said and did in the situation. On the left-hand side, write down any thoughts and feelings you had but did not express. It is not important that you reconstruct the exact dialogue. Your best recollection is fine. What is important is that you write an actual dialogue, as if out of a play.

   Here is an example of the format:

What I thought or felt but did not say	What I actually said
	Me: (what I said)
	Other: (what he or she said)
	Me: (what I said in response)

Analyze the case and dialogue using the Ladder of Inference

4. What was it about the incidence that surprised you? What did you expect?
5. What aspect of the conversation did you focus on? Why this aspect?
6. What assumptions do you hold about the person?
7. Why do you think the person behaved the way he did? Why did the person decide to share that piece of information with you?
8. What conclusions did you draw?
9. How did you respond? What actions did you take? Why did you respond in the way that you did? Is this how you wanted to respond? What would you have liked to say or do? Why didn't you?
10. How did that individual respond?
11. How did his response change your beliefs and assumptions about him? About what he was telling you?
12. Have you changed your beliefs or opinions? If yes, how?
13. If you had another chance, knowing what you know now, would you select other information to attend to? Would you act differently? If yes, how?
14. What would you look for to see whether your response was appropriate? Effective?

At its most basic level, *nursing observation* refers to the following:

> An objective evaluation made by a nurse of the various aspects of a client's condition. This often includes the person's general appearance, emotional affect, nutritional status, habits and preferences. It also may include assessing the patient's body temperature, skin condition, and any abnormal processes, including those of which the client complains. The person's religious preference, ethnic backround, and familial relationships are also noted. (Mosby, 2009)

In SBC, the nurse would also intentionally observe for the person's strengths: what makes him unique, what is working, how he is coping, aspects of the environment that supports innate healing, and the like (see Chapter 9 for a more complete assessment of strengths).

Visual system: Sight and images. Sight is a sensory system on which nurses rely most to begin their observations. First and foremost, nurses spend a considerable amount of their time just watching, looking, and noting. They take in a substantial amount of visual information, from which they create a first impression of what is happening. For example, when the nurse first meets a person, she may note how the person is dressed—appropriateness, grooming, and any distinctive style. She also will note the way the person approaches her: hesitantly or confidently. In addition she will observe the person's facial expression—happy, relaxed, calm, sad, tense, apprehensive, the like—as well as the person's general physical demeanor (i.e., position, posture, standing upright or stooped over). An important area to observe is patients' energy levels as reflected in the way they walk—with a spring in their gait or slowly and cautiously—or their level of animation—depressed, excited. Nurses make these multiple observations almost instantaneously and without conscious awareness. There are many thought processes involved in creating the whole, including perceptions, representations, memory, interpretation and the like.

Nurses also rely heavily on visual representations or images as a way of getting to know their patients (Barnard, 2009). Monitors, computer screens, and scanning machines produce visual representations of the body's interior. These technological images provide information about the person's internal organs that is not visible or accessible to the naked eye. Nurses spend considerable time integrating these different visual forms of information to arrive at as comprehensive and complete a view of the person as possible. They are constantly observing at different levels. For example, a mammogram may have revealed the existence of breast cancer. The nurse may have visually seen the tumor on the X-ray and have observed how the patient reacts to the news of a breast tumor.

Nurses also rely on what they see to assess the person's environment and how the environment affects him. What the nurse selects to attend depends to a large extent on the purpose of the observation. For example, if a person is being discharged from the hospital to her home following a stroke, the nurse might opt to visit the patient's home to gather information about its safety and suitability, or meet with a family member who has firsthand knowledge of the patient's home. He would note or ask about the number of stairs to get into the house and the number of stairs inside the house, the location of the patient's bedroom in relation to the bathroom and kitchen, and the presence of handrails and any other physical features that might affect the patient's mobility.

He would also note any safety hazards, such as a loose floor rug; whether there are rugs on the stairs; the amount of clutter; the height of the toilet seat; and the accessibility and ease of use of the sink, shower, or bathtub. He would ask about the person's support system, such as who will be doing the caretaking and, if the caregiver is present, what the nature of her involvement will be and whether her level of openness, commitment, and skill are suitable to care for the patient. Table 7.2 provides some examples of areas to which the nurse may attend when observing a patient or family.

Auditory system: Hearing and sound. Nurses rely on listening to learn more about the patient as a person and how he is coping with his condition and challenges. Consider what a nurse listens for at different levels. At the physical level, the nurse listens to the person's chest to determine patency of air flow in the bronchi, or she may listen for bowel sounds after abdominal surgery as an indication of bowel functioning. To determine the person's emotional state, the nurse listens to what the person says and the way he expresses himself. The nurse listens to, among other things, the tone, pitch, volume, and intensity of the patient's voice. A person who is sad and depressed often speaks in a monotone, with a low pitch and flat cadence. Or consider a mother or an experienced pediatric nurse who is able to interpret an infant's cry just by listening to its timber and rhythm. They are able to differentiate a hungry cry from a bored cry; a bored cry from a cry of pain; and a cry of pain from a squeal of delight indicative of pleasure—an I "want-to-have fun-with-you-now" signal.

The nurse also listens to what people say and how they say it and whether what they say matches their tone of voice and nonverbal gestures. For example, the person may recount a painful incident that happened to her years earlier, and the deep sadness in her voice gives the nurse insight into the impact the event has had on her life (for a more detailed discussion of attentive and deep listening, see Chapter 8). Table 7.2 provides some examples of areas that the nurse listens for and to.

Olfactory and pheromonal systems: Smells and odors. Smell is discerned by the olfactory nerve, which is located above the nose and is used to detect odors. Smell is often the first sensory organ to be activated, and it provides the nurse with cues that all may not be right. The nurse may smell something that is unusual, unexpected, or out of place. For example, on entering a patient's room, the nurse may detect a putrid smell. It is noting an unexpected odor that often leads a nurse to investigate further. There are different odors that nurses need to decipher. Before they can accurately distinguish smells, they must train their noses to detect and discriminate among many different odors. Although there are 260 different descriptors and 88 classes of odors (Arctander, 1961), for nursing's purposes the range of classes is much more limited. The nurse needs to have learned what is a "good" body odor and what odors indicate that something may be amiss. Nurses need to retrain their senses and develop a "nose" for distinguishing abnormal smells. For example, they need to decipher unpleasant odors that may indicate an infection, a problem in the respiratory, digestive, or elimination systems. Nurses detect odors emanating from any of the body orifices or body surfaces (e.g., nose, mouth, anus, or skin pores). Table 7.2 provides some examples of smells that nurses look for.

Gustatory system: Taste. Taste is the least frequently used sensory system in clinical practice. Although nurses may use taste infrequently, they do need to know its elements to understand what their patients are telling them. For example, if a patient complains that a medicine is bitter, the nurse may disguise the taste by suggesting

TABLE 7.2

Observations: Examples of areas that the nurses attend to through their sensory systems of vision, hearing, smell, taste, and touch

Sensory Systems	Examples of Areas
1. Visual system: Sight and Images	
Body behavior	Posture (turning away, turning towards, leaning, standing straight or bent over), movement, gestures, hands open or closed
Eye behavior	Eye contact (eye gaze, eye aversion), staring, focusing, eye movement
Facial expression (evidence of emotion)	Smiles, frowns, raised eyebrows, mouth and lips, indicators of sadness, elation, withdrawn, engaging, happy, uncertain
General appearance	Well-groomed or disheveled
Habits	Tics, unusual gesturing
Head movement	Nodding, turning away
Nutritional state	Well nourished, obese, anorexic
Physiologic response	Quickened breathing, blushing, pallor, pupils, fidgeting
Physical features	Fitness, height, weight, complexion, skin tone
Response time	Hurried or slow
Space and proximity	Distance or closeness
2. Auditory system: Hearing and sound	
Physiological sounds	Breath sounds, gurgling, hollow tympany, assessed by palpation and auscultation
Voice behavior	Tone, pitch, volume, intensity, inflection, emphasis, pauses, silence, fluency, pressure in speech
3. Olfactory and pheromonal systems: Smell, odor	Pleasant (sweet, fruity), foul, acrid, smoky
4. Gustatory system: Taste	Distinguish among different tastes (sweet, sour, salty, bitter, and umami [savory])
5. Somatosensory system: Touch (somatic sense), temperature, proprioception (body position), nociception (pain)	
Hydration	Firm or dry, moist or dry, cracked
Temperature	Hot, warm, cool, cold
Peripheral pulse	Bounding/faint pulse
Tissue integrity	Lumpy or smooth, mushy or firm, elastic or flaccid
Pain	Quality Intensity Descriptors: S—sensory (e.g., stabbing); A—affective (e.g., cruel); E—evaluative (e.g., intense); M—miscellaneous (e.g., nagging)

that the medicine be taken with a sweet liquid, such as orange juice. As part of a neurological assessment, a nurse may ask a patient to taste a food to see whether the patient's gustatory system is functioning. Table 7.2 lists the areas of which nurses need to be aware to understand how taste is experienced and described.

Somatosensory system: Touch. Touch usually involves skin-to-skin contact to assess the patient's internal state and physical status. For example, the nurse feels the warmth or coolness of the skin to assess for body temperature, the skin's turgor to assess hydration, its dryness to assess for risk of bedsores, the strength of the pulse to detect strong or irregular heartbeats. The nurse may apply touch to assess for the presence of pain, such as its intensity and quality. The most widely used pain assessment tool is the McGill Pain Questionnaire (Melzack, 2005). Pain descriptors are classified into four major groups: (a) sensory (e.g., tender, taut, hot, lacerating), (b) affective (e.g., sickening, wretched, frightening), (c) evaluative (e.g., annoying, intense, unbearable), and (d) miscellaneous (e.g., piercing, cold, nagging).

Nurses also use touch as a therapeutic intervention to soothe, calm, and comfort patients as well as touch, to communicate affection, nurturance, and support. The nurse often uses touch in combination with information gathered from other senses. Table 7.2 provides some examples of areas of information gathered by touch.

Observation as an Integrated Perceptual Experience

Observation encompasses the way sensory inputs and sensations come together as an experience. It is about situating the experience within a larger context of how others respond (O'Regan & Noe, 2001). Consider a nurse's experience on the first day of working on an outpatient oncology unit where chemotherapy is administered. What is the "feel" of that unit compared to other units where she has worked? (She could compare the "feel" of this unit with that of a postpartum unit.) To answer this question, the nurse would probably note the amount of activity on the unit and what the nurses are doing. She would observe the expressions on the faces of the patients waiting to have their name called for chemotherapy compared to the faces of new mothers waiting for their infants to arrive from the nursery. She would register the concerned look on a partner's face compared to the elated and excited feeling of new fathers, partners, siblings, and grandparents on the postpartum unit as they get their first glimpses of the newborn. She would watch how nurses approach and speak to anxious patients returning for another round of chemotherapy compared to how nurses speak to anxious new mothers about breastfeeding problems. She would listen to announcements on the loudspeaker, being more primed to hear a code call on the oncology unit than on the postpartum unit.

These observations are not about the activation of the visual and auditory sensory systems but how the nurse registers these activities as an experience—experiences that are qualitatively different in feeling, tone, and message. Thus, all sensations—visual, auditory, tactile and the like—are more about the *experiential*—the nature of the experience created from all the sensory input—rather than about what sensory systems are activated and the type of input being transmitted to the brain.

Criteria to Judge an Observation

A quality observation is ultimately judged by the degree to which the information gathered contributes to an understanding of the situation and, in the case of clinical work, contributes to the nurse's sound clinical grasp of the situation on which he can base judgments, decisions, and actions. For this to happen, the observation must encompass the following:

- Salience
- Relevancy or pertinence
- Relatedness

Salience refers to that which is most important and most urgent in a particular clinical situation (Benner et al., 2010). Salience is about identifying the most important features of a given experience related to understanding the issue and making sense of the problem. It is about assigning importance to one piece of information over another piece of information on the basis of general knowledge of the condition or phenomenon combined with specific knowledge about that specific patient.

Relevance refers to that which is significant and pertinent and has bearing in a given situation. The assessment of relevance is subjective and depends on what the nurse believes to be pertinent relative to other pieces of information. It is about attending, being attuned to, and selecting data to help the nurse discern what is at stake in a given situation, as well as weighing and balancing different pieces of information and deciding which set of data, which cluster of information, and which patterns of responses are most likely to help the nurse grasp or understand what is going on.

Relatedness refers to the interconnectedness among different observations that are brought together to help the nurse understand the whole situation. Nurses are concerned with identifying patterns, information that can be linked. They are always looking to see how information fits, to note which behaviors are consistent with past ways of behaving, or ways of responding across similar situations, and which behaviors are out of character for the person.

Saliency, relevancy, and relatedness are associated with a second set of criteria needed for an observation to be useful:

- Accuracy
- Detail
- Clarity
- Timely

Accuracy refers to the skillful use of the senses—seeing, hearing, smelling, and touching—to capture what has *actually* happened. It involves exactitude and rigor, and the information reported approximates, as closely as possible, what actually occurred and when it occurred. Accuracy involves validity, which means that the observation is communicated using unambiguous terms and is described in ways that are roughly similar to those of other trained observers (CRNBC, 2009).

Detail refers to an observation that contains enough specific information that another person can imagine what has been seen, heard, and experienced, as if she had been there. Detailed observations provide a comprehensive picture of the person: her condition, complaints, concerns, and issues. Detailed observations are always situated and contextualized. For example, a nurse may take a patient's temperature only to discover that it is elevated. A "good" observation would include a description of the patient's skin—flushed, reddened, pale, hot to touch, and associated signs of fever: perspiring, dry, chilled, shivering, and so forth. In addition, the nurse would situate the observation in context by noting the temperature outside and inside the patient's room, whether the patient is dressed appropriately, is in bed covered with blankets or with just a sheet, or has been exposed to a pathogens such as in contact with others with infection. The nurse would systematically look for other things commonly associated with an elevated temperature, such as signs of inflammation— redness, edema which may or may not associated with an infection and signs of infection, skin lesions, exudate, and unusual odor. The nurse categorizes, classifies, and groups observations to identify patterns that can help interpret these data.

Clarity refers to how well the observation has been articulated, described, and explained. An observation is a reconstructed account of an actual event, encounter, or experience. Observations need to be clearly described to allow for different interpretations. Nurses need to be able to speak and write about their observations of patients' physical and emotional responses to their medical condition and treatment and equally well about their narrative understanding of their patients' illness experiences and the issues that are of concern and to communicate clearly to others their patients' wants and needs. In their role of patient advocate, nurses are often asked by patients to be their voice. To do this, they need to be able to clearly describe to others what the patient and family have told them and what they have observed. They need to link their observations to other evidence, including what is known in the literature. They are responsible for synthesizing the information and communicating it clearly to others to ensure that patients are listened to and, more important, heard. Consider the story told in Exhibit 7.3 by Nurse Maryse Godin of Amy Fuller and how Maryse had to make the case on Amy's behalf to Amy's parents and the staff regarding what she wanted in terms of further treatments. Maryse had spent time getting to know Amy, understanding who Amy was, including Amy's fears and concerns, and gaining Amy's trust. Combined with Maryse's belief in a patient's right to self-determination (an important SBC value; see Chapter 3), Maryse was able to act as Amy's advocate and help Amy get her voice heard.

The word *timely* refers to when an observation is made. For an observation to be useful, it must be made and communicated in a timely manner, so if something needs to be done, it can be done. Sometimes the nurse needs to wait for events to unfold before he can fully understand the issues and what is at stake. Other times, the nurse needs to intervene quickly to stop an untoward event from happening or to prevent deterioration in the patient. With practice, nurses learn when to wait and when to go into action.

Now consider the story told by Nurse Marie Grace Espinosa about Stephanie Shore, a young postpartum mother who was not interested in having contact with her newborn infant. It was Marie Grace's astute observations that led to a discovery

EXHIBIT 7.3

Personal experience *Amy Fuller: A story of suffering and resolve and advocacy*

Told by Nurse Maryse Godin

Amy Fuller was a young woman in her early 30s with very limited family support. She had suffered since childhood with an extreme form of juvenile arthritis. Amy was wheelchair bound, and her condition deteriorated to a point where she could no longer function at home. Many of the other children with juvenile arthritis whom she had met during her repeated childhood hospitalizations had died. She was admitted to the hospital with infected joints that required megadoses of prednisone. The antibiotics were not working. Amy had reached a point where she was saying, "I don't want to die, but I can't go on suffering like this." Despite the intractable pain, she kept agreeing to treatments—surgeries, more blood tests—and after each painful procedure, she cried —"I can't take this anymore." She didn't want to disappoint the surgeon by saying no to further treatments. She was really concerned that if she said no to a surgical treatment, the doctor with whom she now had almost a father–daughter relationship would just walk away because he'd have nothing left to do for her. Amy was ambivalent; as she said, "People keep telling me to fight, but I'm tired of fighting." Her mother was busy searching for the next new treatment and would never give up. Amy didn't want to tell her family that she was giving up because she was afraid of what it would do to them. She had come to the conclusion that the disease was going to kill her, but still she decided that she was going to call the shots. She was not afraid of dying; she was afraid of suffering: not only physical suffering but also mental suffering. As the time passed, Amy reached a point where she didn't want them (the staff) to do things to her. As she said, "I don't want this anymore, and how do I make that happen." So she decided to move into palliative care. She asked Maryse to talk to her family, not about making the decision, her decision was made, but to explain her decision and make sure that they were okay with it. And over the weeks, she looked more peaceful, not pain free, but her pain was tolerable. She seemed to perk up. But as she waited for death, it didn't come. As Maryse related, *"Now she finds herself kind of in limbo. She expected to die, but she didn't. Now she is busy planning her next step."*

that had eluded others because they had prejudged this young mother and labeled her behavior incorrectly. In telling the story, Marie Grace illustrates all the criteria for quality observations: salience, relevancy, and relatedness. She also describes the unfolding events accurately, in detail, and with clarity that well captures the role that time played in a missed diagnosis and a delayed treatment that had dire consequences for this young mother. *"Stephanie showed no interest in seeing the baby. She was into herself. She was only thinking about herself. And she was telling me 'I don't understand, they're telling me that I don't care about my baby, but the truth is that I really feel weak.' So I paid attention to her and I said 'It's something that's very subjective.' Everyone else was saying 'She's manipulating us' and everyone—the nurses and staff and even her doctors were getting fed up with her."*

Marie Grace recounted how the staff described Stephanie: *"She's being manipulative, she's the youngest of all of the family, and she's always been manipulative, she tends to get her way."* And yet Marie Grace knew this was wrong. She decided to follow up on what the patient was telling her: *"It became for me that I have to listen to her and find out how she feels. I have to listen to what she says regardless of everyone saying that she's manipulative. We have to listen to what the patient is saying to us."*

What Marie Grace noticed alarmed her: *"Increasingly she was getting more symptomatic, short of breath, and she was swelling up. She looked edematous. I noticed a rash, like a butterfly rash, and I was looking at her and she was telling me about her symptoms, that she hasn't been feeling well, and was very tired, and then something clicked for me 'This patient has lupus.' And I thought then that there's something not right about this patient."*

At Marie Grace's urging, Stephanie was not discharged. Marie Grace continued with the story: *"They did some tests. At one point Stephanie's blood pressure was quite low and she would just lie down in bed and say 'I feel weak, I don't have energy.' And even though they did tests, they were inconclusive. . . . Stephanie deteriorated. One evening, I was working evenings and Stephanie just became psychotic. She was screaming in the hallway. She had an IV and she pulled it out. She started throwing everything: She threw the phone and we had to call stat for the orderly, code white. And then a psychiatrist had to come and he had to give her medication. She deteriorated within five weeks' time. But . . . looking back she had the symptoms [of lupus]. There were days she said she couldn't get up. And then now the stress of having a baby, that caused stress in her body, and it (the lupus) flared up. She had some shortness of breath. It seemed that it (lupus) had already attacked her lungs. Then the confusion when it attacked the brain. So by then they had consulted the [intensive care unit] to see if there was something wrong, to investigate, and that's when they transferred her to a medical floor. And they said that she's very sick."*

Marie Grace first recognized inconsistencies between what Stephanie said about her baby and how she felt about being a mother by *relating* two ideas. Because she knew this patient, she knew that what she was observing in Stephanie was not manipulative behavior, as interpreted by the staff, but something else. Marie Grace recognized the *salience* of the rash. She understood that it was important to listen to patients and realized that what they are telling the nurse is usually *relevant*.

Documentation and Strengths-Based Care

Florence Nightingale understood the importance of communication and knowledge dissemination. She was a master at recording what she observed, documenting her observations supported by data, facts, and research. She recorded her thoughts and ideas in letters, briefs, newspaper articles, books, position papers—and communicating detailed descriptions in a timely manner to influence and plan care. She wrote to educate, such as when she wrote the book, *How to Care for the Ill for the Laboring*

(Working) Class. She also wrote position papers for members of parliament to develop public health policy. She carried on an extensive correspondence with family, friends, and people of influence, including Queen Victoria and Prince Albert. She recognized that it is insufficient just to train nurses to be astute observers: Nurses also needed to be trained to systematically record and communicate their observations accurately and in a language that was accessible and usable. A patient's health, safety, and even his life depended on nurses and doctors having timely and detailed information to guide them in making clinical decisions, deciding what action to take, and what treatments to prescribe.

> Learning to observe is a beginning. Nurses also need to be trained to systematically record and communicate their observations accurately and in language that is accessible and usable by all health care providers.

There is a YouTube video made by Jennifer Murdock reading from *Notes on Nursing,* Nightingale's words on the importance of documentation. See http://www.youtube.com/watch?v=_ID5vQiwI-M&feature=related

Nursing documentation has traditionally included Nurse's Notes, Kardex, shift reports, critical incidence reports, and care maps as the more common forms. More recently, nurses have begun to use electronic records, electronic tablets, iPhones, and the social media to document their observations and share with others what they know about the person and family.

Nurses have generally preferred oral communication to written communication (Jefferies, Johnson, & Griffiths, 2010) and have been more adept in communicating detailed observation in this mode. By relying heavily on oral communication, much of what nurses do and how they do it has been lost, because information that is orally transmitted takes its meaning from the immediate situation (Jefferies et al., 2010).

Written communication, on the other hand, has many advantages. It provides the profession with a repository of nursing knowledge. It helps document nursing's development and nursing's unique contribution to patient care and patient outcomes (Jefferies et al., 2010). Unfortunately, nurses have not used written communication effectively or to their advantage. In fact, a consistent finding across studies is that nurses tend to use written communication as little more than an "accounting mechanism" to record the minimum about the patient's condition and the tasks they have undertaken, to fulfill their legal obligation rather than to record details about the patient's condition and the care provided (Allen, 1998).

Nurses have a responsibility, both professionally and legally, to document their observations accurately, in detail, with clarity, and in a timely manner. Nurses' documentation has been used in court as a source of evidence and has played a role in determining the innocence or guilt of defendants.

In 2003, the American Nurses Association introduced its Principles for Documentation based on their Code of Ethics for Nurses (Ferrell, 2007; Monarch, 2007). In Canada, many provincial Colleges of Registered Nurses, including Nova Scotia (CRNNS, 2005); Alberta (CARNA, 2006); British Columbia (CRNBC, 2009); and, most recently, Ontario (CNO-OIIO, 2008) have developed standards and guidelines for documentation. There is a remarkable consensus among these practice standards in terms of the purposes served by documentation and suggested guidelines to improve the quality of nursing records.

Nurses generally are required to document their observations, actions, and patient outcomes to record and communicate client and patient information. Documentation serves multiple purposes (Cheevakasemsook, Chapman, Francis, & Davies, 2006; CNO, 2010; CRNBC, 2009; Jefferies et al., 2010), such as to (a) define what nurses actually do and their contribution to patient care; (b) communicate patient status and ensure patient safety and to help others in their decision making; (c) demonstrate knowledge, judgment, and critical thinking; (d) promote good nursing by ensuring continuity of care, quality of care, and planning of care through communication; (e) furnish legal evidence of the process and outcomes of care; (f) provide evidence for research, and financial and ethical quality-assurance purposes; (g) provide databases for future planning; (h) provide benchmarks for nursing's development, and so on.

Nursing organizations at both the national and at state/provincial levels have suggested ways to improve the quality of various documentation systems. They have devised some documentation tools and suggested strategies to increase accuracy to help nurses communicate in a clearer, more focused, and concise way. These suggestions have ranged from improving how best to record patient narratives to charting using a structured system such as SOAP (*S*ubjective data, *O*bjective data, *A*ssessment, and *P*lan) and PIE charting (*P*roblem, *I*ntervention, and *E*valuation). In addition, there are other tools to help improve communication to become more focused and to detail specific types of information targeted to specific readers and audiences. These include such systems as critical pathways, care maps, and incidence reports.

> Quality observations are acquired as the nurse learns what is clinically important (saliency), pertinent and significant to that client/patent/family (relevance), and how observations are interconnected to reveal patterns (related).

In summary, quality observations require that the nurse take time to make detailed observations by attending to and being attuned to what is happening and how the person is experiencing her situation. If the observation meets the criteria of salience, relevance, and relatedness, and, more specifically, is accurate, detailed, and communicated both orally and in written form in a clear and timely manner, then the information should help nurses, doctors, and other health team members who rely on these observations in developing insights into the nature of the clinical problem and become the basis for sound clinical judgment and ethical decision making.

TOOLBOX

Tools to Become an Astute Observer

Becoming an astute observer requires being trained to attend to what is happening all around and, most important, to register these observations.

It begins by doing the following:

- *Being mindful.* Recall from Chapter 5 that mindfulness involves being fully present in a situation. It requires that the person switch from functioning on automatic pilot to being fully aware of what is going on inside herself—those bodily sensations that may sabotage efforts—and in one's surrounding environment. A nervous person is unlikely to attend to input from the environment. Simply taking a deep breath before going into a patient's room may calm the nurse's nerves, thereby opening him to see things afresh. You may want to review the strategies and techniques that were suggested in Chapter 5 for improving mindfulness.

- *Attending to* elements of a given situation requires focused and sustained attention, alertness, and effortful control (Siegel, 2007). The nurse needs to ready her mind by being fully alert and constantly on the lookout. It begins making a conscious decision to train all the senses to what is happening. Nurses can use a number of strategies and techniques to train the mind so they can be fully present. All nurses can benefit from such training. Specific techniques have been found to improve recording details and encourage listening in a more attentive manner. These techniques are described below and elaborated further in Chapter 8.

- *Alerting.* The nurse needs to be at a moderate level of alertness as well as be vigilant by preparing for the expected and being on the lookout for the unexpected. The nurse needs to ask himself, "What am I seeing (observing) in this situation? Is this what I expected?"

- *Attuning to* refers to becoming aware of and in tune with what is going on inside oneself (i.e., one's bodily sensations, emotional states, feelings, and thoughts) in order to be attuned to another person's state. Nurses can do this by monitoring what is happening inside themselves by asking the following questions:
  - What am I feeling?
  - What am I thinking?
  - How does that patient make me feel?
  - Am I comfortable or tense with this patient?
  - If I am tense, why is this the case?

- *Adopting a reflective approach to practice.* An important technique to add to the nurse's toolbox is learning to become a reflective practitioner. Reflection-before-action, reflection-during-action, and reflection-on-action involves constantly and continuously asking oneself questions about what one is seeing, hearing, smelling, and touching. Specific techniques for developing reflective skills have been covered in Chapter 5, Essential Nurse Qualities to

Practice SBC and are elaborated in Chapter 10, Approaches for Working with Strengths.

- *Asking for and learning from feedback from others.* Feedback is essential for learning. It is important to listen to what another person has observed. A good mentor will first listen to what has been observed before offering her own impressions. It is important to listen to feedback and learn from constructive suggestions. It also is important to entertain alternative ways of seeing and experiencing the same situation and to learn from others' experiences. More experienced nurses will quickly attune themselves to the critical elements of a situation. Peers are an important source of support and feedback. It is important to ask another person to observe the same situation and then to share these observations (Davys & Jones, 2007). It is in listening to what other people saw, and understanding why they selected to attend to what they did, that will sensitize the learner to what is salient in a given situation.

Developing Tools to Improve the Quality of Observations

Nurses need to develop a number of strategies and techniques to improve the quality of their observations and add to their toolbox. Quality observations are acquired as a nurse learns what is salient and relevant and how observations are related. These tools are summarized in Table 7.3 and described in more detail below.

A. Developing a sense of salience *requires that the nurse:*

become actively engaged in learning. You need to understand your own thinking behind what you attend to and why you select what you do.

TABLE 7.3

Toolbox: Tools for developing quality observations

Experiences For Retraining the Senses	Suggested Tools for Maximizing Learning
1. Salience	• Prepare for clinical practice • Compare observations with an experienced nurse • Learn from clinical narratives and cases • Become curious; ask questions • Listen to how others describe their nursing • Learn by exchanging information with experienced and less experienced clinicians • Read broadly: Use formal knowledge to help interpret the clinical situation
2. Relevance	• Learn to ask "what if" questions • Rehearse how to respond • Listen to your own inner voice
3. Relatedness	• Construct a concept map • Write or tell about the clinical incident in the form of a case study, story, or narrative • Adopt an "unknowing" stance • Keep your eyes and ears open at all times

The following are strategies nurses have used to develop habits of the mind (Benner et al., 2011) and develop their sense of salience (Benner et al., 2010):

1. *Prepare for clinical practice.* As a nurse, you need to
   - Read up about the patient's diagnoses and treatment.
   - Find out as much as possible about the patient beforehand by reading the chart. Ask about the patient's responses to treatment and the impact of the condition has had on him and his family.
   - Make a list of what you expect to see. During and after the clinical experience, record what you actually saw that was on your list. If you have time, return to the patient and look for the items on your preclinical list. If additional things you observe were not on your preclinical list, you can add them even if you had not expected them.
   - Explain why you think those items were or were not on the list.
2. *Listen to how others describe their nursing.* Become actively engaged in the discussion by considering whether you would have attended to the same information. What information would you have selected instead, and why?
3. *Compare observations with those of an experienced nurse.* To begin, list five observations and rank them in terms of importance. Explain the reason for your rank ordering. Now ask an experienced nurse who has also been caring for your patient to do the same. Then compare your list with hers and discuss what was on your list—what was the same, what was missing, and why.
4. *Learn from clinical narratives and case studies.* Attend to what the nurse who is sharing the story or describing the scenario chose to focus on. Question her choice of events and features and listen carefully to her underlying rationale.
5. *Become curious.* Learn to ask questions and learn from others. Try to understand the thinking behind another's thinking. Ask such questions as
   - How did you know that?
   - What did you look for in that situation?

B. Developing a sense of relevance *requires that the nurse:*

1. *Learn to ask "what-if" questions:* Prepare for different eventualities by asking "what if" questions, for example, "What if the patient experiences a sharp drop in blood pressure when I am getting him out of bed for the first time post-op?" "What if the patient is agitated?" Think of the information you will need to gather to be prepared for that "what-if" scenerio. For each scenario you think about ahead of time, the better prepared you will be to anticipate and respond effectively in a relevant manner.
2. *Rehearse how to respond appropriately.* Review different responses to the possible different scenarios and, if necessary, role play with others. In particular, make sure that your response is relevant. Provide your rationale for its relevancy.

CAVEAT

Nurses who practice SBC are always responsive to the situation and never prescriptive. A nurse can be responsive only if she is open to many possibilities and if she has developed a large repertoire of skills, strategies, and tools to deal with a wide range of issues, diagnoses, and treatments.

3. *Listen to your own inner voice.* Take time to and find a quiet space to attend to your inner voice, a "gut" reaction, or unpleasant bodily sensations. When you get in touch with your inner feelings and know that not "all is right," it is important for you to follow up and deliberately ask yourself— "What am I feeling, and why do I think I am feeling this way?" "Is my response relevant to the situation that I am dealing with?" Explain your answer. It is important that you not ignore what your body is telling you. The body often registers ideas, messages from the subcortical region of the brain, before it forms them into rational thoughts in the cortical regions of the brain.

C. Developing a sense of relatedness *requires the nurse to:*

1. *Construct a concept map.* A *concept map* is a diagram or graphical representation of how different ideas and concepts are related. It is a useful tool for synthesizing vast amounts of information and finding relationships among them (Novak & Canas, 2008).

> There are many excellent resources on the Internet that explain how to construct a conceptual map. A most useful website is http://www.ihmc.us

2. *Write or present the clinical or critical incident in the form of a case study, story, or narrative.* In writing or telling the story, you can become aware of what you know and what you do not know, what is present, and what might otherwise go unnoticed (Frank, 2004). In creating the person's story, remember the patient's concerns and how they relate to events such as the chronological sequence of how events unfolded, the different actors or players who have been involved, the nature of their relationships, and any change in their roles. The patient may also want to discuss people who were conspicuously absent. The story should include changing circumstances and contexts. In creating the story, put together the interconnections among different events and pieces, those aspects that fit and those that matter. Note what aspects do not fit or make sense. Constructing stories and retelling the narratives raises questions that need to be answered and identifies information that is lacking or missing. Also summarize that which is known and that which still needs further observation. Remember, everyone has a story, and it is by learning their story that their uniqueness and strengths are revealed.

Additional tools to improve the quality of observations are summarized in Table 7.4.

1. *Make and take time to observe.* Learning comes from observing. It is important to think of the practice setting as the nurse's learning laboratory. It is while caring for patients that you will develop and hone your skills of accuracy. Moreover, the more information you takes in, the more you will understand and come to know, and the more complete and comprehensive your observations will be. Take your time observing and learn how to accurately observe. You need to

TABLE 7.4

Additional tools for developing and improving observations

Experiences For Retraining the Senses	Suggested Tools for Maximizing Learning
1. Make and take time to observe	• Make direct observations • Choose a way to record observations • Make time to observe • Set aside specific time per shift • Use SBC values as a guide
2. Undertake training programs	• Use original art and focused training • Use reflective and structured questioning to guide observations
3. Develop exercises to improve accuracy, detail, clarity, and timeliness	• Learn to scan the environment • Train your memory • Use peers to compare observations • Reflect on observations • Develop skills of clear documentation • Practice situation-responsive nursing

become aware of and in tune with your thoughts and feelings and the way you are experiencing the activities surrounding you.

Russell and Ng (2009) suggested a number of strategies to improve the quality of an observation:

- *Make direct observations.* An important part of observation is to note the climate and culture of the unit and how you develop your practice with or without the assistance of your peers.
- *Choose a way to record observations.* Events can be videotaped, and conversations can be audiotaped. Incidents, dialogues, and interactions can be re-created in written form, as in a journal, or in note form. What is important is that you create a record of your experiences and documents these observations. You need to have a written record to share with others, to reflect and analyze what has been experienced, and to come up with new insights.
- *Make time to observe.* Patients are always being observed. Nurses can set aside specific time to observe indirectly, that is, when they are not providing direct care. Practice observing even from outside the patient's room, for example, when the patient is interacting with a family member, a roommate, another nurse, a physician, and the like.
- *Set aside time to watch what is going on.* If and when possible, put aside a specific amount of time each day just to develop skills of observation. Such time slots can range from a few seconds to a few minutes or longer.
- *Use SBC values as a guide.* You should use the values underlying SBC to guide you as to what to watch and listen for. For example, a nurse who values readiness and learning will attend to and record any statement or behavior that is indicative of the patient's readiness. You should list the values underlying the framework you follow, as described in Chapter 3, and devote time to identifying what the patient said or did that would provide data about those specific values.

2. *Undertake training programs that improve skills of observing.* A number of studies have found that nurses can be trained to become better observers:

- *Use original art and focused observational training.* Structured, short, focused observational experiences can improve the quality of observations. Nursing students, when given original works of art and asked to visually itemize everything in a short period of time, not only improved their skills of observation but also were able to successfully transfer this training to the clinical situation (Pellico, Friedlaender, & Fennie, 2009).
- *Use structured and reflective questioning about what you have observed.* For example, medical and nursing students from the University of Texas Health Center who participated in a three-week workshop offered by the McNay Art Museum in San Antonio improved their observational and communication skills (press release from McNay Art Museum, January 20, 2011) and demonstrated measurable improvement in their visual observation and communication skills that translated into improvements in patient care.

3. *Develop exercises to improve accuracy, detail, and clarity.*
To improve accuracy:

- Scan the environment, noting physical surroundings, smells, unusual sounds, and so forth.
- Make a mental note of what you saw.
- At the first opportunity, reconstruct key observations by writing them down, clearly and concisely.
- Reread notes at a later date for detail and to see whether they are understandable.
- Add a clinical note by filling in gaps and omissions.
- Ask a colleague who is familiar with the situation to verify your observations by asking, "Is this what you observed?"
- Ask a peer to observe with you. One person should focus her attention on observing, and the other person should take notes to aid in feedback—then reverse roles.

To increase detail:

- Choose an inanimate object or a situation that is relatively stable to observe, such as a patient's unit, the nursing station, or a patient who is alone. Spend five minutes looking and listening. Now record your observation. Return to the area and compare what you have noted with what is actually there. Repeat this the next day to see whether your memory and recall have improved.
- Reflect on the observation as recorded in your notes. Ask yourself, "What caught my attention? Why did I attend to what I attended to?"

To increase clarity:
When communicating observations both orally and in written form:

- Keep sentences short. Avoid complex sentence construction with coordinating conjunctions such as *because*, *nonetheless*, and *therefore*.
- Write about one idea at a time.
- Introduce the point you want to make in the first sentence of the paragraph, and then elaborate what you mean. Illustrate the point with a concrete example. Use the patient's actual words.

- Avoid interpretation and labeling. It is best to describe the event and verbal and nonverbal behavior without interpretation.

To increase timeliness:

- Be guided by knowledge of the phenomenon and the person. This is called *situation-responsive nursing.*
- Get to know the patient. Observe for and listen to cues of readiness.
- Learn the difference between choosing to wait with intention and doing nothing because you don't know what to do.

Key Summary Points

- Each profession has a specific professional gaze that is their practitioners' orientation that directs observations.
- Nurses need to train and retrain their senses to become astute observers. Accurate and detailed observations are required for clinical reasoning and clinical decision making.
- Clinical inquiry is about gathering information from many sources to identify and clarify the issues, define the problem, get to know the person, and discover ways to work with the person and family. On the other hand, critical inquiry also is the act of analyzing the information to make sense of the information gathered.
- Siegel (1999) identified four streams of awareness under the acronym SOCK: Sensation, Observation, Concepts, and Knowing. Each stream is involved in clinical work.
- The art of observation involves mastering the what, why, who, when, where, and how of observation. Observations require perception, memory, and interpretation.
- Information is experienced through the five traditional, "outer" sensory systems, namely, the (a) visual system (sight and images), (b) auditory system (hearing and sound), (c) gustatory system (taste), and (d) somatosensory system (touch), and through the three "inner" senses—(a) awareness of that which is happening inside oneself, (b) awareness of one's feelings and thoughts, and (c) awareness of that which is happening outside oneself in the surrounding environment and its impact on oneself—that are key to self-awareness and other sources of information about the patient's condition. Information is then processed by relating it to memory, interpreting it, and registering it.
- The criteria to assess the quality of observations are (a) salience; (b) relevancy; (c) relatedness. They in turn are affected by the accuracy, detail, clarity, and timeliness of the observations.
- Observations need to be documented. Documentation serves to communicate to others what has been observed.
- Nurses need to have in their toolbox a large repertoire of strategies, approaches, and techniques to develop and improve the quality and comprehensiveness of their observations.

Reforming Skills of Social Involvement: Attunement, Authentic Presence, Attentive Listening, and Clinical Conversation

8

LEARNING OBJECTIVES

After reading this chapter, you should be able to:

- Explain what social involvement is and why it is important to reform and retrain one's social involvement skills to become a professional nurse
- Discuss the relationships among inspired knowing, therapeutic relationships, professional caring, and Strengths-Based Care
- Define *attunement, authentic presence*, and *attentive listening* and explain their importance in nursing
- Describe the tools to develop attunement, authentic presence, and attentive listening
- Compare ordinary conversations and clinical conversations
- Discuss the differences between dialoguing and interviewing and the various tools to develop and improve these skills
- Explain behaviors that can derail clinical conversations and some repair tools

> Nursing is an art: and if it is to be made an art, it requires an exclusive devotion as hard a preparation, as any painter's or sculptor's work; for what is the having to do with dead canvas or dead marble, compared with having to do with the living body, the temple of God's spirit? It is one of the Fine Arts: I had almost said, the finest of Fine Arts.
>
> —Nightingale, n.d. as cited in Donahue, 2011, p. 349

Nursing is a complex profession, highly trusted by the public yet poorly understood by most people. Everyone knows that nurses play a central role in the health care system, but most are not quite sure what nurses do and why nursing is so important. The perennial question—asked by administrators, the public, other professionals, and even nurses themselves—is this: "What is nursing?"

Part of the difficulty in answering this question lies in the complexity of nursing's role, a role that few fully appreciate. As Lee Schulman, past president of the Carnegie

Foundation, astutely observed, "Nursing is a hybrid profession, an interdisciplinary and inter-professional nexus of roles and obligations made up of many roles and obligations . . . a hybrid of advocacy and medicine, engineering and ministry, teaching and caring. . . . " He went on to observe, "Hybrids are often particularly robust because they combine the strengths of several species into one. But they may also be particularly vulnerable" (quoted in Benner et al., 2010, p. xi).

Nursing is robust. It has grown, evolved, and transformed while still being rooted in values of caring and making the patient the focus of care. It is the glue that holds institutions together. It has also experienced vulnerability. Nurses and nursing have been devalued because many, including nurses, often fail to recognize what is involved in professional nursing. Nurses have been treated as expendable. This can be seen when skilled, experienced nurses are replaced by less skilled, less educated workers.

When nurses and others are called on to answer the question "What is nursing?", most respond instead to an easier but different question: "What do nurses do?" They will list the multitude of tasks that nurses do. Almost everyone has observed or experienced the "doing" skills of nursing: nurses monitoring machines, taking vital signs, administering medications, coordinating activities related to patient care, assisting doctors, advocating for the patient, taking charge during crises, and the like. Yet these tasks are only part of nursing.

Julie MacDonald, a nurse and the chief operating officer of St. Joseph Mercy Healthcare System, classified the work of nursing as falling into two categories: (a) "doing" and (b) "being" (Koerner, 2011). The "doing" category of nursing is visible and measurable. The "being" category is often invisible and difficult to quantify but is at the heart of nursing and captures the spirit of what it means to care. It is also the aspect of nursing that protects and safeguards patients from harm.

The "being" dimension of nursing is about how the nurse actually *is* with the patient and the nurse–patient relationship. Nursing is a relational phenomenon because everything a nurse sees, does, and experiences arises from that relationship (Koerner, 2011). The "being" dimension thus transforms nurses from technicians into professionals, from nursing as a technical trade made up of just "doing" tasks into a profession with a focus on understanding the person to provide person-centered, holistic care. It is only when the "doing" and "being" are brought together seamlessly that Nightingale's (n.d.) observation of nursing as she wrote in the quotation above, "It is one of the Fine Arts: I had almost said, the finest of Fine Arts" is possible.

Unfortunately, the "being" dimension of nursing has been rendered invisible, in

> The "being" dimension transforms nursing from a technical trade of tasks done to a person into a relational profession in which the nurse and person/family/community enter into partnership to promote the person and family's health, alleviate their suffering, and facilitate their self-healing.

> It is when the "doing" and "being" of nursing are brought together seamlessly that sensitive, responsive nursing is possible and that patients are guarded and protected from harm.

part because it has eluded precise description or has been accorded less value. All too often, "being" is difficult to quantify and measure. When the "being" dimension is recognized and acknowledged, there is also a tendency to downplay, dismiss, downgrade, or degrade it. It is not accorded the same weight as the "doing" function of nursing is. Yet it is nurses' skills of "being" with patients that is the art of nursing and can make the difference between substandard care and superior care. Being is the power of presence:

- It is the "being" skills that give rise to compassionate, empathic, knowledgeable nursing and define the caring work of nursing
- It is the "being" skills that protect patients, minimize risk of harm, and protect patients against becoming a "failure-to-rescue" victim
- It is the "being" skills that nurses give voice to working with person and family strengths
- It is the "being" skills that have the greatest impact on patients and families and help patients and families navigate through their health–illness journeys
- It is the "being" skills that facilitate healing; promote growth; and enable people to profit from, and be transformed by, their life and illness experiences

WHAT IS THE "BEING" DIMENSION OF NURSING?

The "being" dimension is about *how* nurses give meaning to what is involved in caring for another person. In fact, the majority of nursing theories place the nurse–patient relationship at the core of nursing, with the dimension of "being" as its defining feature. Consider the middle range theory of caring developed by nurse theorist Kristen Swanson. She views nursing as informed caring that involves five essential elements: (a) maintaining beliefs, (b) knowing, (c) being with, (d) doing for, and (e) enabling/empowering (Swanson, 1993). *Maintaining beliefs* involves a fundamental belief in the person's capacity to make it through events and transitions and deal with challenges. *Knowing* is about how the nurse comes to understand the person and his situation and the meaning it holds for him. *Being with* involves being emotionally available to the person by listening, attending to, and disclosing without burdening. *Doing for* involves doing things for patients that they would otherwise do for themselves in ways that communicate respect and preserve dignity. Finally, *enabling/empowering* refers to the skills nurses give patients to better equip them to deal more effectively with their challenges by explaining, advocating, supporting, and the like. Taken together, these five elements contribute to patient well-being. In Strengths-Based Care (SBC).

In Strengths-Based Care:

- *Being* is the way the nurse is with the patient. It encompasses the nurse–patient relationship.

> The "being" dimension is about how the nurse engages, interacts, connects, and is involved with the person. "Being" is about giving the other voice. "Being" is about being committed to and caring for another with compassion, respect, and dignity.

- *Being* is how the nurse engages, interacts, connects, and is involved with the person.
- *"Being"* is about giving the other voice.
- *"Being"* is about being committed to and caring for another with compassion, respect, and dignity.

Remember, from Chapter 3, Nurse Frank Carnevale, who cared for Marty, a 12-year-old boy suffering from intractable pain caused by intestinal ulcers. Marty's pain was further exacerbated by the conflict between his estranged parents. He was referred to Frank to manage his pain. In one of their initial encounters, Frank gained Marty's trust after a session in which he successfully helped manage Marty's pain by using relaxation techniques. Frank did this by explaining what he was going to try, talking to Marty, giving him choices, and involving him in his treatment choices.

"I basically explained to Marty, and I guess, indirectly, the mom was present, that I work with children and teens that have pain and suffering from other kinds of things, and what they've found helpful. I described briefly the kinds of things that I use. I talk about it in terms of exercises, things we can do to help you relax, to help you feel better, to help you gain control, and then I actually described them. And I said we can try them and find out which ones you like, which ones you don't like, which ones work, and which ones don't work. Reluctantly he said 'Okay.' What I said was: 'I'd like to try a little bit right now, to give you an idea of what this is like.' I just did a brief relaxation exercise...I put on New Age music and it was really amazing...He relaxed really well, he slouched in his chair, and his face just seemed to drop with the gravity. I could see that the mom was smiling, too. So after about five minutes, the mom said 'He looks so relaxed.' And I asked him if he liked it and he said he liked it."

Frank recalled that a few weeks later he met Marty again at a follow-up appointment: *"[I wanted] to find out a little bit more about Marty—find out what were the kinds of things he did for comfort, the kinds of things he liked. What I learned from him and his mom was that he was a passionate and skilled artist. He drew sketches that were tremendous, and he pulled a few out of his bag, and I thought 'Wow, what an amazing expressive capacity.' So this is what I was trying to see—what works for this person, what's his particular area of strength, what does this person rely on, what has worked, and then see [what happens]. This [Marty's art] is going to be an area where he'll probably have some confidence, some refuge, where he feels he's the master of that domain. So then I look to see if there's any way that that can be transferred over. I thought that this was great and I didn't really know what to do with it [his talent as an artist] at the time, but as it turned out a couple of days later he was hospitalized...because his inflammatory bowel was really spiraling out of control and it looked like he was going to have to have some surgery."*

Frank recounted that Marty was very upset. As Frank explained, *"He felt like people weren't treating him seriously. He had a sense that [the staff] felt he was exaggerating (about the severity of his pain)."* Frank asked Marty if he wanted to have another relaxation exercise session, and Marty agreed.

First, however, Frank created a safe, healing space by ensuring they would not be interrupted: *"I went out to tell the staff what I was working on with him: 'This is what I do, and it's important that when I'm working in this way there are no interruptions, barring an emergency.' So we agreed what kind of signage we could put on the door, because I also wanted to establish a sanctuary for Marty: There is this categorical safe space that you and I can enter and orchestrate. I put the sign on the door and played the music that Marty had selected and Marty really relaxed."*

After the session, Marty wanted to talk: *"And first of all he talked about how he was mad; well, he wasn't mad but he was scared because he felt that nobody was taking him seriously. He was scared about the operation he was going to have. He didn't understand it; he thought it was never going to end because it had been going on for so long. And then he pulled out some sketches that he had drawn... I just thought, 'It's great that if a child is engaged in this reflective, introspective moment and finds a way to express it, then it creates that opportunity for being able to understand it.' But I prefer to try to understand what is going on in the child's own words. I said 'These drawings are amazing; talk to me about them.'"*

Then Frank had an idea that this could be really helpful in how Marty communicated with the staff. Frank shared this with Marty: *"[I asked him,] 'Could you draw for me what it is like for you when you're feeling at your worst and what it's like for you when you were feeling good?' He didn't hesitate. He just pulled out the pencil and he made these two sketches. He seemed to have no problem relating to that; it was something he understood."*

Frank continued to relate his way of being with Marty and his use of a strengths-based approach to care: *"There was one [painting] where he was crouched over, his face was all red and sweat was pouring out of him. And one where he was in his bed, he had glowing sunshine on his belly. Well, I'm wondering if some of these paintings could be used to let the staff know how you are feeling. You could put an image up saying 'This is the kind of day I'm having.' One of my concerns was how to foster communication between Marty and the staff. I also asked him, I said 'Would you like me to talk to [the staff] about the way that you're feeling because you're saying that they don't understand you very well.' I saw myself in a position to be able to take that talent that he had, which was extraordinary, and to really try to bridge that with the understanding the staff could have."*

For Frank, "being" was being there for Marty, getting to know Marty as a person, recognizing his talents and strengths, listening to and hearing Marty's physical and emotional pain, and helping to alleviate some of Marty's pain and suffering. Frank was successful in doing this because when he was with Marty, he was fully present. Frank succeeded in creating a safe space for Marty to express his thoughts and feelings. Frank asked questions in such a way that encouraged Marty to share his deepest concerns. In Frank, Marty had found somebody to connect to because he knew that Frank understood his pain, appreciated his special talents, empathized with his suffering, and had the tools and knowledge to help him relieve his pain and cope with his challenges. Frank believed in Marty and Marty's capacity to self-heal. Frank had found a way to use Marty's talents to help him communicate with the staff so they would understand how he was feeling. Nurse Frank Carnevale practices SBC.

SBC uses many different ways of being with a person that places that person as the focus and center of care and that defines the person by who she is, not by her condition or disease.

On a busy unit, it is easy for a nurse to think and say, "That's all very nice. I would love to take the time to spend with my patient, but that is a luxury. Who has the time to be with patients in the way that is described in SBC given all that I have to do and that needs to be done?" However, if the nurse believes that nursing is about the relationship and that the way the nurse chooses to be with patients can be just as, if not more, therapeutic than any treatment or drug, the nurse will find the time to focus on the patient as a person and practice "informed caring."

A nurse who values "being" will know how "to be" with the patient even while "doing". Consider the nurse who engages in "being" while "doing," who engages with the patient while adjusting an IV, administering a medication, or checking on the patency of the IV line. In contrast, there are other nurses who spend the same amount of time with the patient but who focus almost exclusively on the IV, the medication, or the patency of the IV line. They "nurse" the equipment, not the patient. Nurses who value "being" make time in their busy schedules to create undisturbed time to be with patients. They are the ones who modulate the noise level in the environment, listen to patients, and focus on being present with the patient whenever the opportunity presents itself. Nurses practice "being," which is a core value, an adopted attitude, and a commitment to SBC.

WHAT IS SOCIAL INVOLVEMENT?

Social involvement is the way one human connects to and forms a relationship with another. Humans are wired for social involvement: Their survival depends on their capacity to form, maintain, and sustain relationships. All aspects of being human are shaped by the experiences one has with other human beings (Cozolino, 2006). From birth, the newborn begins to learn about how to survive by learning how to relate to others, and this learning continues throughout an individual's life span.

Although all relationships share common features, every social interaction is different, and each social relationship is unique. Relationships differ in terms of purpose or goals, the degree of commitment, the amount of investment, the nature of the reciprocity between partners, the power structure created, and the circumstances under which the relationship was formed. All relationships come with a set of expectations; are built on history; and require knowledge and social skills to engage, to connect, to maintain, and to sustain the relationship. The features of relationships are listed in the first column of Table 8.1. In the table, two relationships are compared in order to illustrate the similarities and differences between a social relationship (relationship between adult partners) and a professional relationship (the nurse–patient relationship).

TABLE 8.1

Features of social relationships and a comparison between a social relationship and a professional relationship

Features	Partner/Spousal	Nurse–Patient
A. Partners	Two adults: Male–female, same sex	Two adults: Nurse and patient
B. Purpose	Nurturance, protection, procreation, economics. Meet emotional, intellectual, social, sexual, recreational, and security needs.	Purposeful and goal-directed. Helping, caring: Nurse gives help, and patient takes and expects help, to meet health care needs, carry out treatment, and facilitate healing. Nurse helps for a variety of reasons: paid for services, interest in helping others.
C. Commitment, investment, trust	High in commitment. High emotional investment. Trust needs to be earned.	High in commitment within the limits and boundaries of professional conduct. Investment and emotional involvement contained. Trust: Often there is an inherent trust in the profession. Trust in a specific nurse has to be earned.
D. Time	Takes time to develop and to get to know each other and each other's family and friends.	Immediacy and urgency for the nurse to get to know the patient. The patient needs to get to know the nurse in terms of whether he trusts and feels safe with the nurse.
E. Endurance of relationship	Endures a lifetime even when partners are separated by death or divorce.	Time limited until crisis over, problem resolved, patient progresses, improves, or natural termination, when professional has a day off or is on vacation.
F. Reciprocity	Partnership is reciprocal and equal: More give-and-take, mutual benefit. Depends on agreed-on roles and division of labor. Culturally determined, context specific.	Unequal: Nurse's role is caring for and giving to the patient. The patient's role is taking and benefiting from the skills of nursing. Patient reciprocates by becoming a partner in care, taking in what the nurse is doing, getting better, and responding to treatment.
G. Power	Depends on culture, agreed-on roles, division of labor. Ranges from a hierarchical structure in which one partner dominates to a more egalitarian partnership with shared power, roles, and responsibilities.	Position confers power to the nurse. Depends on nurse's theoretical orientation and philosophical belief structure: Some nurses are aware of the inherent power conferred by their role and exercise it by assuming the dominant role and putting into place a traditional hierarchical structure; others share power and work collaboratively, in partnership, recognizing patients' expertise and their right to autonomy and self-determination.
H. Circumstances of engagement	Meeting through mutual friends, accidental meeting, Internet, life-long friends, etc.	Patients accessing health care system for a complaint, concern that requires skilled nursing care.

(continued)

TABLE 8.1

Features of social relationships and a comparison between a social relationship and a professional relationship   (*Continued*)

Features	Partner/Spousal	Nurse–Patient
I. Expectations	Each partner has expectations to meet needs of companionship, economics, reproduction, etc.	Patients expect nurses to "deliver the goods"—to have the formal training, knowledge, skills, and competencies to meet physical, medical, emotional informational needs. They expect safe, quality care and to be protected from harm.
J. History	Each partner brings his or her own history, knowledge, and skills of relationships from their families of origin and extended families.	Public's trust and status in the profession conferred by society. Individuals have had their own personal past experiences with nurses and the health care system.
K. Knowledge	Knowledge and skills associated with the role and responsibility—spouse, parent, etc.—learned from family of origin, observation, reading, taking courses, and being in the relationship. Often no formal training required.	Nursing knowledge and competencies in the domains of safe and competent nursing practice. Formal education and training and years of practice. Building on acquired and accumulated knowledge and skills in personal life.
L. Social engagement skills	Connecting with a stranger for long-term commitment. Enter relationship with varying degree of interpersonal and communication capabilities and competence acquired, including the management and regulation of emotion. Acquired during childhood and through experiences interacting with parents, siblings, peers, and other partners. Both partners need competency in EQ (emotional intelligence) and SQ (social intelligence) for a successful partnership.	Connecting with a stranger. Transferring and using interpersonal and communication skills from personal life to professional life. Additional training and formal education in re-forming and training social engagement and therapeutic skills to be used in a new context and for different purposes. Onus is on the nurse to be trained in social engagement skills. Nurses must have developed high EQ and SQ. Nurses need skills for clinical inquiry, clinical judgment, clinical decision making, and clinical therapeutic intervention.
M. Connecting	Very little acting. Some management and regulation of emotions, thoughts, and feelings. In secure relationships, able to be one's authentic self.	Some acting, putting on a "professional mask and way of being." During crisis or uncertain situation that is frightening, and where the nurse feels unsure, the nurse needs to manage feelings and emotions and must remain calm.

THE NEED TO REFORM AND RETRAIN SOCIAL INVOLVEMENT SKILLS: PART OF BECOMING A PROFESSIONAL CAREGIVER

The act of helping another is complex and challenging and requires specialized knowledge, skills, and experience. Nurses and patients enter into a very special relationship and need to learn how to relate to one another. Nurses need to become involved with people in times of health or when dealing with illness, disability, or trauma in order to provide care that meets their needs and creates conditions to help them meet their goals. Contrast this with the current practices specific to the deficit and mechanistic model, in which nurses are engaged in diagnosis and treatment but are disengaged and distanced from the patient as a person and his experience with illness, disability, and suffering (Benner, 2011).

SBC requires that nurses learn new ways of connecting, engaging, and becoming socially involved that puts people at the center of care, focuses on their uniqueness and strengths, and works in partnership with them. It requires that nurses acquire knowledge and develop communication skills that are *therapeutic*. Because they often meet patients and their families in times of crisis and stress, nurses have to know how to engage them and gain a stranger's trust in a relatively short period of time. Thus, they need excellent interpersonal skills to connect with patients and families so they can gather salient and relevant information (i.e., clinical inquiry) and

> Nurses often meet patients and families in times of crisis and stress and have to know how to engage them, strangers, and gain their trust quickly.

be able to effectively know how to deal effectively with their concerns (i.e., a therapeutic approach) as with the case of Frank in caring for Marty described above.

For Clinical Inquiry

Nurses must learn to gather relevant information. This requires knowing what to ask, when to ask, and how to ask. It also requires knowing what to observe, when to observe, and how to observe (see Chapters 6 and 7). On the other hand, the quality of information that nurses gather is affected by what the patient and family are willing to share. Patients are more likely to share personal information when they trust the nurse. Patients trust nurses who they believe are open, nonjudgmental, compassionate, empathic, authentic, sincere, and respect them as individuals. They also trust nurses who they believe are technically competent—who have the skills and know how to meet their needs, carry out treatments, alleviate their anxieties, allay their fears, and deal with their concerns. Recall that once Frank had shown Marty

> The quality of information that nurses gather is affected by what the patient and family are willing to share. Patients are more likely to share personal information with a trusted, competent, knowledgeable, and compassionate nurse who has demonstrated that she can meet their needs and keep them safe.

that he could manage his pain, Marty was able to trust Frank with his innermost fears and concerns.

As a Therapeutic Tool

Nurses also need special training in how to use communication as a therapeutic tool. *Therapeutic communication* is a broad term that encompasses a wide range of skills—both verbal and nonverbal—that help people meet their goals and put patients in better conditions to self-heal. Therapeutic communication could be a gentle touch that communicates to another person, "I, as nurse, understand or feel your pain." It could be soothing words that calm, reassuring words that lower anxiety, an evocative question that raises awareness, or a probing question that reframes and gives new meaning to a situation. Knowing what to say and when to say it can serve as a catalyst to help patients change.

Therapeutic communication is about giving information, entering into dialogue, knowing when to talk and when to listen. It is about being a good conversationalist, actor, raconteur, and comedian. It involves being skilled in keeping a conversation going, how to be comfortable with silence, knowing when and how to scaffold (i.e., how to support the other person to achieve his goal). It is knowing when to talk and when to listen. It is about being comfortable with both likable and unlikable individuals, being at ease in connecting with good patients as well as difficult patients. It is about connecting with those who are self-assured and competent as well as with those who are vulnerable and marginalized. It is about being sensitive to a patient's subtle and potent cues and timing responses that are sensitive and appropriate to the situation. It is about reading cues of pain and suffering in those who lack the vocabulary to describe the awful and unimaginable details of what they are experiencing.

Therapeutic communication is about being able to communicate with those who have yet to develop the skills of language or who have lost skills of language: the preverbal infants and children; the frail, failing, and elderly; those made mute from trauma. It is about communicating with patients who have difficulty communicating, including patients who are suffering with autism; the visually compromised; the hearing impaired; the stroke victims; or those who have dementia or other mental disorders.

Therapeutic communication is about reading facial cues in people who show little or no affect (i.e., emotion). It is about being able to communicate with people from different backgrounds, cultures, and countries and who speak a different language. It is about finding how to communicate in ways that transcend language and nonverbal expression in order to reach out to understand others and to connect with them at a deep level.

Therapeutic communication is about being mindful and reflective. It is about the nurse being comfortable; having a degree of self-awareness; and being mindful of the effect her behavior and actions can have on another person, whether that other person is a patient, client, fellow nurse, or other team member. It is about the nurse monitoring, noting, and evaluating the effects and effectiveness her own behavior is having on the person and family. It involves noting reactions, actions, thoughts, and feelings as they are taking place in the moment as well as reflecting back and replaying the interaction at a later time.

Therapeutic communication is about being aware that what the nurse says and how he says it has the potential to cause harm. Nurses can, intentionally or unintentionally, cause a patient harm with an insensitive remark, giving ill-timed advice, making an inappropriate comment, being insensitive, providing inaccurate information, violating the person's sensibilities and boundaries, gossiping, and violating confidentiality. When patients feel that they are being judged, criticized, or blamed, and that the nurse does not know them as individuals or understand their culture, circumstances, or situations, those patients will have difficulty connecting with nurses. In these situations, nurses, rather being considered an important resource, will be dismissed and avoided.

Therapeutic communication is about being aware of how a nurse's appearance and actions can affect a patient. Patients are more likely to connect to a nurse who looks and acts professional. Patients are constantly scanning and sizing up the environment and the professionals therein. Patients often feel vulnerable and find themselves in a compromised state; therefore, they are on high alert to protect themselves from anything or anybody whom they perceive to pose a threat. Patients and families can become very self-protective. Their safety and well-being depend on adopting a vigilant stance. They scrutinize professionals and are quick to judge whether the hospital is clean, organized, caring, inviting, and safe. They arrive at such judgments based on their experience—from minor infractions to major incidents that, for some patients, signal a far more serious problem within the organization.

As a result, nurses and all health professionals need to recognize the power they hold in an organization. They communicate to the public the values and cultures of their institution by the ways they interact with patients and with each other, and in their appearance. Consider the personal experience of Alison Loman, an activist in her community who found herself briefly in the role of a patient. Her story is told in Exhibit 8.1. Weeks after she was discharged from day surgery, she found herself returning to an incident that caused her great distress at the time and continued to do so. She needed to share her experience, hoping thereby to raise awareness of the types of staff behaviors that can cause harm to a patient. Such incidents can be easily dismissed or considered minor, yet, in Alison's case, insensitive ways of behaving on the part of hospital staff had an effect on her that need not have happened. Accounts of professionals doing harm often go unreported.

In short, nurses need to learn a whole new way of being, precisely in the way they communicate, engage, and behave. Learning to become a professional is akin to taking up residency in a new country. Just as a new resident needs to learn about the country's culture and values, so too does the nurse need to learn about the new culture of nursing, about other health care professions, and the health care system in general. The nurse needs to become acculturated into the worlds of nursing, health care, and the health care system, as well as the many life worlds of their patients/clients/families/communities. He needs to learn several new languages, including medical and nursing discourse, attune his ears to how professionals communicate with each other and with patients. The nurse needs to recreate and revise his identity to include "nurse," broaden and acquire new knowledge, and learn new techniques and develop new skills, as well as develop new ways of responding to people in need (Benner, 2011).

On the other hand, individuals seeking help also need to learn about the health care system and how to relate to health care professionals. Patients and families need to learn how to trust and depend on a stranger to meet both basic and complex needs.

EXHIBIT 8.1

Personal experience *Alison Loman: Rudeness and a sloppy appearance can cause a patient harm*

Alison Loman, age fifty-eight, was admitted to day surgery for an excision of a malignant tumor on her upper left arm and for a sentinel node biopsy. Her husband had been diagnosed with melanoma three years previously. Her husband's cancer had been caught in time, and he was now in remission. Alison had lost both her parents to cancer when she was in her twenties. The word *cancer* was loaded with meaning for her.

Alison, a teacher by profession, understood all too well what it felt like to be vulnerable. Her years as a grade school teacher sensitized her to the effects of one's environment. A teacher's appearance and manner of speaking on the very first day of class could transform a nervous child into a calm one. She knew that a warm smile, a pat on the shoulder, calling a child by his name, and inquiring about his summer vacation were small gestures that had big impacts.

Alison was an activist in her community; she was committed to causes and making a difference. She took pride in her local hospital. The high standards she had set for herself in her own personal and professional life she also expected of others, and so she was upset by a staff member and a nurse when they behaved in a manner that she considered to be unprofessional. She felt it reflected poorly on the hospital she loved. If she could play her part in changing the hospital's culture and improving standards, she wanted to find a way, so she told her story to the hospital's ombudsman with the aim of sensitizing professionals to how hospital staffs' behavior affect patients.

Alison vividly recounted her experience as a patient. She arrived at the hospital on the day of her surgery, a "bundle of nerves." Although she had a diagnosis, she did not know the prognosis. She did not know whether the cancer had spread, whether she would need follow-up treatment, and how much tissue the surgeon would have to excise. The uncertainty was matched by her heightened alert state. She noticed everything: the good, the bad, and the ugly.

One of the first things that annoyed Alison was the behavior of the receptionist at the registration desk. As she stood at the registration desk, nobody acknowledged her. The receptionist was engrossed in conversation with another staff member about a personal matter. She never turned to Alison to tell her that she would attend to her shortly. Alison waited. With each passing minute, her annoyance increased. She felt ignored and inconsequential—an object, a number, hardly a patient, and certainly not a person.

Alison finally registered and was prepped for surgery. While she noticed all the activity in the room, few seemed to notice her. Suddenly, a nurse entered the unit who caught Alison's attention. It was not that the nurse smiled or tried to connect to Allison. In fact, it was just the opposite. What Alison noticed was the

(continued)

EXHIBIT 8.1 (*Continued*)

nurse's disheveled and unhygienic appearance—her long, unwashed hair that hung past her shoulders and a short, unironed uniform. Alison also noted that this nurse did not wash her hands—neither on entering the unit nor after seeing another patient. The very thought that this nurse would approach her or perform any procedure made Alison cringe. To make herself invisible, Alison put her head down and remained very still. This nurse's very presence added to Alison's already high level of anxiety. Without even exchanging a word, Alison wanted to have nothing to do with her. Unbeknown to the nurse, she had caused Alison harm and had undermined the reputation of the hospital and her profession.

They need to learn how to open up—often to a complete stranger—to share their insecurities, fears, and vulnerabilities as well as their hopes and dreams.

Patients often meet nurses in settings that are unfamiliar and even terrifying—the hospital—where nurses are employees and patients are visitors. Patients, who come to hospitals in times of need, are often intimidated. Each hospital has its own climate, a different culture, set of rules, and etiquette that both patients and nurses must learn. Certainly, the onus for initiating and maintaining the relationship and communicating the organizational and unit rules falls on the nurse. Therefore, nurses not only have to learn new social engagement skills but also must come to appreciate what is involved in becoming a patient. They need to learn to put themselves in the patient's position and appreciate their perspective. Nurses need to help patients learn their role and manage their expectations of what the system can offer and what its professionals can provide. Whether during a brief encounter or a prolonged interaction, nurses often find themselves having to explain the hospital culture, translate its rules in ways that are understandable, teach patients about how to navigate through the system, instruct them in skills of negotiation, advocate on their behalf, and the like.

A person who chooses nursing as a career often does so out of a desire to help. Being in a helping profession requires that a person be empathic, compassionate, open, and responsive to others' vulnerability and suffering. They begin their education and their training having already developed interpersonal and social skills to connect with family, friends, colleagues, people in authority, and strangers. However, some of the people who choose nursing as a profession are more socially adept and emotionally skilled than others.

A significant part of time spent in learning to nurse is devoted to re-forming and retraining one's social involvement skills. This involves learning how to capitalize and mobilize on skills that the student currently has in order to use them for a different purpose, under new circumstances, to bring about new outcomes (Hames & Joseph, 1980). To practice SBC, students must hone their current skills and acquire new ones.

INSPIRED KNOWING, THE THERAPEUTIC RELATIONSHIP, AND PROFESSIONAL CARING

In Chapter 5, I described eleven essential qualities that nurses need to have to practice SBC. In addition to these qualities, nurses need to have the skills to build knowledge. Through formal education and reflection on personal and practice experiences, nurses develop their own theoretical perspectives, guided by the values and principles of SBC. This process of building knowledge is referred to as *inspired knowing*. Inspired knowing helps nurses to evaluate situations, make judgments, and guide actions. It requires certain emotional and cognitive qualities that are required to form a therapeutic relationship.

What qualities do nurses need so that they can practice inspired knowing and thus form therapeutic relationships? Reed (2009) listed some of the qualities:

- Sense of trust
- Openness and flexibility
- Appreciation of contradiction and conflict
- Comfort with and tolerance of ambiguity
- Honoring of others' wisdom and experience
- Nonjudgmental attitude
- Creative construction of patterns
- Validation of observed patterns with another
- Reflective thinking
- Self-transcendence
- Spiritual and emotional intelligence

Many of these qualities are also involved in caring. Although there are many caring theories and theorists, Milton Mayeroff's (1971/1990) conception of caring is consistent with SBC. Mayeroff believed that caring for another person is about creating conditions that foster that person's growth. With this in mind, caring means relating to another person in a very special way. It involves encouraging the development of the person's humanity and personhood by helping her find her own direction. Caring requires devotion and involvement. Many of Mayeroff's qualities, which he called *ingredients*, are SBC values (described in Chapter 3) and nurse qualities (described in Chapter 5). These ideas apply equally well to caring for the family. They include the following:

- Knowing
- Alternating rhythms
- Patience
- Honesty
- Trust
- Humility
- Hope
- Courage

Knowing requires knowing many things about the person, his powers (Mayeroff's word for what SBC considers strengths) and limitations. It also involves knowing the person's needs and how best to respond to those needs, as well as being aware of the clinician's own powers and limitations. It also requires knowing about other factors that shape a person's development and how to make things happen.

Alternating rhythms involves moving back and forth with another person between her specific issues within the context of a wider frame of reference. It is in knowing that the nurse understands whether to attend to a particular detail while ignoring the background or context or whether to consider the whole—both the detail and its context. Alternating rhythms is required for getting into sync with another person. It means entering that person's mind space and seeing the issues from her perspective.

Patience is needed to allow the person to grow at his own rate. The patient sets the pace and determines the direction. The pace and direction may or may not coincide with what the nurse may want. Patience involves respecting the other person's sense of time and timing and giving him the space he needs. The nurse also needs to allow sufficient time to get to know herself as an individual and now, in her role of nurse. Self-knowledge is a prerequisite to developing a relationship with another person.

Honesty is about being truthful; taking the person as she is and not as one would like her to be. It is about accepting the facts, no matter how unpleasant or distasteful. It is also about being honest in understanding what works and hinders another's growth. It is about being open to another person.

Trust. Trust involves seeing the other person as a separate entity and allowing him to make mistakes and to learn from those mistakes. Trust involves "letting go" and includes an element of risk. It is about allowing the person to be who he is and giving him the space to do what he has to do. It also is about trusting oneself as nurse and one's own capacity to care.

Humility. Caring involves recognizing that there is always something new to learn. It requires that one be humble and open to the idea of learning from another, no matter how young and inexperienced or how ill and infirm. It does not preclude taking pride in a job well done or satisfaction in one's own contribution to another's growth.

Hope. Hope occurs in the moment, whereby one appreciates the present and is alive with a sense of possibilities. Hope is not about wishful thinking or unfounded expectations. Hope rallies energy, whereas despair drains energy. It is not about being passive, waiting for things to happen but about finding something worthy to commit to.

Courage. Courage is required to venture into the unknown, the uncertain, and the unfamiliar. Courage is not blind but is informed by insights gained by knowledge and past experiences. It is based on a trust of the other person's capacities and one's own capability to care. The greater the uncertainty, the more courage is needed to venture into the unknown.

THE RELATIONSHIP AMONG INSPIRED KNOWING, THE THERAPEUTIC RELATIONSHIP, PROFESSIONAL CARING, AND STRENGTHS-BASED CARE

Inspired knowing, the social involvement of the therapeutic relationship, caring, and SBC share common elements. They are highly interrelated and interconnected, and they come together to form an integrated approach to care. How do these elements fit together?

SBC requires that the nurse comes to know the patient as a unique individual. It is through knowing the person that the nurse connects with him. When nurses connect with patients, they enter into a special relationship with patients and families that, it is hoped, will be therapeutic. The therapeutic relationship is a type of social involvement that the nurse creates with patients/clients/family to help promote health, help them deal with suffering, recover from insults, and facilitate self-healing. In the process of nursing, nurses develop insights, new understandings, and knowledge that, when interpreted and explained in light of knowledge, shape clinical judgment and direct decisions and actions. Inspired knowing is involved as nurses build and create their practice-related knowledge. When nurses invest in patients and show that they care, patients connect with nurses and become engaged in their own care and healing. Similarly, nurses connect and become involved with patients and form a relationship. It is in this relationship—the way of "being" with patients—that nurses offer knowledgeable and compassionate care. When nurses become involved with patients and get to know them as individuals, then patients, clients, and families can truly be helped. When patients feel safe and secure in the relationship; when they feel understood and accepted for the individuals they are; and when nurses capitalize, mobilize, and develop their strengths, then the potential for health and healing has the best chance of being realized. The innate mechanisms of healing that reside in every person can be released (Koerner, 2011).

> When nurses invest in patients and show that they care, patients connect with nurses and become engaged in their own care and healing.

Many of the qualities required for SBC, inspired knowing, and caring are similar and yet different. Even a similar quality, such as openness, can be used in new ways to accomplish different objectives. For example, inspired knowing requires that the nurse be open to learning new things from patients to construct knowledge about nursing. On the other hand, when the nurse is open to the patient, he demonstrates caring because the patient feels accepted. In Table 8.2, a reflect and connect exercise, compare and contrast the qualities, characteristics, and ingredients and explain how each is used to serve different purposes.

CAVEAT

By focusing on strengths, the nurse communicates deep caring and inspired knowing.

RE-FORMING AND TRAINING FOR CLINICAL INVOLVEMENT: THE ESSENTIAL "A"s: ATTUNEMENT, AUTHENTIC PRESENCE, AND ATTENTIVE LISTENING

In the course of a day, a week, or a month, a year, individuals come in contact with many people. Most contacts go unnoticed or, if they are noticed, there is no acknowledgment or social exchange. With an exchange, the interaction can be pleasant, brief, or soon forgotten. Unpleasant or irritating exchanges, on the other hand, are usually remembered. Then there are encounters, perhaps also brief, during which two parties feel an instant connection and are able to establish some rapport. This is the nature of social encounters and involvement.

TABLE 8.2

Reflect and connect: Comparison of nurse qualities of strengths-based care, characteristics of inspired knowing and therapeutic relationships, and ingredients of caring

Nurse Qualities of Strengths-Based Care[a]	Inspired Knowing/Therapeutic Relationships[b]	Professional Caring[c]
• Mindfulness • Humility • Open-mindedness • Nonjudgmental attitude (i.e., acceptance) • Curiosity • Self-reflection • Respect and trust • Empathy • Compassion and kindness • Courage • Self-efficacy • Advocacy	• Sense of trust • Openness and flexibility • Appreciation of contradiction and conflict • Comfort with and tolerance of ambiguity • Honoring of other's wisdom and experience • Nonjudgmental attitude • Creative construction of patterns • Validation of observed patterns with another • Reflective thinking • Self-transcendence • Spiritual and emotional intelligence	• Knowing • Alternating rhythms • Patience • Honesty • Trust • Humility • Hope • Courage

[a]This book: Chapter 5; [b]Adapted from Reed (2009); [c]Adapted from Mayeroff (1971/1990).

Reflect and Connect Instructions:

1. Compare and contrast the qualities, characteristics, and ingredients in each of the three columns.

2. Which ones are common to all three elements? Which are unique?

3. Describe each quality and explain the role it plays in its specific context. (i.e., SBC, Inspired Knowing/ Therapeutic Relationships, Professional Caring).

Social involvement looks very different when an encounter occurs in the course of a nurse's work. Nurses come into contact with many patients. For the most part, the nurse will acknowledge the person with a smile, a gentle touch, a nod, or some combination of all three. The nurse will pay greater attention to the persons assigned to her care. In these situations, depending on the circumstances, she will deliberately attempt to establish a rapport. Some connections will extend beyond an initial encounter or brief interaction and could last through the course of the nurse's shift; others could extend throughout the person's stay in hospital or while the person is in need of health care services. The onus for establishing a rapport, making the connection, most often is on the nurse.

Some nurses have an uncanny talent for knowing just what to say and how to say it that puts a patient and family immediately at ease. They know how to calm an anxious patient or family member with a reassuring look, a gentle touch, and by saying just the right thing. They know how to ease their suffering by their very presence, in the way they move, and how they go about nursing, often without giving too much thought to their way of "being."

Not all nurse clinicians are aware of the effect that their presence has on patients and families. What is it that makes one nurse able to connect easily to a patient?

Nurses who are able to connect and establish a relationship with patients usually are high in emotional and social intelligence and have had formal education and special skill training in interpersonal relationship and counseling.

WHAT IS SOCIAL INTELLIGENCE? CAN IT BE LEARNED?

The term *social intelligence*, also known as a *social quotient* (SQ), was first defined by Edward Thorndike, a founding father of intelligence testing, as the "the ability to act wisely in social relationship" (1920, cited in Goleman, 2006). In recent years, with new insights from scientific studies of social relationships, an enhanced understanding of the social brain and the neuroscience of relationships has occurred.

Scientists have recently come to consider the competencies and skills involved in forming and sustaining relationships as a form of intelligence. Intelligence has traditionally been thought of as a single entity involving cognition—an individual's capacity to know, think, and solve problems. For example, when most laypeople hear the word *intelligence*, they immediately think of how smart the person is.

During the past twenty years, to clarify the underlying structure of all human behavior, the notion of intelligence has broadened. Well-known psychologist Howard Gardner (1999) introduced the idea of multiple intelligences. It is now accepted that humans require many different types of intelligences. Multiple intelligences are involved in an individual's growth and development. Gardner identified eight intelligences that operate in concert (see Table 8.3 for the list). His last three intelligences—interpersonal, intrapersonal, and naturalistic—are made up of capabilities, competencies, and skills that, when grouped together, are commonly known as social intelligence (Goleman, 2006). Because social relationships always involve emotions and their regulation, humans also need to develop their *emotional intelligence*, also known as *emotional quotient* (EQ), which has now become subsumed under social intelligence (SQ) (Goleman, 1995). All forms of intelligence are required to interact, connect, form, and sustain personal and professional relationships. SQ is made up of two components: (a) social awareness and (b) social facility. *Social awareness* is made up of what one senses about another person; *social facility* enables this awareness (i.e., what one does with it; Goleman, 2006). Each component requires specific competencies and skills (described in greater detail later in this chapter).

The short answer to the question "Can SQ be learned?" is yes, it can be learned. Whereas some individuals have an almost innate, inborn talent for connecting with others, others are less socially adept. In fact, there is a biological basis for SQ. From the first few months of life, some infants are by nature extroverts, and others are introverts. Introverts are often shy. Some infants are responsive to their environments, whereas others seem less aware and are less reactive. Some infants are slow to warm up and are wary of new situations, whereas others embrace new situations and feel comfortable in the presence of strangers. In other words, each person is born with a set of "social" genes that define their temperament, their personality, and their constitutional makeup (Rothbart, 2011). It should be noted that genes are designed to be modified by experience.

TABLE 8.3

Howard Gardner's (1999) eight intelligences

Types of Intelligences	Competencies and Skills
1. Linguistic intelligence	• Capacity to use words and language
2. Logical–mathematical intelligence	• Capacity to analyze problems logically • Carry out mathematical operations • Investigate issues scientifically • Detect patterns, reason deductively, think logically
3. Musical intelligence	• Skill in the performance, composition • Appreciation of musical patterns • Recognition and composes musical pitches, tones, and rhythms
4. Bodily–kinesthetic intelligence	• Use of one's whole body or parts of the body to solve problems • Ability to use mental abilities to coordinate bodily movements
5. Spatial intelligence	• Ability to recognize and use the patterns of wide space and more confined areas
6. Interpersonal intelligence	• Capacity to understand the intentions, motivations, and desires of other people
7. Intrapersonal intelligence	• Capacity to understand oneself, to appreciate one's feelings, fears, and motivations
8. Naturalist intelligence	• Capacity to recognize, categorize and draw upon certain features of the environment

Source: Adapted from Gardner (1999).

The meaning of this is clear: Shy individuals, from birth and throughout their life span, will have a tendency to feel awkward in new situations. Sensitive parents, however, can help a shy infant develop social skills to navigate strange situations and regulate and control uncomfortable feelings in new situations. On the other hand, even the most extroverted infant can become withdrawn or learn to avoid social situations later in life if his early social interactions and relationships are negative. People learn how to interact and create relationships by the way they learn to regulate their emotions, become attuned to others, read potent and subtle verbal and nonverbal facial and bodily cues, develop empathy, take another's perspective, learn how to communicate effectively, and the like.

Humans are wired to learn throughout their life span and, with education and training, can improve their EQ and SQ.

All relationships begin with establishing rapport. Making that special connection involves three elements: (a) mutual attentiveness, (b) positivity, and (c) coordination (Tickle-Degnen & Rosenthal, 1990). Goleman (2006) grouped these three elements under the umbrella of *empathy*, an overall measure of good feelings. Nurses can be trained to develop rapport:

• Patients are most likely to feel nurses are empathic when they attend to their concerns and communicate an understanding of what they are experiencing

- Patients are more likely to experience positivity when nurses focus on their strengths
- Patients are more likely to feel understood when nurses tailor their behavior to fit theirs. Nurses can do this by picking up on cues and responding in ways that respect the person's space and matches her pace. For example, if the patient is depressed, the nurse should modulate his voice to match the patient's mood. There is nothing more disconcerting to a patient than when the nurse is overly "perky" after the patient has been given bad news

These three elements require a set of competencies and skills that allow the nurse to attend to and be attuned to a person's signals. Therapeutic relationships are built on nurses being trained in the essential "A"s:

- Attunement and awareness
- Authentic presence
- Attentive listening

CAVEAT
These elements are highly interrelated, to the point that they overlap. Together, they make up the skills that are critical for creating a therapeutic nurse–patient relationship.

The major competencies and skills in re-forming clinical engagement and involvement are summarized in Table 8.4.

Attunement and Awareness

Successful relationships are built on one person being attuned to another's thoughts and feelings. Attunement is the cornerstone of SQ; the development of skilled, professional involvement; and the acquisition of interpersonal skills required for compassionate and professional care.

Attunement is the dance that takes place between individuals who sense each other and respond in ways that are in sync. Consider a mother who is attuned to her infant. When holding her infant, she hears a barely audible sound and moves her face closer to her infant's cheek. She senses his slightest change in movement and adjusts her position accordingly. She detects a change in his breathing and examines him more closely. She thus is successful in settling her infant even before anyone is aware of a change in her infant's internal state. Also consider a newborn infant who senses his mother by moving closer to her, molding his body into hers. Or consider the beautiful choreography that takes place between two dance partners as they reposition their bodies one to the other, readjusting their pace and rhythm to match the other's. Consider, too, a nurse who detects a "certain" facial expression, or slight change in skin color, or faint odor on the patient's breath, or an alteration in the quality of the voice, and then turns around to investigate the patient more closely. Or consider a nurse who has information that

TABLE 8.4

Toolbox: Summary of major tools to reform social involvement skills for clinical involvement: Attunement and awareness, authentic presence, attentive listening

Major "A"s	Tools
Attunement and awareness	• Adopt an "I don't know but I want to learn more" stance. • Train to attend to subtle cues: Practice. • Develop a mindful presence. • Retrain the senses by becoming an astute observer and attentive listener. • Become more self-aware and attuned to oneself. • Increase awareness of the effects others have on you. • Imagine and rehearse different scenarios.
Authentic presence	• Be mentally and physically fully present. • Communicate interest in the person and communicate openness through your nonverbal behavior. • Make the person the focus of your attention. • Show respect. • Adopt the stance of a learner.
Attentive listening	• Learn the difference between real listening and pseudo-listening. • Minimize conditions of pseudo-listening. • Become aware of filtering or stereo-typing while the person is talking. • Become comfortable with silence. • Allow the person to complete her thoughts without interrupting. • Listen for the message underlying the person's words without prejudgment and bias. • Use an open-ended form of questioning. • Avoid premature closure.

she knows will cause suffering and looks for the right moment to share it. Many of these changes are subtle and barely perceptible, yet they are detected, interpreted, and used. Nurses who do this are attuned to their patients, clients, and family.

What is attunement?

Attunement is about sensing another person's internal state as well as one's own. It is about being open to another's needs and wants. In the case of nursing, it is about being open to the person's suffering, about reaching out to connect in order to help alleviate or mitigate that suffering through acts of compassionate caring.

Attunement is about paying attention to both potent and subtle cues and interpreting them as signals emanating from the person's internal states. It is about the information that nurses take in and consider salient.

Attunement is about noticing and discerning what information is important, what needs immediate attention, and being able to respond accordingly.

Attunement is about making a connection by uncovering a person's essence. This is the subjective work of attunement (Siegel, 2010). The nurse who is attuned, pays attention to any signals that may provide him with insights and understandings about the patient as a person—who she is, where she is in her journey, where she is coming from, and where she would like to go.

Attunement is the act of taking in information, appraising it, and interpreting it. It happens at the "low road," or subcortical level of the brain. It often passes for intuition, as is the case when a nurse, when asked how she knew a patient was in difficulty even before there were visible changes in the patient's behavior, answers: "I just 'sensed' something was wrong".

Attunement is about being open to, sensing, and monitoring one's own internal state and bodily sensations, either consciously or intuitively.

Skilled nurses know the importance of getting in touch with their "gut" feelings. This process of getting in touch with internal sensation is called *interoception* (Siegel, 2010). Many intuitive individuals attend to even the smallest changes happening inside of themselves. They understand that the first signal that something is amiss registers in their body: "I had a knot in my stomach," "My heart was really racing." They also appreciate that they can rely on bodily sensations to inform them when the crisis has been averted or that everything is fine by monitoring the state of their muscles: "I felt so relaxed; I could feel every cell in my body slowly fall asleep." Often, the body registers a feeling before the mind has had a chance to process and understand what is going on. In every interaction there is a delicate balance between getting in touch with one's inner world and trying to understand another person's world.

Awareness: Mindful practice

It is important for the nurse to develop greater self-awareness and become more mindful. This means that she needs to get in touch with her own thoughts and feelings as well as increase her awareness of how another person's behavior is affecting her. The effects of an encounter, both difficult and pleasurable, are first registered in the form of bodily sensations—in the intestinal, abdominal, and cardiorespiratory systems. When the nurse feels that she has met another's needs, she comes away feeling good about herself. She feels a lightness of spirit. However, if the nurse feels scared or anxious in a situation, she may shut down or shut off, to protect herself. Think of what happens when a nurse is scared because she believes the patient is going to be violent or is afraid when there is a sudden worsening of a patient's condition. In these cases, the nurse switches into automatic pilot. With a potentially violent patient, the nurse may avoid the patient and, in a case of sudden deterioration, the nurse's autonomic system may kick in—which means that the nurse is in fight-or-flight mode, hoping to survive herself. It is only when the nurse gets in touch with her thoughts and feelings that she can turn things around. She may know how best to regulate her own emotion by engaging in self-talk, that is, talking to herself until she has calmed down or by seeking help from a colleague.

When the nurse focuses on becoming more aware of what is going on inside himself, he can then shift his attention to what is going on in his immediate environment and with his patients. He will then find himself becoming more open and more attentive to the thoughts and feelings of others. This is what is meant by practicing in a more mindful way.

Practicing in a more mindful way means to practice with greater awareness and intention. It means that the nurse practices in a way that allows her to pay greater attention to what the patient says and does and what is happening as events unfold. It also means that the nurse practices in such a way that she can be more thoughtful, creative, and open to possibilities (Siegel, 2010).

Part of retraining involves developing greater self-observation. This requires getting in touch with one's feelings and then accurately identifying and labeling emotions. Putting into words what one is experiencing is very helpful, for it concretizes the experience. When a nurse looks inward, she begins to learn how to connect to her thoughts. She learns to discriminate between negative and positive emotions and thoughts and to understand how each may evoke a different set of responses.

Consider Nurse Marie Slovick.* who avoids Mrs. Mathews, a demanding patient. The more that Mrs. Mathews calls her, the less Marie wants to do for her. The less Marie does for Mrs. Mathews, the more demanding Mrs. Mathews becomes; thus a vicious cycle is set in motion. The cycle has a chance of changing once Marie stops to reflect: "How do I feel about Mrs. Mathews?" Marie may answer her own question by thinking, "I really can't stand her." Now Marie has to ask the most important question: "What is it about Mrs. Mathews that I can't stand?" It could be that Mrs. Mathews reminds her of her own mother, who was always very demanding and critical of her. Or it could be that Mrs. Mathews makes her feel inadequate and incompetent because no matter what she does it is still never good enough. Alternatively, Marie may believe that Mrs. Mathew's demanding behavior is a sign that she is deteriorating, making her feel helpless and inadequate. Once Marie gets in touch with her own feelings and thoughts and determines the reason for her reactions, she can then begin to consider different ways of responding.

Change begins by getting in touch with what is going on inside oneself, labeling the emotion and then intentionally trying to change the thought. This is the basis for cognitive–behavioral therapy. To understand this idea, let's return to the example of Marie and her interpretations of her reactions to Mrs. Mathews. Once she has discovered the link between the demanding patient and her own critical mother, Marie may begin to remind herself that Mrs. Mathews is not her mother but a woman in need of help. Marie may also engage in some detective work. When do Mrs. Mathews' demanding requests occur? Is there a pattern to her behavior; for example, does she become more demanding in the evening than in the morning, or when the shift changes? If so, what else is happening at the time? Once Marie understands the dynamics at work then, instead of avoiding Mrs. Mathews, she can make a concerted effort to get to know Mrs. Mathews and her concerns.

Siegel (2010) reported on a process that he labeled SNAG, an acronym for *S*timulate *N*euronal *A*ctivity and *G*rowth. Within the human brain, there are specific neuronal circuitries (residing predominately in the prefrontal area) that are responsible for how an individual regulates his body, becomes attuned to others, and finds the right emotional balance between low and high arousal (see Figure 10.1). SNAG is the process used to stimulate neuronal activity and growth in areas of the brain that are dedicated to calming fears, developing insight and empathy, acting out of moral conviction, and getting in touch with the emotional and intuitive side of being (Koerner, 2011; Siegel, 2010). These activities are required for mindfulness. Mindful and reflective practices

---

*Hypothetical nurse.

help the nurse become more nonjudgmental, more in tune with and in touch with his own bodily sensations and aware of what's happening in the immediate surroundings. These practices also help him identify and then correctly label emotions and thoughts. Finally, they help the nurse become more skillful at self-observation.

TOOLBOX

The tools for attunement and awareness are summarized in Table 8.4 (page 272).

Tools to Increase Attunement and Self-Awareness

1. *Adopt an "I don't know but I want to learn more" stance.* The key to attunement is being open to what the person is saying. It is adopting a position of "unknowing" to get to a place of greater "knowing." It begins when you adopt the attitude "I don't know but I would like to learn more so that I can be of help in a way that you want." You can use phrases such as "Tell me more," "Help me to understand what you are going through," or "What has the experience been like for you?"
2. *Train to attend to subtle cues.* Only when you know what to expect and what is "normal" will you be able to discern and pick up on the unexpected, the unusual. This comes from academic learning, practical experiences, feedback, and reflection. Think of the amount of time dancing partners spend practicing, learning about their partner, as well as about their own response to that other person. It is by reviewing a recording of an event (video) or benefiting from what another person tells somebody about their performance, and then reflecting on what has been said, that the person gains insight into his own and the other person's behavior and the nature of their interaction.
3. *Develop a mindful presence.* Attunement requires that you be fully present in the moment during the interaction (see Chapter 5). Minimizing distractions when you are with the patient will help you be in the moment. Nurses can be trained to be fully present (for a fuller discussion see, later in this chapter, the section labeled "Authentic Presence").
4. *Retrain the senses by becoming an astute observer and an attentive listener.* To be attuned requires that you retrain your senses. You need to become a more astute observer (see Chapter 7); listen more attentively (discussed in more detail later in this chapter); and hone your sixth, seventh, and eighth senses (see Chapters 5, 6, and 7).
5. *Become more self-aware and attuned to one's own self.* One way you can be attuned to yourself is to do a brief scan of your own internal bodily state. Take the test called Inner-Voice, Body Sensation checkup, found in Table 8.5. Any sensation indicates a level of arousal and indicates one's arousal level and state (i.e., from alert to comatose).
6. *Increase awareness of the effects of others.* Some interactions are more comfortable than others. In the course of an interaction, your responses are often shaped by what the person has said or how that person has behaved.

TABLE 8.5
Inner voice, body sensation (IVBS)

Where would you rate your bodily sensation at this moment?			
State of arousal	Calm	0 1 2 3 4 5 6 7 8 9 10	Nervous
Breathing	Natural	0 1 2 3 4 5 6 7 8 9 10	Panting
Heart	Unaware	0 1 2 3 4 5 6 7 8 9 10	Racing
Muscle state	Relaxed	0 1 2 3 4 5 6 7 8 9 10	Tense
Abdomen	Relaxed	0 1 2 3 4 5 6 7 8 9 10	Tense, knotted

Reflect and Connect Instructions:

Step 1: A first step to getting in touch with how a particular person affects you is to ask yourself: "On a scale of zero to ten, how comfortable am I feeling?" (10 = *very comfortable* to 0 = *very uncomfortable*).

If your rating was lower than a "4," then continue to the next step.

Step 2: Describe the incident and, more specifically, when you felt uncomfortable.

Step 3: Answer the following questions:
- What did the person say or do that made me feel uncomfortable?
- What did I feel? Label the emotion, for example nervous, tense, anxious.
- How did that emotion affect my attitude toward the person?
- How did I feel after the encounter? What was I thinking about myself? About the person?

Step 4: Compare this interaction with a pleasant encounter.

Describe the incident with the following:
- What did the person say or do that made it easy to connect?
- Describe how you felt after the encounter

7. *Imagine and rehearse different scenarios.* Another important strategy to add to your toolbox is to imagine and rehearse different scenarios. Imagine different scenarios and then place yourself in each situation. Think about what you are going to feel and how you may react. Try to visualize yourself in the situation. Put into words what you are feeling and thinking.

Authentic Presence

Social engagement requires presence. What is *presence*? The definition depends on how presence contributes to the person and family's health and well-being.

Daniel Siegel (2010) defined presence as the practitioner's way of being with the person who is seeking help. He believed presence is an essential ingredient of any helping relationship because it fosters in the practitioner empathy and an understanding of what the other person is experiencing. Presence requires that the practitioner be able to focus, become more resourceful, and find ways to support the person that are important to him. When practitioners are more focused and concentrate on what is happening to their clients, and their clients' families, they are then in a better position to recognize opportunities to provide help. These ideas support the observation once made by the famed French microbiologist Louis Pasteur: "Chance favors the prepared mind."

Margaret Newman, a nurse theorist, believes that presence is the essence of the nurse–patient relationship (Newman, 2008), which some in the nursing profession consider the "essence of nursing." Newman explained the essence of the process (i.e., of the nurse–patient relationship) in this fashion: "Being fully present in the transformation of ourselves and others, as we search for meaning in the lives of persons who have come to critical junctures in their lives" (p. 51). For Newman, nursing's mission is helping the person find meaning in what is happening to him, particularly during illness and times of tragedy. It is through nursing's presence that the person arrives at new levels of understanding and, in the process, is transformed. Accompanying patients on their journeys can also be transformative for the nurse.

Being *fully present* has come to mean different things, such as having an open dialogue; being open to knowing; being fully engaged, open, and committed to patients; practicing free-flowing attentiveness; understanding what will work; being with the person; taking actions that value the person's dignity, and the like (Doona et al., 1999; McCaffrey, 2009; Smith, 2001).

Another way to understand presence is to examine the different adjectives used to modify this concept. Common adjectives include the following:

- *Authentic* presence (McCaffrey, 2009; Munhall, 2009)
- *Engaged* presence (de Quincey, 2005)
- *Healing* presence (Koerner, 2011)
- *Transformative* presence (Newman, 2008)

Each adjective describes a different focus of nursing, whereas the term *presence* is used to describe "how" the nurse is in the relationship.

Common to all of these views, presence requires being:

- Open to the other person and to other possibilities*
- Nonjudgmental*
- Respectful*
- Concerned with the person's dignity*
- Able to have mutual trust*
- Able to live with uncertainty and unpredictability
- Willing to create meaning
- Transparent in one's intentions*
- Committed, engaged, and involved
- Genuine and authentic

(*discussed in Chapter 5)

All these qualities are required to practice SBC. They also are required to form a collaborative partnership (see Chapter 3; Gottlieb et al., 2006) and to engage in caring practice as a healthcare professional (Mayeroff, 1971/1990: Swanson, 1993).

Strengths-Based Care and Authentic Presence

In SBC, presence is about authentic presence, which encompasses all forms of presence listed above. Thus, it requires that the nurse be present in the moment, become fully engaged with the person and her situation, and progress from a stance of unknowing to one of knowing. It also requires the nurse to be open to the other person and to practice with curiosity. Part of the illness experience is living with uncertainty. Presence is required to help patients deal with uncertainty and cope with their own vulnerability and need for help (Benner, 2011). The nurse needs to be able to do the same, that is, live with the uncertainty of the future and the unfolding nature of the experience in order to fully grasp what is happening (Gottlieb, et al., 2006).

Authentic presence is a precondition for healing. Nurses are responsible for creating conditions that facilitate patient and family self-healing. Presence is the process and the vehicle that allows the nurse to help the patient heal through learning, educating, and finding new meaning. It is also about learning to live with ambiguity and uncertainty, especially during health transitions. The person and family communicate their own presence by the way they respond; take in what is happening to them; become fully engaged in health work in order to repair, restore, change, grow, find meaning; and learn to live with ambiguity when there is an unclear diagnosis or an uncertain prognosis. The process of healing transforms the nurse, the patient and family because of how they choose to be present in the relationship.

Authentic presence is a matter of choice. A nurse can choose to be fully engaged in her nursing, or she can choose to be distant, disengaged, disinterested, and uninvolved. She can choose to be engaged at a given moment or choose to be physically present but mentally and emotionally absent. She can choose to engage with one patient and not with another. She also can choose to be self-aware or to be unaware by being out of touch with what is going on inside herself.

> Authentic presence is a matter of choice. A nurse can choose to be fully engaged in her nursing or can choose to be distant, disengaged, disinterested and uninvolved.

Nurse Ti Phung Hoang described her concept of what it means to be present: *"My philosophy is really just to be there to offer* [*the patient and family*] *what I can in terms of my availability. What I am looking for is to make them feel that they are human again and that life still makes sense for them. When I have this in mind, I am able to hear their stories and I am able to convey my empathy and to talk to them in their own language."*

TOOLBOX

The tools for authentic presence are summarized in Table 8.4.

Tools to Develop Authentic Presence

Presence is a learnable skill. It requires knowledge of what is involved in being fully present. It begins with the nurse becoming aware of her own behavior and the messages she communicates to others by her behavior. It then requires a conscious effort on the nurse's part to develop each of the qualities mentioned above, to understand them and how each contributes to presence. Many of the qualities were discussed in Chapter 5, along with strategies on how to develop them. Here, the focus is on easy-to-implement tools that could make a significant difference to the quality of the nurse–patient client/family relationship.

1. *Be mentally and physically fully present.* When you are with the patient/client/ and or family, you should be fully present even if the interaction lasts only a minute or two. To do this, keep distractions to a minimum by doing the following:
   - Turn off pagers and cell phones.
   - Focus on what the patient/client/family is saying.
   - Stand or sit close to the patient's bed (if at the bedside).
   - Establish eye contact when interacting (if the patient/client/family members feel comfortable).
   - Find a quiet space to talk.
   - Create privacy, for example, draw the curtains around the patient's bed or close the door.
   - Put a "do not interrupt sign" on the patient's door and tell others not to interrupt.
   - Turn your body to face the patient/client/family, lean forward, maintain eye contact, and think, "What is this person telling me?"
2. *Communicate interest and openness through your verbal and nonverbal behavior, such as:*
   - Reaching out and touching the patient's hand when appropriate.
   - Maintain eye contact that is comfortable for the person. Avert your gaze if the person is uncomfortable.
   - Position your body in a way that communicates interest; turning away communicates a lack of interest or lack of time; leaning toward the patient communicates interest.
   - Keep your arms open. Folding your arms across your chest communicates a closedness—"I am not that interested; keep it short"—whereas hands held on a lap or hanging by the side communicates openness—"I am here and open to what you want to tell me."
   - Move your head and interject at appropriate times through nonverbal and verbal gestures (i.e., nod, pause, take appropriate conversational turns).
   - Match your voice and tone to the patient's tempo and rhythm when and where appropriate. This does not apply when a patient is yelling or agitated. In such circumstances, you should adopt just the opposite stance, by talking in a slow, quiet, modulated tone of voice in order to soothe, calm, and defuse the emotion from the situation.
   - Modulate your tone and the volume of your voice to match the person's mood.
3. *Make the person the focus of your attention.* When a nurse is present, she makes the patient the center of attention and communicates interest in him. The following strategies have been found helpful:
   - Inquire about patients' past, their family and personal history—where they come from, what they have been through, their dreams, desires, goals, fears, anxieties, concerns, what is important to them, and of course, their strengths. (see Chapters 9 and Chapter 10).
   - Ask patients how they are experiencing their illness and disability, the meaning of their diagnosis, and how the treatments are affecting their lives.
   - Observe their responses to the disease, medical condition, and treatments. This is an ongoing process of noticing, witnessing, and listening.

4. *Show respect.* As a nurse, you communicate respect in every gesture, action, and behavior when you
   - Listen attentively without interrupting (see below).
   - Ask the person or family about their wishes and how they want to proceed and use this information to take action where and when appropriate.
   - Respect the person's privacy.
   - Adopt a nonjudgmental, open-minded stance (see Chapter 5 for more suggested strategies.) As Nurse Timothy Kavanagh explained, *"Well, it's just sort of being naturally respectful of other people. Everyone's different in their own way. Everyone's got their own strengths and challenges. I know that on our own unit you talk to different people and right off the bat they'll judge someone: 'oh she's terrible at this.' But I always try to keep a very open mind by asking myself, 'Well, why are they terrible at that?' And when I see what approach they're taking, I try to put myself in their shoes, and that often helps a lot because being open-minded to other people's situations allows me to be more compassionate to their situation."*

5. *Adopt the stance of learner.* Pediatric Nurse Timothy Kavanagh recalled this when speaking to parents: *"Compromising, negotiating with [parents] but always being respectful and acknowledging that they know more than I do about their kid. I also know that if the kid's in the intensive care unit, the situation may have changed, and I try to explain my reasoning behind it. And often they're not worried about the medical side. They're worried about things like medication schedules and by expressing thoughts such as "Oh, she takes that pill at nine with her snack, but now we're giving it in IV form."*

Attentive Listening

The final "A" in the list to join Attunement (and Awareness) and Authentic presence is Attentive listening. The way nurses listen to patients and families is different from the way they listen to their own family members, friends, and colleagues. Re-forming clinical engagement and involvement requires training the ear to listen to patients and families, concerns, pain and suffering. Listening is required to create connections and sustain a relationship. Finally, when artfully used, listening can be a powerful therapeutic intervention.

Attentive listening requires that the nurse attend to, be attuned to, acknowledge, and affirm what the person is saying. Listening is key to developing a clinical grasp of the problem. Nurses also listen for opportunities to find approaches to deal with problems in new ways (see Chapters 9 and 10). Attentive listening involves "deep" listening that allows the nurse to go beyond the words and hear the subtext—the message behind the words.

Deep listening and surface listening

Patients' suffering and vulnerability are often too painful to hear and difficult to witness, yet this is what health care professionals are trained to do and why people seek their help and benefit from their training. Nurses need to be trained to go beyond the words and get to the messages, the things that are really bothering a patient. It involves dealing with issues that cannot be easily resolved or that will not go away. They need to be trained in the art and skill of "deep listening." Daniel Siegel (1999) defined *deep listening* as "learning to be open to the many layers of communication" and stated that it "is a fundamental part of getting to know another person's life" (p. 43). Deep listening requires that the nurse learn how to listen for subtle nuances, contradictions, patterns of responses. She needs to have special communication skill training (see toolboxes later in this chapter and in Chapter 7) to help peel away the different layers of communication to get at the heart of the issue and its meaning or significance.

Nurse Maryse Godin is often consulted on difficult issues. However, what the person presents is often not truly an issue, and as an advanced practice nurse she needs to delve deeper until she uncovers the "real" issue.

She explained the process: *"It's presented to you—this is the problem and you deal with it, and after you've dealt with it the problem is gone and the issue is resolved. But what I'm thinking is more in terms that are not so obvious. You're brought in with one concern and as you work on that particular concern, whether it's 'I have a disagreement with nurse So-and-So' or whether it's 'I'm not getting any information, my husband's been here for days and what's happening?', if you explain what's happening then you get the second layer of questions about 'Well, it's not about what's happening now, it's about the global what's happening, it's about what's happening in my life and his life, what's the future, what's this and what's that.' And those are the bigger problems. It drives itself. You have to be listening for the message that's not being said—it's Nursing 101—listen for the cues and listen for the recurring themes, then listen for what is it that's concerning you as opposed to what has been stated as the problem. But you need to ask 'What really is the concern here, what's the bigger picture?'"*

Attentive listening versus nonattentive listening

It is important to distinguish between *attentive listening* (sometimes referred to in the literature as *active listening* or *real listening*) and nonattentive or pseudo-listening (Dossey, 1995; Egan, 2002). Attentive listening is more than just keeping quiet while another person is talking. It requires that the nurse be fully present and listen with intent to the other person. When nurses listen with intention, they come to understand the person's perspective and gain insights into what works best with that individual (Kramer, Melo-Myer, & Turner, 2008). In contrast, *nonattentive* or *pseudo-listening* refers to when the nurse is physically present but otherwise mentally engaged. Nonattentive listening often happens when the nurse is thinking about other things while the person is talking, or when the nurse allows her mind to wander off and think of other things unrelated to what the patient and family are telling her. In these situations, the nurse "listens" but does not hear the person.

Another threat to attentive listening is *distorted listening*. Egan (2002) described different types of distorted listening that can affect the quality of the information a nurse obtains, such as filtered listening, stereotype-based listening, and listening that focuses on fact-centered rather than person-focused information.

Filtered listening happens when nurses filter what a person is saying through their own lenses. These lenses can be their own personal experiences, cultural backgrounds, and values. The danger of this type of listening is that the nurse may negate, distort, or even fail to hear the person's point of view.

Stereotype-based listening is another form of listening that pigeonholes or labels what the person is saying by using stereotypic explanations. The nurse may attribute an adolescent's complaints of tiredness to a particular society's stereotypic view that all teens are lazy, or when a woman of Italian descent complains of pain, the nurse may ignore or discount her pain and fail to investigate further, because the nurse believes that Italian women are overly expressive and tend to exaggerate their pain experience.

Fact-focused rather than person-focused listening occurs when the nurse focuses on collecting facts and gives less credibility to what the person believes, thinks, values, or feels. In other words, objective information is considered more valid than subjective reality (see Chapter 3 for a discussion of this value).

Now consider your own clinical experience and reflect on how you listen. Recall an incident that illustrates the many forms of listening and take time to complete the Reflect and Connect exercise (see Table 8.6).

TOOLBOX

The tools for attentive listening are summarized in Table 8.4.

Tools to Develop Attentive Listening

There are many ways to improve one's skills as an attentive listener. The first task is for nurses to know the characteristics involved in attentive listening. Attentive listening begins with the nurse being fully present and having an open mind to hearing sounds from the patient and her environment, to what the person is saying and how she is saying it, and to different ways of communicating. Listening requires that the nurse be authentically and fully present, with an open, nonjudgmental mind.

CAVEAT
Many of the tools that help a nurse to be fully present will also help that nurse become an attentive listener.

TABLE 8.6

Reflect and connect: Pseudo- and distorted listening

Pseudo- and Distorted Listening	Incident from Your Own Clinical or Personal Experience	Incident You Have Observed
Pseudo-listening	_____	_____
Filtered listening	_____	_____
Stereotype-based listening	_____	_____
Fact-centered listening	_____	_____

Source: Adapted from Egan (2002).

Reflect and Connect Instructions:

1. Recall an incident from your own clinical experience that illustrates the each type of listening.

2. Recall an incident that you observed that illustrates each type of listening.

3. What effect did it have on the interaction?

Consider the story told by Nurse Gisele Melanson, who took the time to get to know her patient, Mrs. Turner, and listen to her story and so made a discovery that had eluded others. Gisele listened to what Mrs. Turner was telling her: *"At first, she said she couldn't come off the ventilator because she had abdominal pain. I really interviewed her about this pain. She had had this pain for years. She had been to every doctor, including her family doctor, a surgeon. She had been gastroscoped. Everybody had tried to figure out what this pain was. She had been on all sorts of medications, and nobody could figure out what it was. So I just went to the staff doctor and I said, 'You know, Mrs. Turner has this pain and when she gets tired on the ventilator, the pain gets worse. If she's on her trach collar the pain gets really bad and she just wants to go back on the respirator because she thinks they're interrelated.' So he went into the room and looked at her. She had had her gall bladder out twenty years ago and she had a little lump in her incision. She had a retained suture. That's what the pain was. So we just did a simple procedure—a little local procedure, and took out this little suture, and her pain that she had had for twenty years went away. So sometimes it's the simple things you do. If you talk about something for twenty years sometimes people just sort of pooh-pooh it (and think) 'Oh, it's just that sort of complaint again.' But her pain was real. She had this pain and nobody could figure out what it was. It boggles the mind."*

Nurses can add the following tools to their toolbox to help improve and develop their listening skills:

1. *Take the time to sit and listen.* Attentive listening begins by communicating to the patient and family that you have the time to listen. This means adopting an unhurried stance. If time permits, sit down and tell them you have the time to listen to what they have to tell you. If standing, stand quietly and through your nonverbal gestures indicate that you are listening to them.

2. *Minimize conditions of nonattentive or pseudo-listening.* Focus your attention on what the person is saying. When you establish eye contact or train your ears to listen deeply, you begin to hear what the person is saying.

3. *Become aware of filtering or stereotyping information while the person is talking.* You need to get in touch with your own beliefs and assumptions. Often, you can do this during or after an interaction by asking yourself, "What am I feeling about the person?" and "What assumptions do I hold?"

4. *Become comfortable with silence.* People have a tendency to fill in and speak when there are periods of silence because silence makes them feel awkward or uncomfortable, yet patients often need time to gather their thoughts. As a nurse, you need to train yourself to be comfortable with silence and to use silence as a tool to enhance nurse–patient communication. Skillful use of silence means becoming aware of uncomfortable feelings during silence and trying to contain them. Some nurses have found that by focusing on their own breathing and slowly counting in one's head are useful ways to deal with the discomfort of silence.

5. *Allow the person to complete his thoughts without interrupting.* When a nurse interrupts a patient, it often is a sign that she is not listening. Indicators of inattentive listening include completing the other person's sentence, predicting what the person is going to say before he has finished what he wants to say, formulating a response while the person is still talking, and the like. You need to train yourself to focus on what your patients are saying. You need to learn how to put aside other thoughts, distracting ideas, and fight against letting your own

thinking intrude or take your attention away from what the patient is communicating. Through training, you can learn techniques to refocus your attention to improve your competencies as an attentive listener.

6. *Listen for the message underlying the person's words without prejudgment and labeling.* This tool involves letting the person tell her whole story, not just parts of it, without interrupting and labeling. Nurse Maryse Godin explained the problem with labels and bias. *"A lot of the time I'm called in to deal with dysfunctional people, such as when a family or person is in denial of their diagnosis or people who are noncompliant. If you go in with the premise that you're dealing with weird people or that their problems are so big that they cannot be solved, it colors your thinking. [You should] go in with the notion that, by and large, most people are not completely dysfunctional and do get through life quite well… And it may not be my opinion of what's normal, and that [family's] dynamics are different in different families. What's acceptable to people, what are their ultimate goals, and what can you work with? That's how I go into a situation and I think that's worked pretty well."*

7. *Use of forms of questioning that encourage talking.* You can encourage patients and families to talk about themselves and their experiences by developing skill in asking open-ended questions, which require the person to describe and elaborate rather than answer with a simple yes or no. Examples of open-ended questions begin with, for example, "Tell me about…" or "I would like to hear more about…" (see Table 8.3 in this chapter for other examples of open-ended questions). If patients are encouraged to share thoughts and feelings, nurses need to be prepared to listen in a mindful way (see Chapter 5 for more on how to develop skills of mindfulness).

8. *Avoid premature closure* by coming to conclusions before listening to the whole story. Stories take time to tell, and you need to develop the skills of helping people talk about their experiences by letting them talk without interrupting and, afterward, asking them to explain and elaborate on different aspects. This includes asking for other details to get a more comprehensive picture by finding out further facts or detailed information, such as
   - Proper context (e.g., "Where did that happen?")
   - Asking about the history (e.g., "When did that begin; can you recall the sequence of events? Is there one specific issue or detail that stands out?")
   - Exploring for other concurrent events (e.g., "Was there anything else happening at the time") and the like.

There also are many other tools nurses can add to their toolbox. These include ways to communicate interest, sustain clinical conversation, and improve accuracy and reduce misperceptions. The skills involved in these tools include summarizing, reflecting, giving feedback, emotional labeling, validating, using effective pauses, and even effective use of silence, and they are summarized in Table 8.7.

CREATING AND ESTABLISHING THE NURSE–PATIENT RELATIONSHIP

All relationships have a beginning, a middle, and an end. What differs is the length of time spent in each phase and how long the relationship lasts. Relationships are made

TABLE 8.7

Strategies to sustain clinical conversations (dialogue)

Strategy	Definition and Purpose	Examples
I. Ways to improve the flow of conversation		
1. Use minimal encouragers	Use brief, positive prompts to keep the conversation going and show the person you are listening and attentive to what he is saying.	"Umm-hmmm," "Oh?". "I see."
2. Give the person your undivided attention	Communicate interest and involvement.	Turn off pagers and cell phones. Do not answer phones.
3. Match your language and style of communicating	Use these to connect with the person and help her understand what is being said by matching your voice cadence with the person's and using the person's words, methods of expression, and metaphors.	Listen to the person's style of communicating. With a person who speaks slowly, slow your speech to match his. Person: "The illness is suffocating me. It is like Hurricane Katrina—Overwhelming and devastating." Nurse: "Talk to me more about feelings of suffocating."
4. Support and give reassurance	Use to communicate empathic understanding for what the person is experiencing.	"That must have been very difficult for you." "I can understand why you might feel that way."
5. Use silence	Allow the person to gather his thoughts and reflect on his answer and to fully express himself.	Silence is usually a pause during a discussion. The length of silence can vary depending on what you observe. If the person is uncomfortable, fidgeting, you may break the silence. If the person is deep in thought, remain quiet and respect the person's need for quiet time.
II. Ways to increase accuracy and reduce misperceptions		
1. Summarizing	Bring together the facts or pieces of the issues to check understanding.	"Is this what you are saying…"
2. Emotion labeling	Put feelings into words, which will often help the person to see things more objectively.	"I'm sensing that you're feeling frustrated…worried….anxious …."
3. Reflecting	Mirror back what the person has said.	Instead of just repeating, reflect the speaker's words in terms of feelings—or example, "This seems to concern you…"

(continued)

TABLE 8.7

Strategies to sustain clinical conversations (dialogue) (*Continued*)

Strategy	Definition and Purpose	Examples
4. Validating	Acknowledge the person's problems, issues, and feelings for the purpose of checking that you have understood and interpreted her message correctly.	Listen openly and with empathy, and respond in an interested way—for example, "This must be very hard for you..."
5. Giving feedback	Let the person know what your initial impressions are. Share pertinent information, observations, insights, and experiences. Then listen carefully to confirm.	"I understand this is what you are saying... Is this what you are feeling?"

up of interactions. Some encounters include all three phases in quick succession, and the interaction is over within a few minutes, but most phases take place over several encounters. Some relationships are short-lived, whereas others span years and are never formally terminated. Even in long-lasting relationships there may be long-term involvement punctuated by episodic encounters. The nurse and patient may know each other over time but come together whenever there is a crisis, when the nurse's expertise is needed. For the purpose of this chapter, the focus is on making a connection with the person and engaging him to provide services that require nursing skills and expertise.

Creating a Connection

Nurses need to engage patients if they are to enter into partnership with them. Making a connection is the first aspect of any relationship. Engagement begins with the encounter, the first meeting, the first impression. (I revisit this topic in Chapter 9 as it specifically relates to uncovering and discovering strengths.)

Importance of First Impressions

In all social situations, first impressions are about the sense with which a person is left (Demarais & White, 2005). It is during the first seconds of an encounter that each party has an opportunity to communicate who they are and to leave a person with a sense of how they will be viewed. Individuals usually form an impression and an opinion on the basis of a limited amount of information. At that split second, that transient moment, patients usually form an opinion of whether to trust the nurse—whether she is sincere, open, and nonjudgmental. On the other hand, nurses form a first impression that is based on the patient's likability. Likability is often determined by a person's personality, openness to engage, flexibility to listen and to respond, and need for nursing care.

 Some people leave a lasting impression, both positive and negative, even when the encounter is brief. Others leave little impression and are easily forgotten. People, by

TABLE 8.8

Reflect and connect: What message do these behaviors convey?

When You Meet Someone for the First Time and He or She Shows the Following Behaviors	What Message Is the Person Trying to Communicate?	What Effect Does This Have on the Other Person?
Smiles and leans toward the person who is speaking		
Avoids direct eye contact; averts gaze		
Shows comfort; does not fidget		
Shows concern or sensitivity by nodding		
Tells the other person about how busy you are		
Asks about what is of concern to them		

Source: Modified from chart on p. 9 in Demarais and White (2005).

Reflect and Connect Instructions:

1. For each behavior, consider what message the person is communicating by their body language or what they say.
2. How does the person who is receiving the message usually respond? How would this message make him feel?

their verbal and nonverbal behaviors, send messages such as "I am interested in knowing more about you and your experiences"; "I am approachable, please approach,"; "I have time to spend with you"; or "Stay away, not now, I'm too busy."

Messages come from the following sources:

- Body language: open versus closed
- Eye contact: direct or averted; shy versus approachable
- Facial expressions: smile versus frown, happy or sad
- Tone of voice: welcoming versus hostile, angry, or letting the person know she should stay away
- Timing of response: delayed versus immediate
- Intensity of response: mild versus extreme

Consider the behaviors in Table 8.8. What message do you think is being communicated by each behavior?

TOOLBOX

Tools to Connect

Nurses can add a number of tools to their toolbox that will help them facilitate engagement. These are summarized in Table 8.9 and include the following:

1. *Be aware of the importance of first impressions.* Nurses need to be aware that patients and families are scrutinizing them and after a few exchanges will decide whether or not to trust them. Therefore, it is important to think beforehand how to approach the person and what messages to convey to the person by what you communicate through non-verbal body language and by what you say.

2. *Prepare for the first encounter.* When nurses are open and communicate confidence and competency by how they present themselves, then when they are "doing" for the patient they are more likely to be trusted. Patients trust nurses who know the facts and have information about their case, have had experience in caring for patients with such a diagnosis, and are interested in getting to know them as a person. People want to be cared for by knowledgeable nurses who know about their medical condition and treatment. You should be familiar, at the very least, with the person's history, medical diagnosis, and treatment by reading the patient's charts and knowing about her condition and treatment before meeting them.

3. *Introduce yourself by your name* and address the patient by his name. Use behaviors that communicate openness as listed in Table 8.8.

4. *Show interest* by adopting behaviors that communicate openness, availability, and curiosity.
   - Spend time with the patient observing, conversing, and dialoguing
   - Ask questions
   - Listen closely

5. *Use the other's surname* when talking to the patient and family for example, "I understand, Mrs. Jones," rather than just "I understand."

6. *Use strengths-based approach to connect.* Get to know the person and focus on uncovering and discovering her strengths (see Chapter 9).

7. *Be authentic and sincere.* Point out qualities that you have noticed and genuinely admire (see Chapters 9 and 10).

Nurse Line Pharand recalled forming a first impression even before she had met the Phillipses. Nurses had talked about them as being a difficult family. Their son, Mathew, had been involved in a motorcycle accident and was in a coma, having sustained a severe brain injury: *"The words that were used sometimes were that this family was 'demanding or difficult.' Well, that's what was said, unfortunately. And we have these cases where there are families with young victims involved. What I try to do is sit down with the chart and read through it, understand what they've been through, understand the complications that have arisen, try to get the gist of what the situation had been in the unit, try to see what the issues are at the moment."*

It is important to note Line's openness. She was not going to let others inform her first impression. She was also thinking ahead about what would help her connect with this family. All her actions focused on establishing a rapport with them:

TABLE 8.9

Summary of tools to facilitate connection

- Be aware of those first impressions.
- Prepare for the first encounter.
- Introduce yourself by your name.
- Show interest.
- Use the other's surname when talking to the person and family member.
- Use a strengths-based approach to connect.
- Be authentic and sincere.

"I thought it's better to be prepared because then it inspires confidence if the nurse knows what they've been through. So I did that." Line also was aware that introductions are important and leave an impression: *"The first thing I asked—well, I said, 'Hello, my name is Line Pharand.' You introduce yourself even though he's not awake, and I think that this first establishes a rapport with the family and that it was important to make contact with them right away."*

An essential strategy Line recognized was that it was important to enter the room with an air of confidence rather than avoiding eye contact. To connect with the patient or family, it is important to encourage them to tell their story and describe what their experience has been like for them both individually and as a family. This requires both curiosity and an interest in wanting to learn.

As Line explained, *"Some nurses and health care providers are worried about entering rooms like this because they're nervous that somebody's going to ask them questions. I think, on the contrary, you have to do the opposite and be confident and secure. And there are things you may not know. But when you try to offer as much information as you can, and you honestly say 'I know you've been in the hospital for a month and it's been difficult, and tell me about it in your own words,' I think that really helps—and they really appreciate it, and Mr. and Mrs. Phillips had a lot to say. Good things and not so good things. It was balanced."*

Line explained her rationale for why she adopts these strategies to engage families: *"I just want to have an open relationship. I want to build up trust with them. I want to facilitate the care down the road. It's kind of selfish in a way, isn't it? It sounds selfish now that I think about it. It's to facilitate the process for me but it's also for them and it's a two-way street. But I think, yeah, they sense that the energy I put into it will make things that much easier afterwards. I maybe have the sense that people do care that the nurses are not just there doing techniques and interventions. They're important, and what they say is important and has value."*

ENGAGEMENT

Some relationships require many interactions to engage. Depending on the situation and needs, nurses and patients get to know each other over a period of time. Their involvement at times may be intense and, at other times, less so. Some interactions may require hours, whereas others may be brief. Some may be episodic, others more long-term. However, to sustain involvement nurses need to consider how the relationship is created and what will sustain it.

Nurses need to consider the environments they create. Recall from Chapter 3 that one of the values of SBC is that the person and environment are integral. The nurse is an integral part of the person's environment, so she need to pay attention to how she creates environments that make people feel safe and secure in order to gain the person's

> The nurse is an integral part of the person's environment. Nurses create healing environments when they are attuned, aware, authentically present, and attentively listen. They create a healing environment by setting a positive tone and working with person and family strengths.

confidence and trust. She can create the right environment by setting a positive tone in the way she communicates her understanding of what the patient and family are experiencing.

Setting the Tone

The manner in which the nurse interacts with the person and family sets the tone for the interaction and the development of their relationship (see Chapters 9 and 10 for a fuller discussion). *Tone* refers to the emotional climate that the nurse creates or attempts to change. The emotional climate can be characterized as friendly and warm or cold and distant, open and accepting or hostile and confrontational, caring or noncaring, or involved or indifferent. The tone of an interaction is created by subtle behaviors the nurse communicates often without even being aware of the message that she sends. All nurses must to be mindful of the way their behavior affects others.

Consider a story told by Nurse Diane Lebeau of a situation that could have ended in disaster but instead ended on a positive note because of Diane's correct reading of the emotions and behaviors involved, her sound judgment and clear actions in creating a safe and secure environment for the Jardine family. Mr. Jardine, age seventy, was dying. Although he had been estranged from his first wife for many years, she was the mother of his three children. She had been caring for her former husband on the palliative care unit. Their 30-year-old daughter, whom the family had not seen for many years, called to announce that she planned to visit her dying father over the objections of her mother and the other two siblings. The family had told the staff on the unit that this woman had a difficult personality and was mentally unstable: *"We were told that this daughter could create a big commotion. The family had warned us that she was terrible, that she could scream, that she could be awful, and they were scared. It was a tense situation for the family and I remember feeling scared as well: 'Oh my God, I have to handle the situation the best that I can.'"*

Diane recounted how she assessed the situation and the actions she took not only to defuse this emotionally tense situation but also to help the Jardine family repair: *"I could see this not very old girl, not yet thirty, with a hat on but also looking fragile and as scared as I was feeling myself. She walked in, and I kind of let things develop just to see how things would go. The family was there and had asked what they should do when she came in. I remember that I took some time to say 'well, she needs to be there with her dad. So maybe give her some space so that she can be with her dad.' So that's what they did. When she came, they left to sit in the solarium."*

As chance would have it, shortly after the daughter's arrival, Mr. Jardine took a sudden turn for the worse.

The daughter came to tell Diane about the change in her father's status, and Diane saw an opportunity for this estranged daughter to be a part of this family experience. *"I remember thinking . . . that she'll be the one going to say to her family that he's dying, she had a role to play, a part in it because she was the one at the bedside and this gave her a place. I was thinking 'She's calm, I sense there's something.'"*

Diane instructed the daughter to call the family back to the bedside. Together, they stood vigil as Mr. Jardine slipped away. Diane's last memory of this family was positive: *"The memory that I have of this family leaving the floor is the mother having her arm around the daughter's shoulder, and I thought 'Gee, that is great.' I didn't know from here what would happen, but I felt that this estranged daughter was part of something that she deserved, and thank God it went well."*

Because Diane was aware of her own feelings and could identify with the family's feelings, she was able to step back to observe objectively. She was able to use this information to create a safe and secure environment for all concerned that in turn opened up new possibilities for them as a family to begin to come together once again. (For further descriptions of creating safe and facilitative environments, see Chapter 10.)

THE IMPORTANCE OF CLINICAL CONVERSATIONS

Nurses have many opportunities to talk with patients and their families. It is during a brief encounter or a lengthy conversation that nurses can learn more about the person, the family, their situation, their concerns, their medical condition and treatment, how they are coping, and the impact that their condition or illness is having on their lives. The nurse can learn new information and gain new insights into how the person and family think and feel about their situation during a clinical conversation.

Nurse Margaret Eades described the importance of talking with patients: *"Over the years I've had the wonderful opportunity of meeting so many people that it's reinforced the idea that every person has a wonderful set of strengths and resources. It's up to me, as their nurse, to get to know them by just asking them questions about what is important to them, what they have brought to other situations, and what's happened to them before. For me, it's about building on this information so that they can move forward."*

Margaret values the importance of getting to know the person in order to know how best to work with him.

Thus, clinical conversations can take many forms: a dialogue, a narrative, a discussion, a form of questioning, or any combination. The clinical conversation can serve many different purposes, including gathering specific information, getting to know the patient and family as individuals monitoring the situation, having social exchange, and providing a therapeutic intervention. Yet the clinical conversation does differ from the ordinary conversation in several ways, and it is these differences that provide some understanding into what skills need to be modified and which new skills need to be acquired.

SIMILARITIES AND DIFFERENCES BETWEEN ORDINARY CONVERSATIONS AND CLINICAL CONVERSATIONS

All conversations are a form of dialogue. Infants engage in conversations with their mothers when they signal to their mothers that they want to interact with them. They do so by crying or cooing and once the mother is near them, they try to capture their mother's attention by looking at them, and even throwing them the occasional smile. They learn quickly how to engage their mothers, capture their attention, and keep the "conversation" going. They also send messages to their mothers when they have had enough by averting their gaze and looking away—in other words, sending out disengagement cues (see Table 8.10). Similarly, toddlers learn how to engage siblings and peers by tracking their whereabouts, imitating them, and engaging in social exchanges. They do so when they want to play, learn about the world, seek companionship, develop a sense of belonging, and are bored and are looking to fight. Conversations include taking turns: sharing and grabbing, talking and listening, asking questions and responding, and having periods of strenuous activity punctuated by periods of quiet activity.

To understand what is involved in re-forming and retraining social involvement skills as one learns to become a nurse, a good departure point is to understand what is involved in an ordinary conversation and then to understand how ordinary conversations can be modified and new skills added to transform ordinary conversations into clinical conversations.

What are the characteristics of an ordinary conversation?

- *Ordinary conversations* provide a forum for sharing and exchanging information, usually, but not always between two or more people who know each other (Rubin & Rubin, 2005).
- *Ordinary conversations* begin with small talk and contain other elements of communication, such as control talk, search talk, and straight talk (Miller et al., 1998).
  - *Small talk* is when people exchange information of little consequence, such as talking about the weather.
  - *Control talk* ranges from light to heavy, with the purpose of persuading the person to think in a specific way.
  - *Search talk* is when information is sought and elicited.
  - *Straight talk* is when information and facts are exchanged in a direct, straightforward manner.
- *Ordinary conversations* have an emotional climate that is set by the topic of the conversation. For example, when the talk is characterized by banter, such as when two parties share a joke, the emotional climate is light and happy; however, when the topic deals with a serious or painful issue, the emotional climate is likely to be heavy, sad, tense, or even confrontational.
- *Ordinary conversations* require that people have basic conversational skills to initiate and sustain conversations. Conversational skills often involve being interested in and attuned to and aware of the other, attentive listening, turn-taking, synchrony, and so on.

Clinical conversations share many of the characteristics of ordinary conversation but with some variations:

- *Clinical conversations* require that the nurse and patient, who meet as strangers, get to know the other in a relatively short period of time.
- *Clinical conversations* focus less on control talk and more focus on search talk.
- *Clinical conversations* usually find the nurse usually spends more time listening to the person and family than on talking. The onus is on the nurse to quickly attune to key events, recurring themes, and difficult issues and to listen and identify the emotional tone of the conversation that may indicate how the person and family are experiencing their situation.
- *Clinical conversations* look to the nurse to set the tone and maintain an emotional climate in which ideas can be exchanged in straightforward ways. The nurse "regulates" the emotional climate by listening to suffering, absorbing painful feelings, and by down-regulating and defusing volatile situations.

- *Clinical conversations* have varied focus. They often begin with the nurse trying to understand the patient/ client/family concerns, issues, symptoms, or complaints. Later, the conversation may focus on the person and her experiences with illness or tragedy. It can then involve focusing on health goals and health work, and the person and family strengths, in order to know how best to assist them.
- *Clinical conversations* find the nurse focused on getting the story by listening to the sequence of events, the key players, the plots and subplots of the person's experience, and the influence of these elements on the person and family. Nurses learn the person's story by talking with him, asking questions, and piecing together the different pieces of information.

Clinical conversations require that nurses have a broad repertoire of interpersonal and communication skills.

THE ART OF CLINICAL CONVERSATION

Having a broad repertoire of clinical inquiry tools to gather quality information, however, may be insufficient. For SBC, the key to obtaining relevant information is not only to know what questions to ask but also to know when and how to ask them. Thus, clinical conversations require that the nurse be an excellent communicator, with a wide range of competencies and skills. As discussed above, excellent communicators have high EQs and are emotionally intelligent (Goleman, 1995). They are also score high on SQ (Goleman, 2006). SQ incorporates EQ and is the basis for how well one person is able to relate and interact with another person's overt and subtle verbal and nonverbal behaviors. Individuals who have a high SQ know how to navigate and negotiate complex social relationships. They have the competencies to accurately read their environments and to adapt their reactions and subsequent behavior accordingly. In short, they are successful with people.

Nurses must have high EQs and SQs. Some nurses will already have well-developed emotional and social skills, whereas others will be less socially adept. Some will be excellent communicators in carrying out ordinary conversations, and others will not be as skilled in this. Regardless of how socially adept one is when engaging in ordinary conversations, anyone who wants a career in one of the helping professions will have to undergo specialized training in the art and science of clinical conversation. Some helping professions place more importance on developing a relationship with the patient and family than do others. If the educators value the importance of being good at talking to patients, they will commit more time to training students regarding social involvement and clinical conversation. Nursing is a relational profession that places emphasis on the nurse-person/client/family relationship and on relationship skill building.

As introduced on page 269, SQ requires two broad sets of skills: (a) social awareness—what the person can sense about others and (b) social facility—what the person then does with this awareness.

Social awareness skills involve sensing nonverbal emotional signals (primal empathy), being attuned to overt and subtle verbal and nonverbal behaviors (attunement), accurately reading the situation and what is going on (empathic accuracy), and knowing how the social world works (social cognition).

Social facility builds on social awareness and results in smooth and effective interactions. Social facility skills involve interacting smoothly at the nonverbal level (synchrony), presenting oneself effectively to invite conversation (self-presentation), knowing how to shape and influence the flow of interaction (influence), and showing compassion and concern (Goleman, 2006). Skills in these areas result in sensitive, responsive, and appropriate nursing.

Nurses begin to develop social awareness and show facility skills when they learn how to be attuned to people's individual ways of communicating.

Being attuned to a Person's Way of Communicating

Each person has a unique, personal style of communicating. Some people are open and share their life story readily, whereas others are closed, preferring to keep to themselves. Some people like to talk, whereas others prefer to listen. Some people readily warm to new people, whereas others are shy and slower to warm up. Some people are approachable, whereas others keep their cards close to their chest, being more inaccessible and distant. People communicate their style of interaction primarily through nonverbal behaviors, such as their facial expressions, bodily posture, and gestures. It is imperative that nurses learn to read potent or obvious cues as well as subtle cues. Learning the meaning of a behavioral cue is even more important with individuals who have limited language capability, as in the case of the preverbal infant or the person whose speech has been affected by a stroke or dementia.

Nurses need to train on how to read the person's behavior and interpret cues. Dr. Kathryn Barnard and Georgina Sumner of the University of Washington, founders of the NCAST organization and developers of their materials and tools, identified behavioral cues that preverbal infants use to communicate their interest to engage in interaction and the cues they use to communicate "I've had enough" and disengage. Engagement and disengagement cues are further divided into those that are easy to interpret (potent cues) and those that are more difficult to see and "read" (subtle cues). These cues also can be observed in nonverbal adults, such as patients with dementia and can be used to interpret what the person wants to communicate. A list of engagement and disengagement cues, both potent and subtle, are found in Table 8.10.

Health care practitioners often need to explore sensitive or private issues. Patients sometimes feel obligated to answer the nurse's questions even though they may not want to do so or are not ready to disclose information. It is important that nurses remember that their patients have a right to privacy and the right not to answer questions.

CAVEAT
It is important that the nurse not use any form of coercion to have the person divulge information.

There are only a few rare occasions when patients are obliged to answer questions, such as when the person poses a threat to himself or to the health and well-being of others. In these circumstances, health care professionals may be obligated by law to

TABLE 8.10

Infants' potent and subtle engagement and disengagement cues

Behavioral Cues	Potent (Easy to See)	Subtle (Not as Easy to See)
Engagement	• Stilling (stops moving) • Looking at your face • Smooth movements of arms and legs • Reaching out • Turning eyes or head toward you • Smiling • Feeding sounds • Cooing • Babbling/talking	• Eyes wide and bright • Face bright • Raising head
Disengagement	• Turning head away • Crying/fussing • Coughing/choking • Back arching • Falling asleep • Squirming/kicking • Pulling away • Pale or red skin • Spitting up/vomiting	• Turning eyes away • Fast breathing • Yawning • Wrinkled forehead • Dull-looking eyes • Frowning • Hand to mouth • Hiccups

Source: Adapted from Barnard, Sumner, and Spietz (1990).

report such information to protect society. This may happen in cases of suspected abuse or when the patient has a disease that can be transmitted to others and can endanger their lives (e.g., AIDS, HIV positive, syphilis). In many countries, each level of government has its own legislation concerning matters when protection of its citizens takes precedent over individual rights.

Nurses need to be aware when patients are uncomfortable or reluctant to discuss an issue. Patients may communicate their feelings indirectly, through subtle, nonverbal behaviors, such as when they change topics, avoid answering a question directly, shift sitting positions, fidget, turn away, avert the nurse's gaze, and so forth. The nurse needs to be attuned to these cues and respond accordingly. He may go with the flow of the conversation by following the patient's lead. Alternatively, he can elicit information simply by asking, "Does this question or discussion make you feel uncomfortable?"; "Is this discussion difficult for you?"; or "If you feel uncomfortable or are not ready to talk about it, you don't have to answer that question if you don't want to."

Some people may be more direct and forthcoming with the nurse and may simply say, "I prefer not to discuss this with you" or "I prefer not to answer your question." It is important that the nurse respects their wishes and changes the direction of the conversation to an area that is less charged, preferably one that the person chooses. The nurse can simply ask, "Is there something you would like to talk about?" If the issue is still of concern at a later date, the person may raise the issue when he is ready or feels that the nurse has gained his confidence and can be of assistance.

Timing of Questions

SBC's approach to clinical conversation is situation-responsive. Situation-responsive nursing underscores the importance of the nurse responding to and being directed by the person and family. It is not predetermined; instead, the nurse customizes and tailors her line of inquiry on the basis of what emerges from her interactions with the person and the family, as well as the nature of the situation. The nurse may have some predetermined areas that she wants to explore with the person, but the timing and the way she explores these areas should be directed and dictated by the person.

A skilled nurse knows when to ask a question because he has a sense of the situation and has picked up signals from the person, specifically, whether the person wants or is ready to discuss an issue and share information. Consider a situation, though, when a doctor has shared the results of a patient's biopsy, which is malignant, or has to come to tell a family member of a loved one's critical condition. This would not be a good time for the nurse to intervene by introducing a new subject.

Even if a patient indicates that she would like to engage in such a conversation, the nurse should be aware that the person may be physically present but will probably not be listening. If she is listening, she most likely will be able to absorb only a small fraction of the information that the nurse is telling her. Thus, it is important to recognize cues of readiness, as discussed in Chapters 3, 9, and 10.

FACTORS THAT INFLUENCE THE QUALITY OF CLINICAL CONVERSATION

Several factors can affect the flow of conversation. These include the creation and use of space and time. Nurse–patient qualities and characteristics can also affect how well they join together to engage in meaningful conversation.

The Physical Environment

The environment can be considered in terms of physical space and personal space. Physical space includes the layout of the physical environment, the type of furniture, the placement of chairs, the size of the windows, and the color of the paint on the walls. It also includes the noise level, the lighting, the temperature, and the quality of air (Fontaine, Briggs, & Pope-Smith, 2001). Let's consider a few of these features and how space can affect the direction and flow of the conversation.

Consider how the size of the room affects access to privacy, which indirectly affects what can be discussed. When there are several individuals in the room, including visitors, it is difficult to engage in a meaningful conversation with the patient. Moreover, in small, enclosed, crowded spaces there may not be enough chairs, or even room, to hold a patient conference or talk to family members. When there are many people in a small, enclosed space, the room may become stuffy, hot, and uncomfortable. Individuals may become preoccupied with their physical comfort and getting their physical needs attended to instead of talking with a nurse about things other than changing the physical conditions of the environment.

Consider the noise levels in hospitals and their effects on conversation. In most health care settings, the physical surroundings are very noisy environments, with call bells, intercom announcements, alarms from equipment, and even the noise made by staff shoes. Research has revealed that the decibel level from a gunshot or a jet taking off, two of the loudest sounds, produce sound levels of 140 dB (Cmiel, Karr, Gasser, Oliphant, & Neveau, 2004). Compare this with the decibel levels of noise made in hospitals: the change of shift (113 dB), hallway phones (84 dB), bedside monitor alarms (79 dB), and conversational speech (60 dB). It is therefore not surprising that often the person and family have trouble finding a quiet space to collect their own thoughts let alone talk about sensitive issues. The nurse needs to create a quiet and private space to talk by closing the door, turning down the volume on monitors whenever possible, or putting up a "do not disturb" sign.

Take Time to Converse with the Person and Family

Finding out about a person requires spending time with him. A person will be more likely to divulge sensitive information if he feels that the nurse has the time for him and is not rushing to do the next thing on her list. When nurses tell their patients that they are very busy, the patients are often reluctant to ask for anything for fear of being a burden or taking up too much of a nurse's time.

Taking the time to establish a rapport has been found to be one of the most important factors that encourages patients to self-disclose. Moreover, one of the most challenging areas around which to gather information is regarding secrets and painful experiences such as abuse. It is even more challenging when the person is a child. Consider the empirical study described in Exhibit 8.2 of expert nurses who identified the factors that allowed them to help children self-disclose about being abused, (Finn, 2008).

A COMPARISON OF CONVERSATIONAL STYLES: TRADITIONAL APPROACH TO CLINICAL INQUIRY AND THE STRENGTHS-BASED CARE APPROACH TO CLINICAL INQUIRY

Recall that one purpose of clinical conversation is clinical inquiry. The ways in which nurses gather information determine the nature and quality of the information they obtain (see Chapter 7). There are two major approaches to gathering information: the traditional approach and the clinical conversational style approach. The former uses a preset format with structured questions, whereas the latter is more informal and occurs as part of engaging in conversation. These two approaches can be compared in terms of the following (see Table 8.11):

- Structure of the interaction
- Roles assumed by the nurse and person
- Scope of inquiry
- Methods to obtain information

Structure of the Interaction

In a more traditional approach to gathering information the focus is on the information, not on gathering information in the context of a relationship. The nurse meets the patient, asks the questions following a specific protocol and, once the information has been obtained, terminates the conversation.

EXHIBIT 8.2

Empirical study *Examining how nurses obtain self-disclosure from victims of child abuse*

The Problem

One of the challenges in clinical work is how to get children to disclose that they are being abused. A child's self-disclosure of abuse is a critical component in initiating intervention to stop the abuse, address its effects, and decrease the likelihood of long-term negative outcomes.

The Issues

The purpose of this study was to describe the context in which child abuse victims have disclosed their abuse to expert nurses. Knowing more about how the nurses' interviewing styles and techniques resulted in disclosure by children of abuse may help nurses move children from silence to disclosure.

The Study

This descriptive qualitative study targeted expert nurses who had been able to get children to disclose that they had been abused. Thirty expert nurses who practiced in the United States and Canada were interviewed and described how they were able to get children to share their experiences of abuse with them. Interviews were transcribed and qualitatively analyzed.

The Findings

Five key factors played a role in the child's self-disclosure: (a) interviewing in a child friendly environment, (b) connecting with and building rapport with the child, (c) engaging in "real" listening, (d) believing the child unconditionally, and (e) being aware of the potential for false disclosures. The single most important factor that affected whether a child self-disclosed was building a rapport and connecting to the child. The researchers recommended that one-on-one listening is the best way to build the type of rapport necessary to facilitate a child's sharing of such a secret.

The Bottom Line

The child's perception of the nurse having unlimited time and the nurse's engaging in real listening were critical to the disclosure process. Nurses need to be ready to spend the time to build rapport and establish trust and then be fully present when a child is ready to disclose or share a secret.

Source: Adapted from Finn (2008).

In contrast, SBC subscribes to an approach in which clinical inquiry is an integrative and integral aspect of all conversations that occur between patients and nurse and is embedded in the nurse–patient relationship. Clinical inquiry is enhanced when the nurse and patient engage in a collaborative partnership that involves a mutual and reciprocal process of give and take, with both the nurse and person sharing and exchanging information. The nurse is open to what the person has to

---

TABLE 8.11

A comparison to clinical inquiry between the traditional approach versus strengths-based care

Facet of Nursing	Traditional Approach	Strengths-Based Care Approach
Structure of clinical inquiry	Separate and distinct activity in the interaction	Integrative, integral, ongoing collaborative partnership
Roles of practitioner and person	Nurse takes the lead and asks questions; person answers	Person and nurse both ask and answer questions. The nurse is directed by the person and their situation. Nurse assumes the role of learner.
Scope of inquiry	Narrow, targeted	Breadth and depth Situated context and culturally aware
Approach to clinical inquiry	Standardized questioning, a priori	Flexible, responsive, tailored

---

say and tries to understand the situation from the person's perspective, even if they have different perspectives and subscribe to different values. The nurse believes that every encounter and interaction affords an opportunity to learn more about the person and her family. Nurses should look for opportunities to spend time talking with patients as well as for other opportunities to get to know the person by, for example, talking with other people, such as family members, friends, or other team members.

Roles: Monologue versus dialogue

In most traditional clinical situations, the practitioner assumes control over the process of gathering information and conducting the clinical inquiry. It is often the practitioner who initiates and then directs the conversation. Many times, the nurse and person engage in a monologue in which the nurse asks the questions and the patient is expected to provide an answer. It is more of a one-way conversation. The nature of the conversation is that nurse speaks to the person, not with the person.

In SBC, both partners are involved in sharing and exchanging information. The conversation is a two-way dialogue. An encounter may begin when the nurse initiates conversation by asking a general question designed to get to know the person and explore what is of most concern to him, or it may be that the person initiates a dialogue by asking the nurse for specific information. Regardless of how the interaction begins and who initiates the dialogue, nurses take their cues from the person and the situation. They observe, listen to, and ask questions that are based on what they have seen, heard, learned, as well as what they know from experience. It is these sources of information that then direct the nurse's next response and subsequent action. In other words, the nurse's approach to clinical inquiry is situation-responsive.

Scope of Inquiry: Focused or Broad

Another characteristic that distinguishes SBC's approach from the more traditional approach to gathering information is the scope of the inquiry. In the traditional approach, the scope of clinical inquiry is focused; targeted; and limited to understanding the patient's medical condition, presenting symptoms or concerns, and monitoring the response to a treatment regime. This may be appropriate, in particular when the issue is circumscribed and specific information is required to make a decision.

In SBC, the nurse may begin with exploring an issue or concern and then "drill down" to gain a deeper understanding of the issue by asking more specific, targeted or focused questions. This approach is often referred to as an inverted "funnel" approach. Like a funnel, it begins with a general line of question and then narrows in focus. At the same time, the nurse's scope of inquiry is also broad. SBC requires that the nurse gain as complete and comprehensive picture of the whole person and her situation as possible. The nurse may venture into different areas of the person's life, working with its many threads and how these threads relate and are woven together to create the person's story. The nurse understands that people are complex, their lives are complex, and their experiences are complex. People can best be understood when their concerns are situated within their proper context and understood from the patient's perspective and culture. It is only by understanding the person's culture, with its unique beliefs, values, and meanings, that the nurse can begin to understand the significance and importance of a concern and the person's choices in dealing with it.

Style of Questioning: Preset Versus Open Ended

Nurses often use a standardized set or list of questions to explore a given issue. The approach is to ask the same question of every person admitted to that unit who is suffering from a specific medical condition, to follow a specific treatment protocol. The nurse is told that every question must be answered, and there is little improvisation or deviation from the structured format.

In contrast, SBC subscribes to a more flexible approach to gathering information. The nurse may have developed a series of questions or areas of inquiry over the years. These questions or areas may derive from knowledge of the medical condition or problem, from past nursing experience of caring for patients dealing with a similar condition, or from having faced similar issues in the past. Although the nurse may know the areas to explore, she should listen to what the person is saying and then tailor her next line of questioning accordingly. With patients for whom the nurse has cared for before, she may listen to new issues and for specific concerns that indicate they are of special significance to that patient and family.

Nurse Margaret Eades's approach to gathering information and getting to know her patient encompasses all four characteristics of this approach. Margaret explained what happens during every encounter: *"I listen for the person and ask myself, 'So who is Mr. Smith? What's important to Mr. Smith, and where has he been?' What's happened to him is a very important part of his story because the context that he's living right now is who he was before this illness happened. I am interested in knowing what makes him tick, what does he want to do, who is his family, how does he see himself moving forward, and what's standing in his way."*

It takes time for Margaret to gather all this information. She also listens for areas that will shed light on the general questions guiding her clinical inquiry. In effect, she keeps those questions in the back of her mind, and during every clinical conversation, or whenever she interacts with the person and family, she remembers them, filling in the details until a picture of "Mr. Smith" takes form. Margaret listens in order to learn more. This can happen at different times, such as when the person is discussing something else, or when Margaret senses that the person wants to share more about himself and his life. Margaret's approach to clinical inquiry is flexible and responsive. She takes her cue regarding when to ask a question and how to ask it from her patient or the situation. Note that Margaret does not enter into the conversation with a "blank slate." She has in mind general topics to explore that come from formal knowledge, past clinical and personal experiences, and her nursing orientation.

FORMATS OF CLINICAL CONVERSATION: UNSTRUCTURED AND SEMISTRUCTURED

Two formats are most often found in a clinical conversation: the (a) unstructured format and (b) semistructured/focused format.

In an *unstructured format* the conversation contains few specific questions, and the person is encouraged to talk about whatever she wants to talk about. The nurse is directed by the person and takes the lead from her.

In a *semistructured format*, on the other hand, the nurse begins to ask more focused questions in the course of the clinical conversation. The format is still conversational, but there is an interviewing process going on, even if it is less formal. During this part of the conversation nurses may take the lead and ask the person more specific questions to gain a clearer understanding of the situation.

In most clinical conversations, both formats are used. The nurse may begin with an unstructured format, move into a semistructured format when specific information is required, and then move back to an unstructured format.

FORMS OF CLINICAL CONVERSATIONS: DIALOGUING AND INTERVIEWING

All conversations contain elements of dialoguing and interviewing. The dialogue is at the heart of communication between nurses and the person and family. The interview is usually used to gather information that is more specific. Both have their own characteristics and their own types of questioning.

Dialoguing

Dialoguing requires that the nurse tune in to what the person is saying by being attuned to the person's potent and subtle nonverbal and verbal behaviors. The nurse also needs to have developed skills of turn-taking, which involves knowing when to speak and when to listen. It requires that nurses be aware of their own behavior and how their behavior affects the other person. It further requires that nurses reflect on their own way of communicating. This involves becoming more self-aware of how they present themselves and how well they attend to the patient's behaviors and then match their own behavior accordingly.

Dialogue begins when the nurse invites the person and family to engage in conversation for the purpose of gathering information by being visibly attuned to what each person is saying and how he is saying it, as well as skilled in the use of open-ended questioning.

Inviting Dialogue: Visibly Tuning to the Person

Dialoguing requires that the nurse be visibly tuned in to the person by becoming aware of how she behaves when engaging in dialogue. Egan (2002) identified five skills or techniques to help practitioners communicate that they are interested in the person. He grouped these skills under an approach that he titled "visibly tuning to the person and family" using the acronym SOLER:

S: Face the person SQUARELY
O: Adopt an OPEN posture
L: LEAN toward another
E: Maintain good EYE Contact
R: Try to RELAX with the person and family

These five skills are described in Table 8.12, along with suggested techniques of how to accomplish them.

Inviting Dialogue: The Use of Open-Ended Questioning

There are many ways to initiate dialogue and create a rapport with the person, just as there are many ways to begin a conversation. Often, the interaction begins when a nurse introduces himself, engages in small talk, and then asks an open-ended question

TABLE 8.12

Egan's (2002) five SOLER skills of visible tuning to the person

Skill	Clinician's Behaviors
S: Face the person SQUARELY	Adopt a position that communicates interest and involvement. Turn toward the person, not away from him. Sit directly in front of the person, not at an angle or sideways. Position yourself in such a way that the person is comfortable (i.e., at a comfortable distance).
O: Adopt an OPEN posture	Show that you are available, but adopt an open stance. Do *not* cross your arms.
L: LEAN toward another	Lean toward the person when she is speaking. Move backward and forward depending on the situation person's response and level of comfort.
E: Maintain good EYE Contact	Look at the person frequently and exchange eye contact to communicate that you are involved.
R: Try to RELAX with the person and family	Stay calm. Do not fidget, shuffle, or turn away. Show interest to make the person more comfortable.

Source: Adapted from Egan (2002).

that in effect serves as an invitation to enter into dialogue to talk about those things that are of concern to the person and family. What the nurse looks for is guided by his nursing orientation. In SBC, the orientation is about wanting to get to know the person and family to understand their concerns and how they are dealing with them.

Nurse Diane Lowden, who works with persons and families dealing with neurological degenerative diseases, explained that she enters new situations with the following ideas in mind: *"During the first visit with a patient and family, I focus on trying to get a sense of where these people are at, finding out who is in the family, what they are most concerned about, what their experiences mean to them, what they want to know and also, what they don't want to know."*

An open-ended question is often taken by patients as an invitation to discuss what is most important to them. Open-ended questions also allow the dialogue and discussion to be directed primarily by the patient rather than by the nurse. Nurse Virginia Lee summarized this approach: *"I let the patient direct the conversation. What he discloses to me is where I go. And that is what I take as meaningful for his life at that time."*

An open-ended question is designed to encourage a full, meaningful answer using the person's own knowledge, experience, and/or feelings. Open-ended questions typically use phrases such as "Tell me about...," "Help me to understand," and "Could you tell me what happened...?"

Open-ended questions can also be asked in question form, using interrogative pronouns such as *what* and *why*. The important point to note is that the phrase or question is asked in such a way as to elicit a more detailed answer rather than being answered by a single word or simple phrase. For example, if a nurse asks a patient "What did you do today?", one patient may respond by saying "Nothing much," whereas another patient may recount the details of his day. With the first patient it would be necessary to follow up with a more targeted question, such as "Tell me what happened when you first saw the doctor..." In contrast, closed-ended questions are designed to elicit short or single-word answers. These two forms of questioning are compared in Table 8.13.

Inviting Dialogue With a Family

When talking with a family, the nurse should be interested not only in hearing from each family member about their concerns but also in learning how their concerns are affecting the other family members. Thus, the nurse should ask each person to share her knowledge and understanding of a situation, in order to explore differences among family members, including agreements, disagreements, and different meanings (Wright & Leahey, 2009).

Using open-ended questions, the nurse might ask the following questions:

- "Tell me about your family's concern over your mother's stroke" (a family-focused question)
- "How are you feeling and responding about caring for your mother?" (a question directed at individual family members)
- "What do you think your mother would want?" (a question directed at an individual family member's perception of another family member)

TABLE 8.13

Examples of open- versus closed-ended questions

Open-Ended Questions	Closed-Ended Questions
Purpose Designed to invite discussion and promote conversation and dialogue. Intended to help the person describe his thoughts, feelings, experiences, and understandings.	*Purpose* Designed to obtain specific information and not to encourage discussion or dialogue. Does not generally use phrases to gather information.
Examples of open-ended phrases • "Tell me about... [your experiences]" • "Help me to understand what it has been like for you...." • "Describe what these days have been like..." • "Explain what has been going on..." • "Begin where you would like..."	*Examples of closed-ended questions (when, where, and who)* • "When did this happen?" • "Where did it happen?" • "Who was involved?"
Examples of open-ended questions ("what" and "how") • "What have you been experiencing?" • "What has this been like for you?" • "What do you know?" • "How has that experience been?" • "How do you understand what is happening?"	

Even if family members are not actually present, the nurse thinks "family" and asks questions through a family filter. This is known as adopting a *family-minded* lens (Gottlieb & Carnaghan-Sherrard, 2004). The nurse is aware that each person has a family of origin that influences her behavior throughout her life span. The nurse is also aware that the person is part of a family. The person's condition is affecting those with whom the person is linked and, in turn, the person is affected by the reactions and needs of the other family members. In this situation, "family" is whoever the person identifies as family.

Consider Nurse Margaret Eades's encounter with Mrs. Bushey, who contacted Margaret to discuss her husband's condition. Mr. Bushey was being treated for symptom management following diagnosis and treatment for stomach cancer: *"Actually it was Mr. Bushey's wife who came to see me after their follow-up appointment for his symptom management. Mrs. Bushey said to me, 'We need help. My husband's disease is progressing. I can see he can do less. I'm very concerned, and he doesn't seem to know that his disease is progressing and the consequences that that will entail.' And I said, 'Maybe you can tell me a bit about where you're coming from and what has been your experience?'"*

Margaret thus opened up a dialogue in order to discover the needs of all family members.

Interviewing

During an interview, the nurse's goal is to obtain specific information from the person and family by asking specific questions. Most clinical conversations include both dialoguing and interviewing. One format may predominate depending on the purpose

TABLE 8.14

Five types of questions in strengths-based care with illustrated examples

Question Type	Example Questions to Ask
Focused	"Have you ever experienced this before?" "When did this start?" "What makes it better?" "What makes it worse?" "What have you tried?" "What medicines are you taking?" "Has anyone in your family experienced this?"
Clarification	"I am not sure what you mean when you say____. Can you describe it further?" "Help me understand what you mean when you say____." "Can you describe this a little more for me?" "What were you thinking when you experienced this?"
Elaboration	"What was happening just before this started?" "What else were you experiencing when this happened?" "Did anything else happen when you tried this?"
Circular	*Differences:* "Can you help me understand how this experience is different from the last time it happened?" *Hypothetical:* "If you could change one thing, what would it be?" *Future-Oriented:* "What are you hoping you will achieve when this is all over?"

Source: Based on Levinson (1987).

of the conversation. There are times when using an interview format is more appropriate than adopting a conversational style, in particular when the nurse needs specific information about the person, his medical condition, his reactions to his treatment regimens, a follow-up of and evaluation of a treatment plan, or a course of action.

Interview questions are usually grouped into the following four categories: (a) focused questions, (b) clarification questions, (c) elaboration questions, and (d) circular questions. Each type of question elicits specific information, phrased or worded in a particular way, and used at specific times during the clinical conversation. Examples of each type of question and descriptions of their distinguishing features are provided in Table 8.14.

Focused questions elicit specific information or greater details about a situation. They probe into a particular aspect of the person and her experiences. It begins when the nurse identifies an area or issue that he would like to learn more about. For example, in discussing a patient's concern over the loss of appetite, the nurse may ask: "When did you first notice a change in your appetite?"; "Are there times when you feel less hungry? More hungry?"; "Are there certain foods that make you lose your appetite? Increase your appetite?"; or "How is your husband reacting to you?"

Focused questions usually follow open-ended questions. Open-ended questions provide a broad overview of the area of interest, whereas focus questions are designed to be more specific and targeted, "drilling down" to elicit more detail about different aspects of the issue. If the nurse uses only focused questions, she may get detailed information but fail to understand the larger picture in which the details fit.

Clarification questions are used when the person has explained something that may lead to different explanations. In other words, the nurse is unclear about an issue because the person has been vague or imprecise. When nurses use clarification questions, they usually begin by summarizing or repeating what the person has said and then asking the person to explain what they mean. For example, the nurse can ask: "You said...., what were you trying to say?" or "Did you mean...?" In particular, the nurse has to listen carefully to what the person is saying and ask clarifying questions when she is having difficulty understanding what the person has told her, or when the vagueness of what the person has revealed is subject to different interpretations and can be misconstrued or the information misinterpreted.

Elaboration questions are used to further investigate an issue in order to provide a more detailed and complete picture about a particular experience or situation the person has described. For example, the nurse can ask such questions as: "What were you doing before you experienced...?"; "What were the circumstances or situation surrounding...?"; "What else happen when you tried this?"; and "How did you react physically to the news?" The nurse should always wait for the person to complete his answer to a question before asking him to elaborate. It is important, however, that the nurse respect the person's style of talking, how much he wants to reveal, and his readiness to reveal details before asking him further questions.

Circular questions have been designed to help people think about and reflect on the meaning of their experiences (Arnold & Boggs, 2006; Wright & Leahey, 2009). These questions tend to be less judgmental and may have a liberating effect on the person and family (Brown, 1997). They are a form of questioning that can be used both as a clinical inquiry tool as well as a therapeutic approach to help people gain new insights about themselves and a deeper understanding of the issues. However, in the context of this chapter, circular questions are used as a clinical inquiry tool. Keep in mind that when a person and family are asked circular questions they often reflect on their answers. Such reflection may in turn stimulate them to think about their situation differently. There are three types of circular questions: (a) questions that seek comparisons, (b) hypothetical questions, and (c) future-oriented questions.

- *Questions that seek comparisons* are used to help people understand how the context or situation is affecting how they are feeling, thinking, and acting (Brown, 1997). These questions are designed to have the person compare one situation with another, to draw distinctions between them, or highlight their differences. The nurse can ask the person to compare differences in the following areas:
  - **Across time:** "When did this begin?"; "Can you compare this experience to a previous one?"; "What was similar about the two?"; "How did they differ?"
  - **Between people:** "Who in the family is most upset by John's diagnosis?"
  - **Between situations**: "Is he more violent in public or at home?"; "In what situation is the problem worse or better?"
- *Hypothetical questions*, also known as "what if" questions, are designed to help the person and family reflect on the meaning of their experience and to think about the issue in a way that may not as yet have occurred, or, if has occurred,

to think about what happened in differently. The nurse could ask, "What if you could change one thing that has happened: What would it be?" or "What if you could replay that event, would you do anything differently and, if so, how?"

- *Future-oriented questions* help people see patterns or make connections. One way to see the whole picture is to ask questions that draw connections or linkages between events, behavior, feelings, beliefs, meaning, and relationships (Brown, 1997). These questions are designed to tap into feelings, help uncover beliefs, make sense of what is happening, discover patterns, see the whole, create meaning, and help in the interpretation of information. There are six areas in which connections can be made:

    Events: Do you see any connection between how your mother reacted to your diagnosis and the fact that her sister died of the same disease?

    Behavior: "How do you understand why you don't take your medication?"

    Feelings: "When your wife feels upset, how does that make you feel?"

    Beliefs: "When you believe that there is a problem with expressing your anger what effect does that have on your daughter?

    Meaning: "How do you understand why your mother reacted the way she did?"

    Relationship: "When you feel that the family is working together, do you feel closer or more distant to your siblings?"

    Another purpose of *future-oriented questions* is designed to help people describe their goals and hopes for in the future. Such questions are important in understanding what the person and family would like to achieve. The nurse could ask, "Where would you like to be in 6 months from now? How can we work together to make this happen?"

CAVEAT

Nurses need to approach every encounter and patient situation with an open mind in order to consider many possibilities.

Nurses who practice SBC enter into dialogue with patients from an "unknowing" stance with a desire to get to know the person. Although open-ended questions allow patients to tell the nurse what is important to them, it is imperative that the nurse use a variety of other questioning formats to explore as fully as possible the person's situation within the available time. Many times, nurses have to act before they have all the pieces, understand how the pieces make up the whole, or the puzzle is fully understood. However, having a broad repertoire of different types of questions is the nurse's best resource to gather information. The information that she gathers enables her to grasp how the patient's medical condition and his physical, mental, and emotional status interrelate and contribute to the person as a whole. Using different forms of questioning rather than keeping with one format will provide richer, more in-depth information and lead to a more comprehensive, complete picture of the person's situation. By being less prescriptive and more open and situation responsive, the nurse can avoid premature closure by arriving at unsubstantiated conclusions that can lead to inaccurate judgments or to follow a course of poor decision making and ineffective actions.

NURSE BEHAVIORS THAT CAN DERAIL CLINICAL CONVERSATIONS

A nurse can promote effective conversation and become a skilled communicator not only by learning good communication techniques and developing good tools of inquiry but also by becoming aware of errors in communication. These errors, which can result in miscommunication and misunderstandings, fall into the following categories:

- The nature of the question
- The phrasing of the question
- The methods of questioning

The most common pitfalls are summarized in Table 8.15, along with alternative ways of asking questions as well as repair techniques.

Nature of the Question

"Why" questions asked in a negative tone of voice. For most people, asking "why" something has happened stumps them, either because they are unsure of the answer or have never thought about it. A patient may believe she should know the answer and, therefore, may interpret the question negatively. She may feel judged, or feel she is being blamed for what happened to her. For example, the question, "Why did you come to the clinic before waiting to see what would happen?" can be interpreted as criticism because it has a critical tone, implying that the person has done something wrong.

Leading questions. Leading questions anticipate the answer when little is known. Rather than exploring with the person what he is experiencing, the nurse attempts to describe what he is feeling. The problem with this approach is that the person has to decipher the nurse's message and then describe his experience. The nurse's wording may suggest how the person *should* be feeling instead of how he actually *is* feeling. An example of a leading question is "Do you think your shingles is related to the difficulties you are having with your children?"

Phrasing of Questions or Statements

Negative phrasing. Avoid asking a question in a format that downplays, minimizes, or negates the person's actual experience, for example, "You aren't afraid of a needle, are you? Even children with diabetes as young as six test their own sugar levels."

Unfamiliar language. Also avoid using language that is unfamiliar to the person, including medical terminology or technical jargon. A nurse may ask the person about her symptom using medical terminology rather than nonmedical language. The person may answer the question even if she doesn't understand what she is being asked for fear of sounding ignorant. For example, a nurse may state, "Your son is in diabetic ketoacidosis caused by his malfunctioning pancreas that is failing to produce insulin." Many parents would not know that this statement refers to their son's blood sugar levels. It would have been better if the nurse had asked, "Have you noticed any

TABLE 8.15
Nurse behaviors that derail clinical conversations and repair methods

Pitfall to Avoid	Example	Suggested Preventative and Repair Techniques
1. Nature of the question		
"Why" questions	"Why did you not call your family doctor first before coming to emergency today?" (asked in an accusatory tone of voice)	Use open-ended questions: "Tell me what brought you here."
Leading questions	"Do you think your stress caused the rash on your face to get worse?"	Use open-ended, focused, elaboration, and clarification questions: "What is your understanding about what is contributing to your rash?"
2. Phrasing of questions or statements		
Negative phrasing	"You aren't nervous, are you? It's just a minor procedure."	Phrase questions in neutral terms: "How are you feeling?"
Vague statements	"The dressing seems a little funny to me."	Use focused, clear, and specific statements: "I can see that the dressing needs to be reapplied. Tell me what you have noticed" or "Is there more oozing on the dressing since it was last changed?"
Jargon	"Your sinus rhythm seems a little tachycardic on your ECG."	Use the person's language and methods of expression: "Your heart is beating a bit fast."
3. Methods of questioning		
Irrelevant or poorly timed questions	"How is your brother's health?" (asked after the person has revealed he is no longer in contact with his brother following a bitter dispute)	Be attuned to subtle and overt nonverbal and verbal behaviors.
Asking too many questions	Asking one question after another with little time for the person to pause, answer, and reflect.	Keep questions to a minimum. Spend more time listening than talking. Match questions to answers. Match tone to mood.
False reassurance	"Don't worry, your son will be fine." (when all data indicate otherwise)	Be truthful while at the same time look for the strengths to convey hope. Dialogue and discuss further.
Defensiveness	"I know you want to get out of bed, but you are not my only patient today."	Be open, truthful, and transparent.

changes in your son's mood or level of alertness?" or "Did your son complain about not feeling well?"

Methods of Questioning

Irrelevant or poorly timed questions. A nurse can affect the flow of conversation when she asks a question that the person considers to be off topic or ill timed. For example, a person is informed that the treatment is not working and is asked about his plans about it. People often need time to digest information before they are ready to think about other things.

Too many questions. If the nurse asks the person too many questions in rapid succession, without giving her time to answer, she may feel that the nurse is interrogating her rather than having a conversation with her. Excessive questioning sends a message that the nurse is in charge, that her agenda is more important than the patient's, and that she is too busy to listen to anything other than specific information.

Inaccurate or false reassurance. Nurses, in their need to make the person feel better, sometimes provide reassurance when the situation does not call for it. False reassurance occurs when the nurse deliberately gives misleading information to patients in order to reassure them. For example, a mother whose son has suffered a massive brain injury following a motorcycle accident and shows little brain activity asks the nurse how her son will be, and the nurse responds by telling her that her son will be fine. The mother may feel that the nurse is telling her something that is not true. When the person realizes the true situation, she may come to mistrust the nurse and discount other information the nurse gives, believing that the nurse lacks knowledge.

Defensiveness. When a nurse responds defensively—that is, when he tries to justify or defend an action that he knows is insensitive, inappropriate, wrong, or covers up an error—he in effect communicates that he is unwilling to discuss the issue further. When the nurse speaks in a defensive manner, his tone of voice can upset the person and can escalate tensions between them. For example, a person may ask to get out of bed. If the nurse responds by telling the person that he is very busy and that the person will have to wait her turn, the person may become angry and frustrated with the nurse. Ideally, the nurse would tell the patient when he will be available to help her out of bed and explain that he will then give her his full and undivided attention.

Many of the above pitfalls may close off communication. When this happens, nurses will have more difficulty getting to know their patients and developing a trusting relationship. However, by reflecting on what is being said and how it is being said, there are many ways the nurse can repair the conversation.

Nurses should conduct each encounter and every interaction in a manner that honors SBC values by doing the following:

- Talking with the patient, not about him.
- Encouraging the person to talk about herself and tell her story.
- Giving the patient a voice and joining the patient's voice with her professional voice.

Final observation: Florence Nightingale recognized that nurses needed to be trained to nurse. Nursing is *not* innate or inborn. By drawing attention to the effects of the nurse's way of "being" on a patient's healing, Nightingale cautioned nurses in what not to do and instructed them on how to become more effective healers so that the patient could self-heal. A significant part of Nightingale's (1860) *Notes on Nursing* is devoted to instructing nurses in changing their ways of "being" as the keys to improving the person's road to health and healing.

Key Summary Points

- Learning to nurse requires that students re-form and retrain their social involvement skills to engage in clinical inquiry and therapeutic dialogue with individuals entrusted to their care.
- Therapeutic communication accomplishes many goals and fills different purposes. The most central purposes are to enter into clinical conversations and to dialogue with the patient and family to get to know them and understand their concerns so that care can be planned that is responsive to them and their situation.
- Milton Mayeroff's essential ingredients of caring share many of the same qualities of nurses who practice. These ingredients are important if patients and families are to engage with nurses in meaningful ways to work together to promote health and self-healing.
- Re-forming and training for clinical involvement involves developing skills of attunement/awareness, authentic presence, and attentive listening.
- There are specific tools for developing an authentic presence, such as being mentally and physically fully present, showing respect, and adopting the stance of a learner.
- The tools to develop attentive listening include experiences in learning about attentive or real listening, minimizing conditions of nonattentive or pseudolistening, becoming aware of filtering or stereotyping while the person is talking, listening for the message underlying the person's words without any prejudgment and bias, and the like.
- The art of clinical conversation involves developing social awareness and social facility skills.
- Personal and situational factors can influence the quality of clinical conversations, including creating a suitable physical environment and taking time to be with the person and family.
- In a traditional approach to gathering information, the focus is on obtaining specific information, narrow in scope, rather than on getting to know the person, understanding the person and family's concerns, understanding how pieces of data relate, identifying patterns, etc.

- SBC subscribes to an approach in which clinical inquiry is an integrative and integral aspect of all conversations that occur between patients and nurse and is integral to the nurse–patient relationship. Forms of clinical conversation include dialoguing and interviewing.
- Interviewing requires a broad repertoire of forms of questioning that are used to elicit different types of information. Each type of question encourages patients to share information. There is skill in learning to ask questions, to dialogue, and to converse with the person and their families.
- Certain nurse behaviors can derail clinical conversations. The nurse needs to be aware of how her behavior affects patients and to reflect and think prior to, during, and after an encounter. The nurse needs to increase awareness of ways of communicating that can potentially derail a conversation. She needs to have, as part of her repertoire of interpersonal and communication skills, repair tools to facilitate and encourage clinical conversations.

The Spiraling Process for Uncovering and Discovering Strengths

9

LEARNING OBJECTIVES

After reading this chapter, you should be able to:

- Explain the importance of the nurse–patient relationship in Strengths-Based Care
- Describe why Strengths-Based Care requires that the nurse develop a collaborative partnership with the person and family
- Describe why Strengths-Based Care requires both an exploratory and an a priori approach to gathering information
- Identify the four phases of the Spiraling Process and the major activities that take place within each phase
- Describe the strategies and techniques nurses can use to discover and uncover strengths

> The famed artist has that thought alone
> Which is contained within the marble shell:
> The sculpture's hand can only break the spell
> To free the figures slumbering in the stone
>
> —Michelangelo

Famed 15th-century sculptor and painter Michelangelo recognized that within every piece of marble dwells a beautiful sculpture, on which one need only work to reveal it (Zander & Zander, 2000). The challenge faced by nurses who work with patients and their families is not unlike the challenge faced by the sculptor. Nurses seek to discover the person for whom they are caring, not with a hammer and chisel but through the use of their own presence, interpersonal skills of engagement and connection, and assessment tools. Strengths are more apparent and easier to uncover in some people and families than in others. Some people's and families' strengths are hidden or less apparent, and their strengths need to be discovered. These discoveries are often made in the course of nursing for them. Discovering patient and family strengths may not always be easy; however, when nurses discover and focus on a person's strengths, they are able to connect to the person at a deeper level and be more fully present in the relationship. Herein lie both the challenges and rewards of clinical work.

Nurse Jane Chamber-Evans, in her role as clinical nurse specialist in an intensive care unit, told of the Burns family, whose many strengths she uncovered while working with them over the course of over two years as they faced crisis after crisis. As Jane recalled, *"I had a call from the nurses, 'You've got to come right now.'"* A seventeen-year-old boy had been admitted to the unit in grave condition. His name was Scott Burns.

Jane recalled the events of her first encounter with Scott's mother: *"My first impression of his mother, Barbara, was that she was a very beautiful and highly intelligent woman who was completely distraught over her son's condition. Her husband was away on business. Her son had presented the day before with what looked like the flu, so she sent him to bed. During the night he had a seizure. He was taken to the emergency department where he was diagnosed with encephalitis, and his condition quickly deteriorated. They couldn't get the seizures under control. He was very, very ill, and his mother was absolutely beside herself."*

Jane saw Barbara's strengths immediately and, in so doing, must have communicated this to Barbara by being fully present. When Jane first met Barbara, her first thoughts began with the unknown. She wondered, *"'Who is this mother? Who is this family? What does this mother need me to do immediately for her?'"* Jane recalled feeling an instant connection with Barbara, in part because she was also a mother and could identify with Barbara's anguish and fears, and Jane also saw Barbara's inner strength and dignity as she tried to cope and make sense of this overwhelming and potentially devastating situation.

With each encounter, Jane discovered new inner strengths in Barbara: *"Barbara was warm and it was so obvious that she loved her son. It was obvious also that she needed to have some way to take back control of being a mother so that she could be in charge of what was happening to her son. Her philosophy was that there was no stone too big that [it] can't be overturned. So it didn't matter what barrier came in front of her; she rallied the family. I have to say also her husband was a wonderful man but became more defeated by what happened to his son."*

The process of assessing people for strengths is a process of creating new possibilities for health, recovery, and healing because it involves the following:

- Focusing on what is unique about that person and family
- Discovering the human spirit as reflected in the person's attitudes about life and living
- Providing insights into what makes the person and family able to pursue their goals, live life to its fullest as they meet everyday demands, face difficult life challenges, and make difficult health care choices
- Giving the nurse insight into how best to work with the person and family to enable them to become empowered and take charge of the things that matters to them and those they choose to change

Uncovering and discovering strengths does not exist in a vacuum but is part of the larger process of getting to know the person in her current situation, including her history, what is important to her, what she values, what she has been through, the challenges she has faced and is facing, and what she would like to achieve. Certainly, coming to know the person requires clinical inquiry and critical inquiry skills in general as well as how to use these skills in a particular situation (see Chapters 7 and 8, in particular). The quality of the information that the nurse uncovers about the person is related to the quality of the relationship that the nurse is able to establish with the person. Jane was able to appreciate Barbara's strengths almost immediately, and it is this appreciation of Barbara as a loving, concerned mother that helped Jane connect with her and that helped Barbara open herself to Jane's offers of help.

To illustrate further how one comes to know something, consider the story of the fisherman in Exhibit 9.1 (as told by Smith, Persson, & Lynn, 2008). This simple story describes how a father taught his daughter how to learn how to know the whole, not just its parts. The fisherman subscribed to the value of holism, as described in Chapter 3.

THE NURSE–PATIENT RELATIONSHIP AND THE NURSING PROCESS

The nurse–patient relationship. All helping professionals acknowledge the importance of the practitioner's relationship with the person as an important component of the therapeutic process. What differs among professionals, however, is the significance they give to that relationship and the way the relationship is viewed. Social workers, psychologists, and therapists talk about the use of their professional selves to create the *therapeutic alliance* (Berkman & D'Ambruoso, 2006). Nursing professionals talk about the centrality of the nurse–patient relationship as the heart of nursing practice and believe it is nursing's quintessential value (Hagerty & Patusky, 2003). Pioneering nurse scholars understood that the quality of the relationship that nurses formed with their patients was critical to the person's healing and helped the person achieve a higher level of health (Orlando, 1961; Peplau, 1952; Travelbee, 1971). The nurse–patient relationship is essential for caring and gives nursing its identity (Benner & Gordon, 1996; Watson, 1997).

The nursing process. All health care practitioners have a systematic way of organizing their activities to carry out practice. Physicians are schooled in the use of the medical model. Nursing activities are organized and described within the nursing process. The nursing process is a reflective and practical method based on knowledge and experience for understanding and analyzing the health needs and concerns of the person and family; arriving at a clinical understanding or grasp of the situation; and finding ways to work together to promote health, allow for recovery, and facilitate and sustain healing. The nature of the nursing process can vary in form and structure depending on the nurse's orientation and how a nurse uses it to guide clinical judgments and actions. Strengths-Based Care (SBC) requires that the nurse use a process to uncover the person's concerns, get to know the patient and members of the family as individuals, and discover their strengths in order to plan and carry out nursing care.

Nursing activities take place in the context of the nurse–patient relationship, and its effectiveness depends on the quality of the relationship that the nurse establishes with the person and family. Caring relationships are built on knowing the person and

EXHIBIT 9.1

Personal experience *Coming to know the whole: The fisherman and his daughter*

Once there was a seasoned fisherman who was passing his knowledge and wisdom on to his daughter. He told her that the most important teaching he could impart was for her to come to know the fish. He told her to go and return to him when she came to know the fish.

The young girl scampered off and caught a fish. She examined the fish carefully and then returned to her father. She told the father the details of the fish's scales, fins, eyes, and tail. Her father said, "You do not yet know the fish…return to me when you do."

The daughter was puzzled but determined to prove to her father that she could arrive at the knowledge he was seeking. She caught another fish, dissected it, removed its parts, categorized them, and described them with the utmost precision. She returned to her father and presented her findings on the fish, showing him a poster detailing her careful analysis. The father smiled and gently told her, "You do not yet know the fish. Come back to me when you do."

Now she was getting a little frustrated. This time she drew on all the available technology. She used an electron microscope to examine the cellular structures of the fish organs. She conducted chemical analyses of the tissues. Now she returned to her father, confident of her in-depth knowledge of the fish, armed with tables, charts, and graphs. He listened calmly and said, "No my child, you do not yet know the fish. Return to me when you do."

This time she was angry and hurt. She had worked so hard…of course she knew every part of that fish. What was he talking about?! Exhausted, she collapsed by the bed of a slow-moving stream. She began to relax with the sounds of the stream, the odor of the earth and moss, and the light glistening off the water. Her eyes caught a glimpse of a beautiful trout swimming downstream. She watched for a long time as it meandered through the rocks, paused to nibble on a stone and brought its mouth to the surface of the water for a breath. She was fascinated, enthralled by the fish's beauty and uniqueness, how it thrived in its environment. For what seemed like hours she watched and marveled. She returned to her father, humbled by her experience. She told him that she could not know everything about the fish…only what she experienced in the time she was present on the bank. She described the water bubbling, the fish darting and stopping as it swam through the water, the vibrant colors changing in light and shadow. She told him how this fish was different from and similar to others in the stream. Her father smiled, "Now, my daughter, you know the fish."

Source: Adapted from Smith, Persson, and Lynn, (2008).

on being honest, authentic, trustworthy, and a source of hope and courage (Mayeroff, 1971) through the use of presence (Finfgeld-Connett, 2008; Siegel, 2010).

Connections between nurse and patient can be brief—lasting a few minutes, a day or longer, and they can evolve over a considerable period of time (Johnson, 1994).

Often, a relationship develops when the nurse accompanies the person through a major life event, with its ups and downs, its cycles of exacerbation and remission that, at times, lead to death. A long-term relationship often entails the formation of a deeper understanding of the person than that which is possible with a brief encounter.

Let's return to the Burns family and Nurse Jane Chamber-Evans to see how their relationship developed over time: *"It was a long, long haul for Scott and his family. Scott needed intensive rehabilitation following his bout with encephalitis and, after several months of therapy, he regained everything. Just as he was about to go home, Scott suffered a massive stroke. He even ended up having kidney failure [and] needing dialysis. It was just one assault after another after another."*

Jane was intimately involved with this family for over two and a half years: *"In the beginning, I'd see them three or four times a day. And Barbara had my pager number and would sometimes call me, even in the evenings. When Scott was transferred to the unit, I would visit them at least once a day. When he went to rehab, they would call me once a week. But when a crisis happened, they would come back, often in a panic. I would say 'Okay, we've done this together in the past and we're going to be able to do this together again.' Sometimes it would just be a matter of 'Let's remember when Scott had a spike and when he had a slight setback and he was able to move forward again.'"*

By being intimately involved and fully present with this family, accompanying them on every lag of their journey, Jane earned their respect and gained their trust. They sought her out regularly because they knew she understood and appreciated them as individuals and as a family and could meet their needs. Jane, over time, came to learn about this family and what sustained them. They needed hope, hope that was based on reality, not on fantasy, on possibilities, not wishful thinking. She was open and honest with them and was able to establish and sustain a caring relationship with Scott and his parents.

Jane's approach suited the Burns family: *"We talked a lot, and we always talked very frankly. Every once in awhile Barbara and her husband would come into the hospital. They would knock and my door and come in and see me, and one of the things that they always said to me was, 'You never tried to cushion the truth. You never hurt us, but you never tried to hide, you were always straightforward and would keep us well grounded in what was reality. This was very important for us.'"*

COLLABORATIVE PARTNERSHIPS AND STRENGTHS-BASED CARE

An important question to ask is, "If the nurse values SBC, then what type of relationship does the nurse need to develop with the person and family?

In Chapters 1 and 3, I described two approaches to care: (a) a collaborative partnership and (b) the traditional hierarchical approach. Collaborative partnerships are premised on the idea of sharing power (Gottlieb et al., 2006). To become partners and share power with the nurse, the person first needs to feel he has something to bring to the relationship. He has to recognize and value what he brings to the partnership. He also has to value the nurse's contribution. To be a partner in care, the person also has to feel that he has a role to play in directing his own care. He will be able to do this when both he and the nurse identify and recognize and value each other's skills and expertise. The result of such a partnership is that the person gains knowledge, skills, and confidence to assume greater control over his own health and health care decisions by understanding, discovering, and developing personal and family strengths.

Now consider how this approach differs from the traditional hierarchical approach that is paternalistic in orientation. Here, the nurse assumes authority over the patient and is responsible for overseeing her care. The person's primary role is as a passive recipient; she is expected to comply with the medical and nursing regimens and do as she is told. The need to know a person's strengths, therefore, is of secondary or of relatively little importance.

A collaborative partnership is more consistent with SBC than the traditional hierarchical approach to care because it is built on principles of person-centered care and empowerment (see Chapter 1 for a discussion of these two topics).

METHODS USED TO GATHER INFORMATION: EXPLORATORY AND A PRIORI

SBC requires that nurses use both the exploratory and a priori methods to gather information about the person and family. The *exploratory* method requires that the nurse be open to learning about the person and how he is experiencing, responding to, and dealing with his situation. The nurse may have general knowledge about the person's condition but not about *that* person's unique reactions, ways of responding, special circumstances, and history. For example, in the case of diabetes, the nurse knows about diabetes—its signs and symptoms, pathophysiology, and treatment options. What the nurse does not know is the meaning that diabetes holds for this particular person who has been diagnosed with diabetes, or for his family. The nurse needs to gather information from the person and family: the age of onset, the type of diabetes, management control, the person's physiological responses to changing blood sugar levels, reactions to the medication, family history and experience with diabetes, how having a member with diabetes is affecting family functioning, its impact on different family members, and so forth. The former information is a priori knowledge. The latter information concerning that person is acquired through the use of an exploratory approach.

To more fully understand people and their situations, nurses need to recognize that patients, clients, and families are their primary source of information. In the course of nursing people, nurses get to know them by using a broad repertoire of clinical inquiry skills, including using all their senses, making astute observations, engaging in clinical conversations by being attentive and fully present, being mindful and open to their own internal responses and those of their patients, being an empathic listener, knowing how to elicit the person's narratives, and taking a good medical and social history—and this is only a preliminary list! (See Part 2 for a detailed description and discussion of these clinical inquiry skills.)

First and foremost, the nurse needs to assume the role of learner. As a learner, the nurse begins from a stance of "unknowing" (Munhall, 2009). When she adopts this mindset, the nurse appreciates that she may know something about the medical condition but that she does *not* know about the person: who he is, what challenges he and his family face, and how they live with their challenges. When the nurse adopts this mindset, she is open to really learning about this person and this family. The nurse understands that every encounter with the person is an opportunity to learn more about herself, the patient, his family, and his life. The nurse should talk with family members and individuals, consult with professionals, and use any source of information that will lead to greater understanding of the person and family.

Nurse Catherine Gros explained why taking the role of learner rather than expert and using an exploratory method to gathering information about the patient is important in nursing: *". . . It's being a learner versus being an expert who can predict the future and who knows what's best for everybody. When the nurse has an attitude of 'I know what's best for this patient and family,' I find this way of thinking very arrogant. As a nurse, I should be a learner. My job is to learn from the person: who they are, what they want, and what they want to achieve. I also want to learn from them how I might best help."*

An exploratory approach requires that the nurse continuously consider what he needs to know about his patients in order to find the best approach that works for them. Nurse Christina Clausen described the questions she wants to explore with patients: *"I'm looking at how I can work with this patient to help them get to where they want to go. I ask myself: 'What do I need to know about them to help them deal with their emotions that are part of their situation? What do I need to do to bring them to a certain level of understanding? What are those questions that I need to be asking the patient to help them make decisions and also to help them feel that they made the right ones?'"*

In contrast to the exploratory method, a priori knowledge is that which the nurse brings to a given situation. It has been acquired through what the nurse has learned in the academic and clinical settings—in her personal and professional experiences. A priori knowledge can inform the nurse in only a general manner about the issues. A priori knowledge serves to initially guide nurses as to what to expect, what to look for, and what information to explore.

Consider the approach to assessment used by Nurse Cindy Dalton in planning care for Nathan, a 50-year-old man with Parkinson's disease, and his partner, Nancy, whom you met in Chapter 3.

Cindy used an exploratory approach to find out about Nathan and Nancy's life and the activities Nathan enjoys in order to decide with him when the best time for him to take his medication would be: *"I would meet with Nathan and Nancy to assess their home situation and what it was like for them living with this disease. One concern was when he should take his medication. For instance, Nathan liked to swim. So how could we time his medication so that it would be at its peak effect, let's say, by 2 p.m.? I needed to find out what activities were being affected by his Parkinson's and then to time the taking of his medications accordingly."*

Cindy combined her knowledge of Parkinson's disease and when the drug action is at its peak effect (a priori knowledge) with an exploratory approach to find out more from Nathan what is important to him and what he enjoys so that he could still maintain some quality of life despite his physical disability caused by the progression of his disease. The optimal timing of medication would enable Nathan to get the most out of his life.

People feel understood when their concerns have been interpreted correctly and when nurses take the time to listen to them. The nurse listens not only to the facts but is attuned to subtle nuances and nonverbal cues by picking up the underlying subtext and listening to the person's understanding of her situation (See Chapter 8 for a full discussion of attentive listening). Using all his senses—including noticing, listening, attending to, attuning, and asking the person specific questions—the nurse *senses* the meaning and significance of a situation, *perceives* patterns that indicate that something is amiss or that something is working, develops a *feeling* for what he can do, and *knows* when to act and when to wait (Johnson, 1994). This is the work involved in getting to know a patient and in gathering salient information that can help the nurse grasp the situation and piece the puzzle together to direct clinical decisions and formulate actions.

Clinical inquiry and critical thinking skills are the nurse's tools for exploring with patients their concerns and issues and understanding their salience. The essential nurse strengths, basic mindset, know-how, and habits of the mind skills in the nurses' toolbox were presented in Chapters 5 through 8. Once these skills have been mastered, the nurse needs to combine them and develop a more specific set of clinical inquiry skills to uncover and discover strengths so she can know how best to meet her patients' and families' medical and health care needs and challenges with them together, as a team.

THE SPIRALING PROCESS

The *Spiraling Process* is a nursing model developed by Deborah Moudarres and Helene Ezer to guide nursing practice that consists of four phases, as shown in Figure 9.1 (Gottlieb et al., 2006).

Each phase is distinguished by a major activity and the roles that each partner (nurse, person/family) assumes. In Phase 1, called *Exploring and Getting to Know*, the major focus is on exploring the person's concerns and getting to know the person and the family. In the Phase 2, *Zeroing In*, the nurse and person focus on sorting out issues and deciding on priorities and where to direct their energies. In the Phase 3, *Working Out*, the person and nurse begin to try out different ways of dealing with the problems and issues. Phase 4, labeled *Reviewing*, involves stepping back and examining what has

FIGURE 9.1
Diagram of the Spiraling Process.

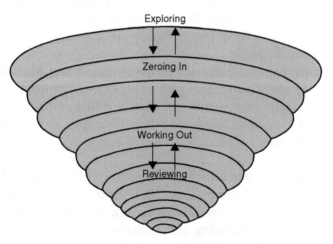

Source: Reprinted with permission from Gottlieb, & Feeley with Dalton, (2006).

happened in order to reassess and evaluate what is working and what is not and deciding what needs further attention. During each of these four phases the nurse is assessing for, discovering, and uncovering the person's strengths. Each of the major phases in the Spiraling Process, as well as the strength characteristics that were described in Chapter 4, are summarized in Table 9.1.

Moudarres and Ezer elected to depict the nursing process as spiral because a spiral has no specific beginning and no particular end point but instead is a continuous flow of activity, similar to the work that takes place in actual clinical practice (Gottlieb et al., 2006). The Spiraling Process does not follow a linear pattern, and it does not consist of a series of sequential steps as other nursing process models do. Although each of the four phases is distinct, they are highly interrelated and intertwined, folding onto and into each other. In other words, during an interaction, the nurse and patient can "spiral" backward and forward depending on the issue with which they are dealing. Several phases of the process may be present during an encounter if the nurse and patient are working on several issues. Consider what happens during a typical nurse–patient encounter. The nurse may review with the patient how well he is doing on a new medication (Phase 4: Reviewing). During the same encounter, the nurse may also inquire about how other family members are coping with the patient's new medical regimen or the changes in his physical condition (Phase 1: Exploring and Getting to Know).

Regardless of the problem or issue with which the person is dealing, nurses always must be aware of their relationship with the person and family and how best to develop and sustain it. As the nurse and patient get to know each other, they develop trust and respect for and in one another. Trust and respect are created when the nurse is authentically present and open to new information, attentively listens, adopts a nonjudgmental attitude, and provides the person with a safe and secure environment in which to

TABLE 9.1

The four phases in the Spiraling Process and assessing for characteristic of strengths[a]

Phase	Characteristics[a]
Phase 1: Exploring and Getting to Know	C3-Strengths coexist with weaknesses and vulnerabilities. C5-Strengths are defined by the context and circumstance. C6-Strengths are multidimensional. C8-Strengths are transferable. C9-Strengths are personal constructions.
Phase 2: Zeroing In	C4-Strengths are related to goals.
Phase 3: Working Out	C1-Strengths are developing entities. C2-Strengths can be learned. C4-Strengths are related to goals.
Phase 4: Reviewing	C7-Strengths can be depleted and replenished. C9-Strengths are personal constructions.

[a] Characteristics of strengths are described more fully in Chapter 4.

explore her issues. Each phase in the Spiraling Process affords the nurse an opportunity to learn something more about the patient and family.

Nurse Jane Chamber-Evans described the relationship that she developed with Barbara Burns during Scott's roller coaster recovery. Several times during the trajectory of Scott's illness, he was at the brink of death's door but somehow managed to rally. His mother, whom Jane described as courageous, realistic, supportive, loving, resourceful, and a strong person, had moments when she *"fell apart."*

Jane described how she made herself available to Barbara during these periods of crises, providing Barbara with a badly needed *"safe haven"* for Barbara to *"unload"* and vent: *"One of the things in working so closely with Barbara is that we really developed a close relationship. I came to recognize those markers that signaled she was becoming anxious. For example, she wouldn't go for lunch or be able to concentrate on her book or talk with Scott. I would see her get a little short with people. All those behaviors weren't usual for her. When I saw these indicators of distress, I would say 'Do you want to come and sit and chat with me for a few minutes?' By being present and being able to recognize those little markers, I could create a safe space in my office for her. We talked frankly as mothers about her dreams for her son and what she was going through. I would say, 'I can't imagine the pain. You need to tell me about what you're going through so that I can understand it.' I really tried to encourage her to tell me about her experience and not to assume that I knew what she was experiencing."*

SPECIFIC PHASES OF THE SPIRALING PROCESS FOR UNCOVERING AND DISCOVERING STRENGTHS

Phase 1: Exploring and Getting to Know

During an encounter, there are always some elements of exploring an issue and getting to know the person and his family better. However, when the nurse's primary focus is on gathering information about the patient/client as a person and his specific issues, then the nurse and patient/client/family can be said to be in the first phase of the Spiraling Process (see Figure 9.2).

Nurses should focus on assessing and understanding the patient and family's concerns and assess weaknesses and deficits that may put the person at risk for illness or prevent healing. At the same time, nurses must look to uncover strengths that contribute to the patient's ability to cope, enable recovery, and facilitate healing. Thus, nurses need to strike the right balance between focusing on deficits or weaknesses while attending to strengths. Both areas need attention; neither can be ignored. Nurses need to remember that no situation, no matter how negative or grim, is without its positive aspects. Conversely, every situation, no matter how positive, contains weaknesses that can increase the person's vulnerability and heighten the risk for illness and further trauma.

When nurses focus solely on a person's deficits or problems and fail to notice strengths, they may develop a distorted or skewed picture of the situation. They may, for example, fail to understand what is keeping the problem or weakness in check or how strengths serve to prevent a problem from getting worse or prevent an illness from occurring.

FIGURE 9.2

Diagram of Phase 1 of the Spiraling Process—Exploring and getting to know.

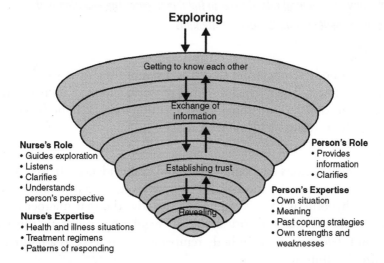

Source: Reprinted with permission from Gottlieb, & Feeley with Dalton, (2006).

There are many innate biological mechanisms, and psychological processes commonly referred to as *defense mechanisms* that help maintain and protect the person's integrity. Too often, practitioners see these as weaknesses and problems that must be fixed. Consider the symptom of fever, which is usually interpreted as a pathological event (the symptom must be treated) rather than the body's natural immunological mechanism to fight infection—as described in the empirical study described in Exhibit 9.2. Or consider when an individual first receives bad news. The news may put her into a state of shock. On the surface, she may continue to carry on with her regular routine because she is not ready to deal with the full impact of the news and its implications. Often, health care practitioners may interpret the person's behavior as indicating that she is in a state of denial, with denial also interpreted as negative, something to be corrected and fixed.

During a first encounter with a patient, the nurse tries to gain as much information as possible about his concerns and issues. People are more likely to divulge information about their concerns with a nurse whom they feel listens to them, is competent and skilled, acts in their best interest, and is a person whom they trust (de Raeve, 2002). Patients trust nurses who spend time with them and show that they are interested in them as an individual and provide more than just physical care (Luker, Austin, Caress, & Hallett, 2000).

There are many different approaches nurses can use to get to know a person. The nurse may begin by exploring the person's concerns, problems, or symptoms. Some nurses talk about the importance of "getting the story." Each individual lives his or her life as a story. To make sense of what is happening to them, people often create a narrative to explain and interpret seemingly unrelated events. They often have many narratives going on simultaneously. When a nurse meets the patient and family, he enters their lives in the middle of an ongoing, unfolding story. The nurse may go beyond the presenting problems and ask the patient/client/family to talk about themselves. When

EXHIBIT 9.2

Empirical study   *The natural role of fever in fighting disease: The importance of symptoms in the context of understanding strengths*

The Problem

An increase in body temperature (fever) is a symptom that is sometimes interpreted as a weakness. The normal response of warm-blooded animals, including humans, to infection and inflammation is a natural increase in body temperature that is strongly correlated with survival.

The Issues

Given these observations and significant biological evidence, there is a need for researchers to examine the mechanism of how fever affects the immunological system. The hypothesis of this study was that the thermal microenvironment (body temperature) plays a critical role in regulating events in the immune response and that an increase in body temperature can serve as a natural trigger to mobilize the immune system.

The Study

To examine the direct effects of fever-like temperatures on immunological parameters (lymphocyte and antibody production), the researchers designed ways to raise body temperature by one or two degrees and measure its effects on the immune system.

The Findings

A safe technique was developed to raise body temperature by one or two degrees and applied to nine individuals diagnosed with solid tumor cancer. All individuals experienced a significant positive effect on their immune system.

The Bottom Line

Characteristics sometimes considered weaknesses, can depending on the circumstances, be viewed as strengths. In this case, fever may be an important and natural way of fighting certain diseases.

Source: Adapted from Pritchard et al., (2004).

the nurse is talking to a patient she may be interested in learning about who she is, where she comes from, what is important to her, and what else is happening in her life. The way the nurse asks questions and how he listens will affect how much information the person is willing to share. It is often through nonverbal communication that the nurse can discern clues about whether the person is ready to explore her concerns. As Nurse John Kayser explained, *"The key is to start a conversation by being as open as possible, with the least structure, so that the person can just talk. Inevitably, people talk about things that are important to them."*

In the nurse's desire to know the patient, she may ask questions that focus on how the patient and family are affected by the problem and how they are dealing or coping with it. It is through observing, listening to, and conversing with them that the nurse begins to gather information.

The following are examples of unstructured statements and questions that a nurse may use:

- Tell me about what has happened that brings you here.
  - Can you tell me more about that? (probing question)
  - Help me to understand what you are experiencing or going through. (probing statement)
- What are you most worried about? What is it that is of most concern?
- How long has this been an issue or concern?
  - Has the concern changed over time? If so, how? (probing question)
- What else is currently happening in your life that you think is affecting this concern?
- How are these symptoms affecting your life?

Specific areas that the nurse may explore

The areas to which the nurse attends and selects are guided by SBC values, described in Chapter 3 and shown in Exhibit 9.3. Reflect on each value and connect it to how a nurse can use these values to get to know a person. How do the values of SBC guide what the nurse attends to, observes for, and inquires about?

Exploring the importance of an issue to the person and family. The nurse needs to understand not only what the issues and problems are but also what they mean to the person and family.

Nurse Christina Clausen explained the importance of attending to what the person initially shares: *"As I'm going through the interview process with a patient, I'm learning what they are sharing with me first. My impression is that whatever they are sharing with me has to have some importance for them. There is something in that first conversation that I have to be very astute about, remember to come back to, and explore further when the time is right because there's a reason they have decided to talk about that (issue) first."*

The nurse may summarize what she has heard to validate her impressions with the person. She may say, "You have told me...(summary of what the person has just told her) and then ask, "Is this what is most important to you?" Their answer will determine whether the nurse should probe the issue more deeply.

Exploring the person's beliefs about the issue. Nurses also need to understand what the person believes. Beliefs are at the heart of how a person reacts and responds to various situations (Wright, Watson, & Bell, 1996). To assess a person's beliefs, nurses can ask the following questions (Murphy, Taylor, & Townsend, 2001):

- What is your understanding about what is happening to you?
- How does your family understand your concerns?
- Who or what is responsible for the problem (e.g., a person, a medication, a treatment)?
- Did you think there is a solution?
- What would be the benefits for you and your family if the concern is dealt with?

EXHIBIT 9.3

Reflect and connect *Assessment guided by Strengths-Based Care values*

Reflect and Connect Instructions:
Reflect on each value of Strengths-Based Care (SBC). Think of how a nurse can use these values to gather information about a patient.

1. Think of what each value means. Give an example of what a nurse could observe for

2. Think of a question to ask to assess for that value.

3. What strengths could a nurse be observing or listening for that would illustrate that value?

SBC value	Example of what to observe for	Example of a question(s) to ask	Example of a strength
1. Health and Healing	Example of healing after a stroke: What does the patient do to regain function?	Tell me what you did before the stroke. What would you like to work on? Where would you like to start?	Observe how the person responds when tired and the efforts made to conserve energy (strength: self-regulation)
2. Uniqueness of the Person			
3. Holism and Embodiment			
4. Objective/ Subjective Reality and Created Meaning			
5. Self-Determination			
6. Person and Environment Are Integral			
7. Learning, Readiness, and Timing			
8. Collaborative Partnership			

Note. The eight values of SBS are described in more detail in Chapter 3.

Exploring the person's coping. Recall that health and healing are reflected in how the person manages their health challenges to promote healing (Value 1: Health and Healing; see Chapter 3). Nurses need to understand how their patients are coping and dealing with their health challenges. With this focus in mind, they should gather information about what patients have already done to deal with the issue, how they have been managing, what has helped and what has not, what has worked and what has not, and how decisions are made that set a particular patient on one course of action rather than another.

Consider the approach to clinical inquiry that Nurse Lia Sanzone uses:

"I try to get them to describe what they're living through right now, what it means to them and how it's affecting them. . . . Having them describe their lives . . . helps me to identify strengths. I also try to find out if they have ever experienced a similar incident in the past. Because if they have, then that in itself is a strength—to say they developed some things in the past experience that allows them to transfer over to this one. On the other hand, I can't just assume that they have developed good coping skills, so I have to explore that with them by asking them, 'When Incident X occurred, did it actually help you? And if it did help you, how did it help?' I often say 'That is a strength, and if it helped you in the past it could help you again.'"

The nurse may further ask:

- Tell me how you are coping with . . . .
- Tell me about a situation that best describes how you cope and how other family members cope
- What have you tried so far?
- How has that worked?
- What has been most helpful? What has made things worse?

Getting to know the person. If the nurse senses that the person is receptive and the timing is right, he may also try to get to know the person better by asking questions such as these:

- Can you tell me a story or something about yourself that best captures the qualities about yourself that you are most proud?
- What would you like me to know about yourself, your family?
- How would others describe you?

Even when the nurse has had a long-term relationship with a patient, there is always something new for the nurse to learn. Age and illness have a way of sometimes masking a person's strengths, yet it is both a person's strengths and weaknesses—the person's essence—that are revealed during periods of challenge and stress. To balance the immediate focus on the weaknesses and deficits so commonly present with age and illness, nurses should seek to discover their

> A person's strengths and weaknesses are revealed during periods of challenge and stress.

patients' strengths. This may occur not through direct questioning but by observing: seeing, noting, and listening (also see Chapters 6 and 7).

Nowhere is this more of a challenge than with elderly individuals with advanced dementia. Because dementia often robs the person of her personhood and dignity, it is important that nurses continuously look for and work with the person's strengths.

It is important to uncover and discover strengths, not only for the patient but also for her family members, who might be so overwhelmed by the losses and changes they encounter that they forget who their loved one is. Some Memory Units (i.e., a unit dedicated to the care of individuals suffering from dementia) in hospitals and residences will ask the family to put together an album of the person's life, or will hang photos of the patient at an earlier period in his or her life to inform the staff and remind the family of the patient's full personhood.

Ora Alberton, a community-based nurse, works with elderly individuals. She explained the importance of being open to new learning and discovering a patient's strengths in order to safeguard that individual's personhood: *"The thing that I try to carry with me is that there's something to learn in every situation, from every person, and in every family interaction. There are even pearls of wisdom from the elderly with advanced dementia when they have very little left of their original capacities. They still have life experiences, coping skills that they've used and that are still somewhat present. They have life values. They have things that they could share about themselves, even if it's just some things in their house, their photos. Even if they're no longer able to cope, there's still something about them that is of value that they could either give to you as a nurse or to society. We have an obligation to protect them, to give them a life of dignity, and to appreciate that they still have experience that they can tell us."*

Ora said it is important to look beyond physical appearances to uncover strengths: *"The elderly can be frightening because they look old. They may smell. Often they don't take care of themselves. They may be hard to understand because some lack of teeth. They my have sores and multiple health problems, but it is important to see them still as an individual who came from somewhere, who is now in transition, who eventually will need protection to go somewhere else at the end of their life. And in that respect you can see their strength. They still have something to contribute and they still have something to receive."*

Setting the stage for collaborative partnership

During the first phase of the Spiraling Process the nurse may also begin to create the condition of partnership by explaining her own role, asking the person about his expectations, and exploring ways that they may work together (Value 8: Collaborative Partnership; see Chapter 3). The nurse may invite the person to join her as a partner in care.

Consider how Nurse Cindy Dalton worked on developing a collaborative partnership with Nathan and Nancy, the couple dealing with Nathan's Parkinson's disease, who you met in Chapter 3. Cindy believes that the patient has to learn how to partner with the nurse.

"It is a slow process that takes work. It begins by addressing the couple's main concerns while at the same time always being open to everything else by asking, 'Is there anything else?' Developing the partnership also involves discussing my role. I usually say, 'As a nurse, this is what I do. I work with families around issues of living with Parkinson's disease. Your physician will also discuss medications. I can talk about how these medications affect your day-to-day life. I'm also here to talk about the impact the disease has on both of you. You're both living with Parkinson's.' I think when I frame the issue in terms of the couple, it is something new for them, to hear that they are both living with Parkinson's. When I ask the question 'What is that like for both of you?,' I ask [it] in the presence of both of them and

also when I talk to them one on one. When I spoke to Nancy, I asked her: 'Now that I'm speaking with you, what is it like living with someone with Parkinson's disease? I'd like to learn more about that.' She's the expert in her situation."

Note that Cindy works hard at creating the partnership. She recognizes that developing such a partnership is a learning process that takes time to develop (Value 7: Learning, Readiness, and Timing; see Chapter 3). She not only explained what she can offer as a nurse and undertakes this role by asking the questions and raising issues that she is willing to address. She is open minded and assumes the role of learner. She genuinely believes that patients are the experts and that they need to help her understand what it is like to be living with the disease.

An important prerequisite for collaborative partnership is establishing trust. Trust derives from many sources of information and develops as the nurse accompanies the person and family through a health crisis and during transitions within the trajectory of an illness (de Raeve, 2002; Jansson, Petersson, & Uden, 2001). Patients and families are more likely to trust a nurse when they feel that the nurse:

- Takes the time to get to know them
- Is truthful, open, and nonjudgmental
- Always behaves in a moral and ethical manner
- Shows respect for their opinions and supports their choices
- Likes them for who they are and not for what they represent or can offer
- Is open to understanding what they are going through, what their experiences have been
- Displays genuine interest and concern for their well being
- Provides them with a sense of safety and security by advocating for them

Nurses are more likely to want to create a partnership with the person and family when they:

- Genuinely like the patient
- See the patient as a special, unique human being and not as a diagnosis or an interesting case
- Believe they have the necessary knowledge and skills to meet the patient and family's needs and can competently address their concerns or deal with their problems
- Are accorded respect by the person and family and treated with respect by their colleagues and other team members
- Feel that their unique contribution to the patient's well-being is recognized, acknowledged, and appreciated
- Have a reasonable workload that allows them sufficient time to get to know the patient
- Within their workplace, are given the opportunities and resources to function to the full extent of their knowledge and competencies

Specific approaches for uncovering and discovering strengths

A crucial aspect of getting to know a person is getting to know her strengths. As I discussed in Chapter 4, strengths reside within each person and family. Nurses should keep in mind that although no person and family have strengths in all areas of their lives, all have strengths and resources in some areas. Some strengths are more apparent than others, and it is the nurse's responsibility to identify, notice, uncover, and discover them.

Nurses need to develop a large repertoire of clinical inquiry and critical thinking skills to uncover and discover each patient's and family's strengths (A fraction of this broad repertoire of skills has been described in Chapters 5, 6, 7, and 8). These skills include using their senses to identify salient information to develop a clinical grasp of the situation and honing their skills of engagement and social interaction by becoming skilled at initiating and sustaining dialogue, interviewing, active listening, and being fully present. The quality of information elicited from patients and their families relies on the quality of the rapport and trust that the nurse establishes. Nurses can also use scales, instruments, and measuring tools to help them assess patients and families for strengths. In the search for biological, physiological strengths, the use of diagnostic tools (e.g., analyzers, monitors, charts, scopes, imaging devices) can yield invaluable data not only for diagnosing disease but also for revealing what is functioning well physiologically (e.g., strengths). Nurses can use scales and questionnaires to uncover strengths in the other domains of functioning: psychological, emotional, cognitive, social, moral, spiritual, and so on.

Nurses can develop approaches to uncover and discover patients' and families' strengths. The list of approaches provided in the following sections is by no means exhaustive.

CAVEAT

With experience, each nurse will develop a favorite set of questions and specific approaches to assessing for strengths, including calling forth and uncovering strengths.

Approach 1: Nurses need to continuously look for strengths

Nurses practicing SBC need to always have strengths on their mind; in other words, they develop a strengths-based mindset in which they are always listening for, observing for, noticing, and being attuned to qualities (e.g., attitude, capabilities, resources, skills) that could be interpreted as a strength.

The nurse looks to uncover and discover strengths when having a conversation with the person, while providing nursing care, performing a physical assessment, giving a treatment, administering a test, and so forth. Nurses should keep the following three specific questions in mind when interacting with the person and family:

- What is working here? What is functioning? What does the person/family do best?
- What can I do to support what is working to help bring forth and maximize the person's innate or acquired health and healing mechanisms?
- How does the person use his strengths and resources to deal with the situation and facilitate his own healing?

When the question "Tell me what is working?" was asked of Jennifer, who had had a knee replacement several years earlier and was now suffering from arthritis in the knee that severely impaired her mobility, she realized that her upper quadriceps were still working. Once she identified this strength, she began planning an exercise program to strengthen her quad muscles to help compensate for her weakened knee. When this question was asked of John, who had suffered a stroke that paralyzed his larynx but left him able to mouth words, the nurse realized that John would benefit from speech-assisted machines to connect with his family and ease communication. She then arranged a referral to the speech therapy department in her hospital.

Nurse Cindy Dalton described what she thinks about and asks herself or the patient when assessing for specific strengths: *"It is very telling how a person has managed on their own without help from the nurse. I look to see whether they are using social support effectively. The strength is not about having help available but rather it is about knowing whether the person has asked for help: Who has helped them? What have they done to help themselves? For me, I look to see whether they are able to use support (a resource) in the right way and at the right time. I also look at their inner strengths. For example, how do they solve problems? How did they deal with difficulties on their own before they met me? Can they think through situations? Do they figure out what needs to be done first, second, and third, or do they allow themselves to be completely overwhelmed by the situation?"*

Cindy has developed an important habit of the mind in that she keeps a set of questions in mind when caring for her patients. Thus, it is important for nurses to develop a few key questions on which they will routinely call when assessing strengths either by asking the patient or reminding herself what to intentionally look for.

Approach 2: Nurses need to get in touch with their own first impressions

Looking for strengths may begin even before the nurse and patient have met. Nurses may begin to form impressions about a person from what they have heard, or over-heard, from other nurses and doctors during reports or rounds; what they have read in the patient's charts; and what they know from their own experience of working with patients who were dealing with a similar condition, disease, or challenge. Without the nurse even being aware that this is happening, these preconceived ideas may influence how he initially reacts to and interacts with the person.

It is during the first encounter that the nurse and person form an impression of each other (also see Chapter 8). They take in initial information—they notice body language, what is said, and how the other responds. Although this is just a small sample of information, it can have a lasting impact inasmuch as people make decisions about other people on the basis of small amounts of information (Demarais & White, 2005). The first impression may affect the degree to which a person believes she can trust the nurse; the extent to which she will reveal her vulnerabilities; entrust the nurse with her private thoughts, fears, and emotions; and share details of their lives and history. This first impression also has an effect on the nurse in that it sets the tone for later encounters. With some individuals and families, the nurse may feel an instant rapport. He may identify with the family, feel compassion and empathy for what they are going through, and respect and admire their spirit and the ways in which they are handling their adversities. Let's return to the Burns family. Recall that Jane's first impressions of Barbara, Scott's mother, were very favorable. Undoubtedly, those very favorable first impressions contributed to the instantaneous rapport they established and that persisted over time.

Some individuals and families are simply likable. When a nurse stops and reflects on what makes them likable, she often realizes that what makes them likable are those qualities that can be considered in terms of strengths. The "likability" factor also may play an important role in how the nurse and person interact and the type of relationship they develop. On the other hand, some individuals and families may have qualities that the nurse does not like, and these may negatively affect how she feels about the person and, subsequently, how the nurse relates to him. The challenge for nurses in these situations is to try to find qualities in the person that will facilitate a positive connection.

At the same time, it is important that nurses get in touch with their own thoughts and feelings by asking themselves some questions:

- What are my thoughts about this patient, this client, this family?
- How do I feel about them?
- How do they make me feel?
- What were my first impressions of them, and was I right?
- What do I like about them?
- What don't I like? Why?
- What feelings, fears, and insecurities does this person and his behaviors trigger in me?

When nurses get in touch with their own feelings and thoughts about the person and family, and when they are able to verbalize the qualities that they like and admire in the person and family, then they have begun to create a list or inventory of that person's and family's strengths. Conversely, when nurses are able to identify the qualities that make a negative impression on them, they are then in a better position to evaluate whether they are being fair, nonjudgmental, and open minded and to explore ways to turn these negative impressions around. Negative impressions have the potential of sabotaging the nurse–person/family relationship, making each partner inaccessible or even hostile to the other and thus preventing the establishment of any kind of helping relationship.

Approach 3: Sensing, recognizing, and noticing strengths

While the nurse explores the person and family's concerns, he also makes note of her strengths. As she tells the nurse about her concerns and recounts the events of her story, he makes note about how she has coped in the past with untoward events such as illness and health transitions, challenges, and tragedies. He also makes note of how she has reacted to her diagnosis and managed her treatment and the ways others have responded and supported her. The nurse listens for the positive aspects in a person's life—areas that are working and are a source of comfort.

Nurse Diane Lowden explains how to recognize strengths and what she listens for in conversations with patients: *"When I first meet the patient and their family, I often begin with the question: 'What happened to bring you here?' This question usually engages them very quickly because they want to tell their story and they want to have somebody who is going to listen. I listen attentively to know what to follow up on. As they talk, I learn about their context and, as I assess their situation, I'm able to identify their strengths. I listen for what's good in their situation and what's positive. I am always thinking of how can we use what's positive to help this patient and family deal with or cope with this particular situation."*

Nurses look for different strengths in different patients. They often listen to determine whether or not a patient is open, optimistic, and hopeful. They are attuned to whether a patient is willing to learn, how he has gone about getting help, what available resources and support he has, and how he has used them. They also observe how patients and families make decisions and how they can solve problems. All nurses should create a list of specific strengths to which they can routinely refer back. The following is a list of some things nurses might consider in identifying specific patient strengths:

- Are they **aware** of what is **working for them**, what they have **going for them** as individuals and as a family?
- Are they **open** to information? Do they **seek out** information? Do they **ask** questions? Are they willing to entertain and **consider different ways** of dealing with an issue?
- Are they willing to **listen** to another person's opinion?
- How do they **cope** with and handle bad news?
- How do they deal with and **manage stress**?
- How do they go about **solving problems** and **making decisions**?
- Do they **persevere** or easily give up?
- Have they kept their **sense of humor**?
- How do they maintain **hope**?
- How do they prevent themselves from becoming overwhelmed and **regulate** their emotions, thoughts, and behavior?
- How do they establish, maintain, and sustain **supportive relationships**?
- How do they use health care providers (nurses, doctors) to **navigate** the health care system to their advantage?
- Do they have adequate **social support**?
- Do they have adequate **financial resources**?

In other words, nurses must look for strengths in the three forces that govern development (Gottlieb & Gottlieb, 2007): how patients (a) regulate and self-regulate their physiological and emotional arousal states (regulation and self-regulation); (b) connect with and relate to others and develop attachments and social relationships (attachment and relationships); and (c) cope with and manage stress (coping).

The same process of identifying strengths should be used when the nurse performs a physical assessment. As she performs a systematic head-to-toe assessment, or focuses on assessing a specific system, she notes the function and integrity of each physiological system (e.g., neurological, cardiac, respiratory). In addition to noting any abnormalities, negative changes in body systems functioning, and potential indicators of vulnerabilities, she also looks for evidence of healthy functioning and positive signs of improvement. Finally, she notices how the patient compensates both physiologically and psychologically when one biological system or social aspect of his life has been challenged or compromised.

Nurse Althea McBean, who works on an intensive care unit, looks for any positive attributes in the person, the family, or the situation that is functioning properly: "*[Such as] those things like kidney and liver function, whether the patient is moving, whether the blood chemistry shows minimal damage or is fairly normal. I look for other things that indicate the degree to which their condition is under control. I also look to see whether the patient has a very supportive family."*

Another approach for uncovering strengths is to look where the person expends her energy. People expend energy to survive, to protect themselves from harm and injury, and to doing things that they value in areas that have meaning and purpose for them.

Nurses also should look for how patients regulate and conserve energy following an illness or health crisis. Healing requires energy. Body, mind, and soul are repaired during periods of rest and sleep, when energy is redirected toward repair processes. Nurses must assess how patients balance energy expenditure with energy conservation:

- Do they recognize when they are tired?
- Do they find the right balance between work and rest, or do they work to the point of exhaustion?
- How do they make use of resources to conserve energy and find the right balance for healing—repair, restore, and renew—in order to regain wholeness?

Approach 4: Becoming attuned to the person

In the course of getting to know individuals and families, nurses become attuned to their unique ways of responding. Attunement requires that the nurse listen for and discover the strengths that reside within each person. This is not always easy, in particular when the person is closed and secretive. Getting to know a patient requires a commitment from the nurse to go beyond the problem and see the person as a unique human being. With difficult patients, the nurse needs to be particularly attuned to behaviors and qualities that could be uncovered, recognized, and labeled as a strength.

Nurse Heather Hart, whom you met in Chapter 3 in her stories about nursing Ellen, also cared for Mrs. Andrews. Heather and the staff found Mrs. Andrews to be difficult because she was very demanding. As Heather described, *"There was just no meeting her needs. It didn't matter what we did for her; she was never satisfied. There seemed to be nothing positive about her. I just hated going into her room."*

> Energy is key to working with strengths. When nurses look at where the person expends or conserves their energy, they may very well find that they have uncovered and discovered a person's strengths.

Mrs. Andrews had a tumor that disfigured her face. One evening, while Heather was giving her basic care and settling her for the night, an incident occurred that changed Heather's feelings towards Mrs. Andrews: *"I went to flip her pillow to change it around and I said, 'Mrs. Andrews, I'm just going to lift your head'—and I wanted to say—"because I am going to flip your pillow"—but instead I said, 'I'm just going to change your head' instead of the word pillow. And out of her mouth came this: 'if only you could change my head.'"*

Heather continues: *"It wasn't that funny, just a stupid slip of the tongue and then it dawned on me, 'here's her light* [Heather's word for strength]. *She has a sense of humor!'"* Heather's ability to notice Mrs. Andrews's strengths altered her perception of this patient and affected how Heather subsequently interacted with her. After this incident, Heather reported that she found herself behaving a bit more *"cheeky,"* feeling more relaxed and less uptight when nursing Mrs. Andrews. Mrs. Andrews's sense of humor helped Heather to see the humanity in her. Heather came to understand that Mrs. Andrews's demanding behavior was her way of maintaining control as she coped with a very frightening disease and dire prognosis.

Approach 5: Asking people directly about their strengths

Another strategy to uncover strengths, in particular during those first encounters of getting to know the person, is to ask the person directly, "What are your strengths?" Some patients may have difficulty not only understanding the question but also knowing how to answer it because they may believe that they have few strengths or are not clear about what the nurse means by the word *strength*. For these people, the nurse may rephrase and ask the following types of questions (Feeley & Gottlieb, 2000):

- What do you think you do well?
- What is working (in your body, your relationships, other areas of your life)?
- What do others tell you that you do well?
- What makes your family unique or special?

The way the nurse phrases the question to get a person to identify his strengths is often affected by a number of considerations, such as how well the nurse knows the person, his condition, and even his age. Consider the line of questioning Lia Sanzone, a school nurse, takes when probing for strengths with teenagers: *"One that I often use with older adolescents, for example, is: 'If I were to ask your best friend to describe you, what would* [they say]*?' And if my client answered, 'They would say, I'm A, B, C, D' I then will use* [that] *description of themselves."*

Lia explained why she uses this indirect approach of questioning with adolescents: *"If I were to ask 'What do you think about yourself?' they may not know how to answer. But if I turn it around and say 'If I were to ask your best friend to describe you what do you think he would tell me about you?' [I get a response]. Getting the perception of their best friend allows them to think about it and it's easier for words to come out. And then I would use these descriptions of their strengths and follow up by asking 'Why do you think they'd describe you as this or that? What have you done that has led your best friend to describe you like this?' So that's one approach I like to use a lot with teenagers; it's sort of a noninvasive way, not asking directly. And I would use this approach with younger kids as well: 'If I were to ask your teacher, if I were to ask your mom, if I were to ask your sister.' So then you get different perceptions. You also get information about their different relationships with that individual."*

In focusing on problems and dealing with crisis and criticism, the person and family may feel so dejected and demoralized that they believe they are useless, inadequate, or incompetent. When patients feel this way about themselves, it is difficult for them to empower themselves to take charge of different aspects of their lives. They may feel they have no choices, have little hope, and thus become anxious and depressed. This is why it is critical that they have a nurse who can recognize areas of strengths. In these situations, the nurse can ask patients more specifically:

- Tell me about an event or an incidence that you felt you did well.
- When did you feel proud of yourself? Tell me about that.
- When was the last time you liked yourself? Tell me about that.

When the person has completed recounting the event or incident, the nurse should review the incident and probe more deeply to gain a better, more comprehensive view of the person. Consider the question Nurse Lucia Fabijan asks patients who are depressed: "*What are things that prevent you from getting depressed or that lift your spirits?*" One of her patients answered that her dog was her best antidepressant. People often have trouble answering these questions about their strengths. Lucia explained that "*Because families come in laden with problems, they are often sad, angry or totally frustrated. They haven't given it any thought for a long time.*" It is a line of questioning that few nurses use if their approach is *not* SBC.

In situations when a patient feels depressed and/or inadequate, the nurse may "plant" a question and ask the person to take the time to reflect on it. This line of questioning may help the person discover her own strengths. At a later encounter, the nurse can return to this early conversation and ask the person if she has had any new insights or made any new discoveries about herself. The nurse could then ask whether the person has ever used these strengths to deal with other situations.

Approach 6: Using a genogram and an ecomap to uncover and discover family strengths

Family genograms and ecomaps are becoming important tools in nursing assessments. They are designed to help the nurse gain insights into family life and family resources (Friedman, Bowden, & Jones, 2003; Wright & Leahey, 2005).

Genogram. A *genogram* is a visual representation of the members in a family and the nature and patterns of their relationship. It depicts relationships across generations (vertically) and within generations (horizontally; see Figure 9.3). It can be an effective tool to learn more about a family, its structure, and the relationships among family members.

In its simplest form, a genogram is used to depict family composition and provide factual information. As the nurse constructs the genogram with the person, he has an opportunity to learn more about the family. The person and family often recount important aspects about each family member, their relationships, as well as about the family unit as a whole.

By mapping out a person's family genogram with him, the nurse may identify specific individual and family strengths. Support is a major factor that affects a person's health and healing and is a crucial resource for patients and families alike (Neufeld & Harrison, 2010). Positive perceived support has been consistently linked to positive health outcomes, whereas negative relationships can cause great harm. Often, family members are unaware of the support they are receiving until they pause and consider the more subtle forms of help given by loved ones (Uchino, 2009).

As patients recount episodes of illness, the nurse can listen for the inner strengths they used to help them deal with the situation; who in the family was helpful; what roles and responsibilities different family members assumed; how other family members responded; how they did or did not support each other; and the degree to which they perceived that support was available and, if it was, whether it was needed as well as whether the help given was sufficient. The nurse can also listen about those individuals in the patient's network who disappointed or, worse, were sources of distress and pain.

Ecomap. Another commonly used tool in family nursing is the *ecomap*, a graphic depiction of a person's social network, including friendships, extended family,

FIGURE 9.3

An illustrative example of a genogram.

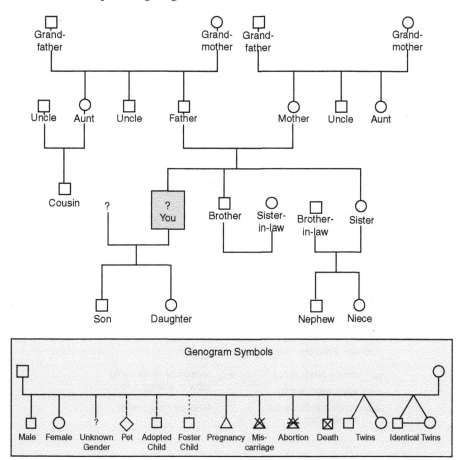

neighbors, work, health care system, religious group, community organizations (Friedman et al., 2003). Straight lines convey a strong, positive relationship; a single line when the relationship is weak, distanced, not close; slashed lines when the relationship is conflictual, difficult, stressful, broken, or dysfunctional; bi-directional arrows when the relationship is reciprocal; and dotted lines to convey erratic and tenuous relationships. The ecomap identifies the depth and extensiveness of a person's network and the availability of social support (see Figure 9.4)

An ecomap is an invaluable tool to help nurses assess patients' actual and potential support systems. In the course of completing an ecomap with a person, the nurse can use this opportunity to explore for strengths and resources.

For Nurse John Kayser, an essential strength that he looks for in people who are trying to deal with problems of addiction (e.g., smoking, drugs) is the nature of their social network, the quality of their relationships, and their ability to ask and look for help. John described what he listens for during an encounter: *"I have in the back of my mind, how do they use the people in their social network? When do they use them? Do they use them when they're feeling great? When they're down, do they call somebody? What type*

FIGURE 9.4

An ecomap.

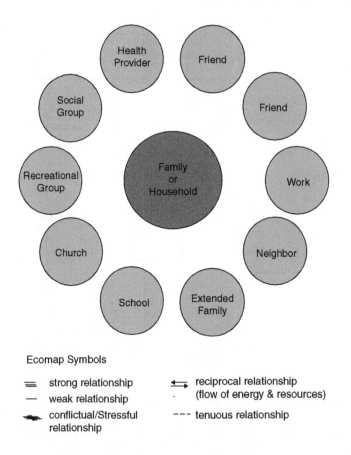

Ecomap Symbols

= strong relationship

— weak relationship

conflictual/Stressful relationship

reciprocal relationship (flow of energy & resources)

- - - tenuous relationship

of connections do they have and who gives them their needed support? Each person in that individual's life will deliver something different to my client."

Once John has a better understanding of the person's social network, he is able to use this information to help his clients understand what type of support they may need from their friends to help them deal with their addiction: *"When the client tells me that many of their friends try to help by telling them what to do . . . I then ask my clients whether they want their friends to give them a solution to their problems or do they need them just to listen or do they need them to take them out and just talk. It's really important to help people get in touch with what they need, and then to coach them on how to help their friends learn how to help them in ways that they want."*

An *ecomap* is an important tool that helps nurses identify the person's strengths and resources. It can also be used to help the person understand how to use her resources more effectively. An ecomap can be constructed with several members of a family to understand what resources are available them as a family unit.

Approach 7: Offering commendation

A commonly used approach to connect with patients, clients, and families is for the nurse to commend the person or family on a specific strength. The nurse can say,

"I notice that you handled that situation with great skill" or "I am impressed by how well you are able to get what you need." What is critical in these statements is that the nurse takes time to note how the person responds to positive feedback. She may attend and be attuned to how the person filters her commendation by observing for and listening to the person's responses to the commendation by noting the following:

- *Changes in the person's body language.* Is the person comfortable with the commendation, as reflected in an exchange of eye contact, smiles when being complimented, and acknowledgment of what the nurse said (e.g., by nodding), or does she feel uncomfortable, averting her gaze, turning away, and/or fidgeting?
- *Verbal response.* Does the person discount what the nurse says or minimize it by saying "It's nothing" or "Everybody does the same thing and even better?", or does she accept the nurse's commendation graciously by thanking the nurse?
- *Fit.* Is there a fit between the person's body language and how well she accepts or negates commendations?

Commending a person is a useful approach to find out how that person feels about himself and his abilities, that is, his strengths (Feeley & Gottlieb, 2000). When the person accepts praise, the nurse may take that as an indicator that this quality is indeed viewed by the person as one of his strengths. On the other hand, if the patient disagrees with the nurse or minimizes what the nurse has said, this may indicate that the nurse has to reevaluate her assessment of his feeling about strengths. Remember, a characteristic of strengths is a personal construction of both the person and nurse (see Chapter 4).

Approach 8. Asking about strengths that were developed through meeting past challenges

Recall in Chapter 4 that another one of the characteristics of a strength is that it can be transferred from one situation to another. Therefore, another approach to discovering strengths is by asking the person about past successes. The nurse can ask the following type of question:

- Tell me about another difficult situation that you have had to deal with in the past. What helped you get through that situation? Any personal qualities? Anyone in your family or network?
- Tell me how your body responded to...?

The nurse can also ask the person to recount past difficulties, challenges, and adversities. The nurse can ask the person and family, "How did you get through this difficulty?" In listening to the answer, the nurse notes how the person and family handled a difficult situation and the personal qualities and resources (financial, friends etc.) they called upon that enabled them to get through it. The nurse also notes how much the person profited from the prior experience: Did she change, grow, and transform, or did she remain the same, regress, or struggle to meet the challenges?

Table 9.2 summarizes the major approaches that the nurse can use during Phase 1 of the Spiraling Process as she explores the person's presenting concerns and problems and gets to know the person and family and, in so doing, uncovers and discovers their strengths.

TABLE 9.2

Summary of major approaches used in Phase 1: Exploring and getting to know the person—specifically to uncover and discover the person and family strengths

Approach	Sample Clinical Inquiry Skills
Approach 1: Nurses need to continuously look for strengths	• What does the person have going for him? • What is working here? What is not? • What and how does the person use her strengths and resources to deal with a situation and facilitate her own healing?
Approach 2: Nurses need to get in touch with their own first impressions	Nurses need to reflect and ask themselves: • What are my thoughts about this family? • How do I feel about them? • How do they make me feel? • What were my first impressions of them, and was I right? • What do I like about them? • What don't I like? Why? • What feelings, fears, and insecurities does this person and his behaviors trigger in me?
Approach 3: Sensing, recognizing, and noticing strengths	Listening attentively for: • What does the person do well? • What are her capabilities, talents, skills? • What does he have going for him? • What areas are working in her life or current health/medical situation? • What do I like about him? • In what areas does she expend energy? • How does he regulate or conserve energy for healing?
Approach 4: Becoming attuned to the person	Observing for, noticing, sensing, and getting to know regular patterns of responding, including observing changes in behavior
Approach 5: Asking the person directly about his strengths	• What do you think you do well? • What is working well in your life? • What do others tell you that you do well? • What makes your family unique or special? • Tell me about an event or an incident when you felt you did well. • When did you feel proud of yourself? Tell me about that. • When was the last time you liked yourself? Tell me about that. Noticing and listening to how the person reacts to nurse-identified strengths: • Body language • Verbal responses • Fit
Approach 6: Using a genogram and an ecomap to uncover and discover family strengths	• Who is a source of support? • On whom can you rely for emotional support and help? • How do they support you? • Are there people in your network who are a burden or whom you find are nonsupportive?
Approach 7: Offering commendation	• I notice that you handled that situation with great skill. • I am impressed on how well you able to get what you need.
Approach 8. Asking about strengths that were developed through meeting past challenges	• Tell me about another difficult situation that you have had to deal with in the past. What qualities helped you get through that situation?

Exploring and getting to know a person takes place in the course of nursing the person and during all phases of the Spiraling Process.

Phase 2: Zeroing In

In most clinical situations, the person and family are often dealing with several problems happening at the same time, that may or may not be related but that affect and are affected by each other. Many of these problems may feel overwhelming to the person and family. As nurses listen to a patient's story, they may feel overwhelmed themselves by the person's suffering and the complexity of the issues. However, there comes a point in the assessment when the best thing the nurse can do is to step back in order to gain some perspective and try to understand how the pieces relate to make up the whole—the whole in this case can be the person's life and their different lifeworlds.

Once both the nurse and patient/client/family have a clearer understanding of the medical and coping concerns, all parties need to consider how best to deal with them. The second phase of the Spiraling Process is Zeroing In. It is characterized by efforts to identify specific, workable goals and then prioritize them (Gottlieb et al., 2006). This phase has two major features: (a) clarifying with the person what she would like to see happen and (b) deciding together (i.e., both nurse and patient or anyone who is involved) which of the goals they mentioned in Phase 1 are most important and most achievable. Thus, the person and nurse need to prioritize goals and explore different avenues to deal with specific issues (see Figure 9.5).

In the case of life-threatening situations, where there are several rapid health transitions, such as during a crisis, when the patient is in critical condition, or where safety is at stake, the goals are obvious and the priorities more easily determined. There may be little time for negotiation, and often the health care team needs to take the lead. That is not to say that patients and families have no voice; there are always decisions and choices to be made. Often, the nurse needs to have some grasp of the situation, assess what is working and what is not, and use this information to set priorities and take action (Benner et al., 2010). For example, when a patient is bleeding, is having difficulty breathing, or is in cardiac distress, the priorities are self-evident. The health care team needs to take charge and do what they can to ensure the patient's survival and safety.

Clarifying goals requires that both the person and the nurse communicate with each other what they hope to accomplish. Once they are clear as to what their hopes and goals are, then they can begin to think about what strengths the person will need to have to accomplish them. Although the nurse may create the conditions to help the person engage in self-healing, it is the person herself who ultimately does the healing work.

When there are multiple problems and the patient's health issues are complex, the person may have many things that are important to him. The issue becomes how to determine where to focus attention. The decision is often helped by an understanding

FIGURE 9.5

Phase 2 of the Spiraling Process: Zeroing Ins.

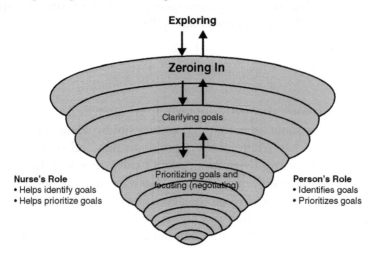

Source: Reprinted with permission from Gottlieb, & Feeley with Dalton (2006).

of what is most important to the person. The nurse may help a person to deal with multiple problems by asking:

- What are you most concerned about?
- What are your biggest fears?

These are the questions that Nurse Christina Clausen asked Mrs. Coreen Kennedy, who had delivered a preterm infant at twenty-four weeks by caesarian section because a month earlier she had been diagnosed with advanced rectal cancer. You may recall from Chapter 1 that the physicians had waited for the fetus to be viable before delivering the infant by Caesarian-Section and start treating Coreen. Coreen had a lot to deal with and much to fear: whether her baby would live, whether she herself would live, and what would happen to her 18-month-old son at home if she were to die. By asking the two questions listed above, Christina gained some insights into this mother's fears. Coreen's most immediate concern was the survival of her newborn daughter.

As Christina describes: *"She always focused on the baby. She never focused on her own health. At the time I asked myself, 'Do I probe the issue of her cancer further or do I just wait, step back and see what's happening?' I decided to step back and focus on the baby. Mrs. Kennedy later told me this was the right approach for her. As she said, 'It was not about my own life, it was about the baby's. I could potentially lose my life, but I had to focus on the baby. That's what was going to get me through.'"*

Christina, by asking the right question and listening to Mrs. Kennedy describe what was important to her and her husband, and understanding their priorities. was able to *zero in* on their main concern.

When a person has several goals, she and the nurse have to decide where to put their energy—what to work on. The following are some sample questions to assess for goals:

- What areas would you like to change?

- What would you like to see happen?
- How can we work with and support what is working, what you do best?

The nurse and person also need to consider the person's strengths that may be required to meet a goal. The following are some sample questions to assess for strengths in light of the person's goals:

- What do you think you need to help you accomplish X?
- What new skills, capabilities, types of information, resources do you think you will need?
- Who can help you make this happen?
- What can I do to make this happen?

In the *Zeroing In* phase of the Spiraling Process, the nurse needs to consider the person's readiness to change (Value 7: Learning, Readiness, and Timing; see Chapter 3). *Readiness* is the degree to which a person wants to change and is prepared to take action. A person may want to get better, try a new treatment, entertain a new way of doing things, alter his lifestyle (e.g., stop smoking, lose weight, change eating patterns, follow safe sex practices), but something or somebody is preventing him from doing so. Many times, the person may want to change but is not ready to change because the timing is not right, the support systems he requires are not in place, the services he needs are not available or are inaccessible, and so forth. When nurses assess a person's readiness, they need to consider the factors associated with readiness, namely, triggers, desire for change, intent to take action, and the costs and benefits associated with change or maintaining the status quo (Dalton & Gottlieb, 2003; Rollnick, Miller, & Butler, 2007).

Nurses also need to have some understanding of what it takes to change and what is involved in change, such as the role that ambivalence plays (i.e., wanting something, but not quite sure how much), belief or lack of a belief in one's ability to bring about the desired outcomes, and the importance of tailoring an intervention that is consistent and congruent with the person's goals. These are some of the characteristics of a well-known, scientifically tested method of counseling known as Motivational Interviewing, which used in the treatment of lifestyle problems and addictions (Miller & Rollnick, 2002; Rollnick et al., 2007; Rubak, Sandbaek, Lauritzen, & Christensen, 2005).

Triggers are indicators of the need to change course. A person may decide to lose weight after she has suffered a heart attack, or a person may decide to stop smoking after learning of a friend's lung cancer. The type of question the nurse could ask is "What happened to make you think differently about the situation?"

Desire for change and intent to take action. A person may want to change. She may talk about what she plans to do in the future or what she expects to change. However, just wishing, hoping, or wanting something to happen is insufficient. The patient must also have a plan to make things happen. The person may want to stop smoking and may even have investigated various smoking cessation programs. She may show signs of readiness, but until she has a concrete plan with specific actions that she has begun to implement she is still in a precontemplative phase of thinking about change and are in a low to moderate state of readiness.

Weighing the costs and benefits. One way of helping a person get ready to change is helping him see that the benefits of change far outweigh the costs of maintaining the status quo or not changing (Miller & Rollnick, 2002). There are many ways a nurse can help a person understand his situation and what needs to be done. These include an appreciation of what strengths are needed to bring about change and an assessment of the strengths that the person already has. If the nurse and person feel that bringing about change requires a specific set of strengths (e.g., attitude, knowledge, skills) and that the person is lacking in any of these, then the nurse and person may use their time together to work on developing strengths. The way the nurse works to develop strengths is described in Chapter 10.

Nurse Jane Chamber-Evans spoke with admiration of the Burns family's ability to modify their goals, create a new focus, and change direction with each setback that befell Scott. To briefly recap: Scott, at age seventeen, had spent six months in hospital recovering from encephalitis and the many complications secondary to this infection, only to suffer a stroke just as he was about to be discharged from the rehabilitation center to home. At one point, Scott was on dialysis after having suffered massive organ failure. The stroke also affected his optic lobe, leaving Scott visually impaired. Scott's parents found themselves continuously shifting priorities and revising their expectations of what Scott could do.

As Jane explained, *"They never said 'We want him to go right back to where he was and he's going to start there and he's going to be exactly who we thought he would be before.' Instead, they were able to make some adjustments that I found quite fascinating—because not all parents are able to do that. In fact, some parents will say, even in the face of a catastrophic head injury, 'I want my son now to be like he was before his illness. I can't accept anything less.' The Burns family's ability to readjust their goals was in part what allowed them to go on. They adjusted their expectations of how they saw their son. But with each new setback and complication they asked me, 'Where do you think our son is going to be? Can he be the best that he is right now?'"*

Mr. and Mrs. Burns' ability to change, accept the new realities of their son's situation, adjust their expectations accordingly, and set new goals are some of the strengths that Jane discovered in her work with them.

Once the nurse and person are clear as to what they want to achieve together, what strengths are needed, whether or not the person has the necessary strengths and is ready for change, they can begin Phase 3 of the Spiraling Process, *Working Out*.

Phase 3: Working Out

Once goals have been identified and clearly articulated, the nurse and person begin the process of trying out different approaches to deal with the problem. *Working Out*, although one of four separate phases in the Spiraling Process, often goes hand-in-hand with figuring out the concerns on which to work. An important aspect of Zeroing In (Phase 2) is thinking about and entertaining different ways of working on an issue. Phase 3 involves putting the plan into action—working out and trying out (see Figure 9.6). Part of the process of "working out" is matching the challenge to be met and the solution being considered with the person's strengths and his available resources. When there is a good fit, the likelihood of success increases. Remember, this is a process and, like all processes, it unfolds over time. It requires regular action on both the patient's and nurse's part until solutions have been found. This process involves rethinking and then shifting direction in light of any new information.

During Phase 3, the person may be required to develop a new capability, learn a new set of skills, or acquire more information. Consider an 18-year-old adolescent girl who has just been diagnosed with Type I diabetes. Her goal may be to live life as usual while incorporating diabetes as just another aspect of herself to be managed, not to be consumed with or controlled by. Doing this requires that she learn about diabetes, including learning about the biology of diabetes and the role in metabolism the pancreas plays in regard to insulin and insulin production. She must learn about the role of nutrition, exercise, and stress; the way they affect insulin levels; and the long-term impact on her health and how to minimize risk. Then she must increase her awareness of *her* own body and the functioning of how *her* pancreas responds to changes in her level of activity, change of diet, and stress. She needs to understand how having diabetes will necessitate changing her lifestyle and adopting new health behaviors. She also has to learn new skills, including how to test and monitor her blood sugar levels, how to recognize signs of hypo- or hyperglycemia, how to regulate insulin levels, and how to self-inject insulin. She may be aware of the long-term effects of diabetes on causing neurological damage, but is not ready to take preventative actions just yet, such as wearing more sensible shoes. She also must increase her awareness of how diabetes affects how she now sees herself (i.e., her identity)—a diabetic person or a person with diabetes. Finally, she needs to understand the impact of her diagnosis on her family and which members seem to be most affected. These different pieces of information need to be integrated. However, it will take her and her family many years to be able to fully appreciate the impact that her diagnosis of diabetes has had on her and on the family. The diagnosis of diabetes will prove to be a turning point in her life, defining her in ways she cannot as yet imagine. In this phase of the process, this young woman and nurse will begin this life-long process of learning and acquiring new skills.

FIGURE 9.6

Phase 3 of the Spiraling Process: Working Out.

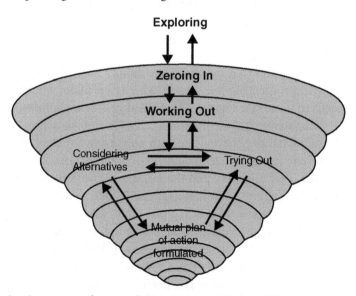

Source: Reprinted with permission from Gottlieb, & Feeley with Dalton (2006).

Recall from Chapter 4 is that one of the characteristics of a strength is that strengths can be learned. Every new situation is an opportunity to further perfect and hone an existing strength or develop new ones.

Let's return to Scott and his need to learn new skills as he recovered from the aftermath of encephalitis and a stroke. Jane described Scott's long journey of rehabilitation and recovery, which he faced with perseverance, determination, humor, and an endearing personality (these are some of Scott's strengths) that helped in working toward his goal of regaining as much function as possible: *"Scott was incredibly frustrated, but he had the same inner strength that his parents had. He just never gave up. He never took 'no' for an answer. He was the biggest joker that you have ever seen and he, of course, just drew the nurses and the orderlies to him like bees to honey. He was always so pleasant, always had a smile, and was always joking. The team was just so totally for him. They created programs for him and helped him with his physiotherapy. He worked on his physiotherapy like a dog. He was so determined."*

Jane described the partnership that developed between Scott and the nurses and other team members: *"When Scott had the stroke, he was devastated. He became very depressed. He was completely devastated because he couldn't see who he was going to be. It was obvious that he had lost his eyesight, one side was quite limited, and the physicians told him that they weren't sure that what he had lost was going to come back. Before his stroke the message had been, 'If you work hard enough we can help you and you're going to regain everything.' That was the incentive to keep going. There were a couple of orderlies on the floor and several nurses who worked nonstop with him. They gave him the strength. They allowed him to be fearful but never wallow in saying that there's nothing good in life. They would work really hard to get him out of his mood and would fight with him until he would do part of it himself. Their message was 'You are a person, and we're not going to let go of you. You're going to keep going.'"*

The loving, caring, supportive, and determined environment that all members of the health care team provided bolstered Scott and his family and provided them with the needed scaffolding until they were strong enough to take over again.

Phase 4: Reviewing

The Spiraling Process requires that the nurse and family set aside time to take stock of where things are, what progress has been made, what is left to do, what has been learned and what still needs to done (see Figure 9.7). Skilled nurses are continuously reflecting on what they are doing while they are nursing (i.e., reflection-in-action), (Benner et al., 2011) or reflecting on what they have done with an eye toward changing their practice or learning from their practice (i.e., reflection-on-action) (Schon, 1987).

The review can be brief, such as when the nurse asks the person during a follow-up visit or telephone call, "Tell me what has happened since we last met. How did your daughter take her medication? Did you try out what we had discussed?" It can also be a lengthier, more involved process such as that which happens when the nurse and person set aside a time to review what has transpired during their weeks of working together. In preparing the person for such a review, the nurse may say: "At our next visit, let's set aside time to review what has been happening. In the meantime, think about where you came from, what you wanted, what you have done, and where you

FIGURE 9.7

Phase 4 of the Spiraling Process: Reviewing.

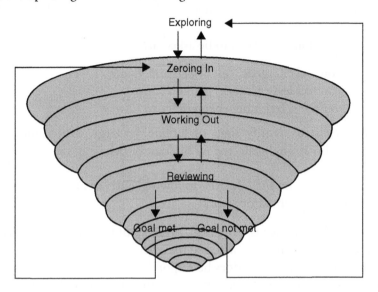

Source: Reprinted with permission from Gottlieb, & Feeley with Dalton (2006).

see yourself going and I will do the same. At our next appointment, we can share our ideas with each other."

Phase 4, Reviewing, affords both nurse and patient/client/family an opportunity to uncover and discover new strengths of which either or both of them had been unaware of or that had gone unnoticed. This is an important time for the nurse to ask the person about his strengths:

- What new things about yourself or others surprised you?
- Did you discover any new capabilities or talents that you weren't aware that you had?
- What new skills have you developed? What have you learned about yourself? About others? About developing new capacities and competencies? How do you think you may use these newly discovered strengths in the future?

During the *Reviewing* phase of the Spiraling Process the nurse should also be assessing the person's *strength resource capacity* (see Chapter 4 for a description of this characteristic of a strength). An important indicator of strength resource capacity is the person's energy level. The nurse needs to observe for any signs of waning energy. Recall that a strength can be depleted if overused or used inappropriately; conversely, some strengths can be replenished by taking time out or time off.

Many goals require some increased expenditure of energy. Energy, a finite capacity, also may be in short supply during times of illness. The innate healing mechanisms themselves are often directed to conserving or restoring energy. This explains why patients sleep a lot during the recovery phase of an illness or after trauma. Energy is required to change direction or alter a habit (e.g., to stop smoking). The nurse appreciates that patients' energy is affected by their mood states and their mood states can influence their energy levels. Thus, when people are happy, busy, and engaged they have more energy than when they are depressed, anxious, and find themselves in the midst of a crisis.

The critical questions that need to be asked are:

- When do you feel energetic, full of pep and vigor?
- When do you feel less energetic?
- What do you do to feel more energetic?

The nurse needs to identify signs of fatigue, lethargy, depression, and anxiety. Energy levels are also strongly affected by biological, personal, family, and situational factors.

Biological factors can include the following and are predominantly assessed through blood tests and laboratory work:

- Is the person's immune response (e.g., presence of fever, elevated white blood cell count) or hemoglobin level affecting his level of energy?
- Is the person in pain? How does he respond when in pain and pain free?
- Is the person feeling well, depressed, or anxious? How does his mental state affect his level of energy?
- What is the person's level of fatigue?
- How is the nature and quality of his sleep?
- What techniques or strategies does the person use to calm himself?
- How does the person self-regulate, that is, find the best balance between activity and rest? Does the person recognize tired cues and pay attention to waning energy before he "falls off the cliff"?
- What is else is going on in the person's life that may be depleting his energy levels?

After the nurse assesses the person's energy status, the nurse needs to take on the role of "pacer" (Gottlieb, 1982). In this role, he needs to help patients learn how to better self-regulate by helping recognize when they need time out. Nurses also can promote rest and help patients better self-regulate by providing comfort measures, such as ensuring that the bed sheets are clean and wrinkle free, or giving a back rub. Comfort measures are required to replenish energy, which is an invaluable strength.

Nurse Jane Chamber-Evans described the importance of recognizing when a person's energy is depleted and finding ways to help them let go. Barbara Burns was the engine that helped her family keep going, yet even Barbara had her limits.

As Jane explained, *"She needed to have some way to take back control of being a mother, so that she could be in charge of what was happening to her son. Her philosophy was that 'There is no stone too big that can't be overturned.' So it didn't matter what barriers came in front of her, she rallied the family. There were times she would let herself feel defeated. During these times, she would ask to see me. I knew that was the day that she needed to sit behind the door where no one but me could see her and she could sob her eyes out. Then she would pull herself back together, use my mirror to 'put her face back on,' and go back to Scott. She would say, 'I have to be Scott's strength. He can't be his own strength; I have to be his strength.'"*

Jane provided her with the space to "let go," to release some of the pent-up emotion.

Jane also recognized that Barbara's goal was to give her son strength through the way she behaved. For Barbara to be Scott's strength, she needed time for herself, time to recharge her own batteries, so to speak. She needed to leave her son's bedside even just for a few hours: *"I talked to her about spending a bit more time on herself. We needed to talk about what that might look like, because she never wanted her son to be alone. We did some trial runs when she left for a few hours because I recognized that she was going to be incredibly anxious to leave him. The first day, she called three times and then the next time she went she didn't call at all. It was a trial and it allowed her the chance to see that Scott was going to be safe."*

Key Summary Points

- The nurse needs to assess for strengths by noticing existing strengths and identifying strengths that could be developed.
- Assessing for strengths is about discovering the person's uniqueness. It is in working with the person's strengths that one finds the key to helping a person achieve her goals.
- Assessing for strengths does not exist in a vacuum but is part of the larger process of getting to know the person.
- Assessing for strengths involves the highest form of caring for another person. Caring is about providing and creating the conditions that enable a person to heal—to recover, grow, and transform.
- SBC is best accomplished when the nurse–patient/client/family relationship is collaborative. SBC and a collaborative partnership are required if the person is to become empowered.
- Uncovering and discovering strengths takes place during four phases of the Spiraling Process: Exploring and Getting to Know (Phase 1), Zeroing In (Phase 2), Working Out (Phase 3), and Reviewing (Phase 4).
- All four phases can occur during the same encounter.
- There are eight major approaches to discovering and uncovering strengths included as part of Phase 1 of the Spiraling Model.
- Every interaction and encounter provides an opportunity to learn more about a person and family's existing strengths, what is working, to discover new ones, and identify strengths that need to be developed to achieve goals.
- The nurse needs to develop a broad repertoire of clinical inquiry, critical inquiry, and assessment skills to uncover and discover the person and family strengths.
- The nurse needs to consider how to work with strengths to support the person's efforts of healing.

Approaches for Working With Strengths

LEARNING OBJECTIVES

After reading this chapter, you should be able to:

- Have a greater appreciation of the conditions and mindset needed to work with strengths
- Create the environmental conditions necessary to work with strengths
- Describe approaches to mobilize and capitalize on existing strengths
- Describe approaches to develop strengths by turning potentials and deficits into strengths

> I've learned that people will forget what you said, people will forget what you did, but people will never forget how you made them feel.
>
> —Maya Angelou

In this quote, famed American author and poet Maya Angelou captured the power that one person's way of relating can have on another. In today's health care climate, where the valuing is on doing and sophisticated technology, there is a tendency to downplay, undervalue, and discount the importance and power of relational interventions. Strengths–Base Care (SBC) restores the nurse–patient relationship to its central place in health promotion and the healing process. The way a nurse interacts with people can be just as, if not more, powerful and long lasting than other forms of intervention. Nurses can make patients feel good and help them become empowered to take charge of their lives and their health care decisions. Nurses can also have the opposite effect and, with some of their actions, make patients feel demoralized. SBC is about making people feel good about themselves and the choices they make, giving them hope, energizing them to take charge, to create change, and have the gumption and courage to explore possibilities in their quest for self-knowledge about themselves and the meaning of life and living.

Many nurses may subscribe to SBC and believe that working with the person's and family's strengths is an important approach. However, they may feel unsure how to work with strengths. In the course of nursing the person, the nurse may have identified the person and family's strengths—but now what? Many nurses may feel more confident in assessing strengths but less confident in how to use strengths to deal with problems.

To work with patients' and families' strengths, nurses need to develop a broad repertoire of approaches and techniques to add to her toolbox. They must know how to mobilize and capitalize on existing strengths, how to develop new strengths, and how to use strengths to counterbalance the effects of deficits and weaknesses. These approaches derive from knowledge of strengths and their characteristics. You may want to review the characteristics of strengths described in Chapter 4 and summarized in Table 4.5. It is through understanding the characteristics of strengths and then working with them that nurses can alter a patient's responses to disease, illness, and challenges; prevent complications; restore that which has been compromised at a physical, psychological, and emotional level; and support the person's innate healing mechanism. In so doing, a nurse is fulfilling the role envisioned by Florence Nightingale (1860) "to put the patient in the best condition for nature to act upon him" (p. 133).

WHAT ARE STRENGTHS?

Recall from Chapter 4 that strengths are a person or family's special and unique qualities and resources that define their personhood. Strengths are needed to meet goals, develop health, meet illness challenges, facilitate and promote healing by restoring wholeness, and assist the person to get the most out of living. Strengths are a person's capabilities, and they come in many forms, including assets, capacities, competencies, resources, skills, talents, and gifts. These can be biological, emotional, psychological, or social in origin and nature. There are internal strengths (e.g., motivation, courage, resilience) that reside within the individual, as well as external strengths, in the form of resources (e.g., finances, connections, support, religion, spirituality). The paradox is that because strengths come in many forms and are expressed in so many different ways, they may be readily apparent in some people and less apparent in others. Moreover, they may be more discernable to the person and the nurse at certain times and in certain situations. The latter is often the case when the issues with which a person is dealing are complex, the problems or deficits are many and quite serious, and when dysfunction and pathology are pervasive. In these situations, the problems may often overwhelm both the person and the nurse in ways that prevent both of them from seeing the person as well as his strengths. Nurses too often become so focused on problems and trying to "fix" them that they may be blinded to those things that are working and helping to maintain the integrity of the person. This is something akin to weeds in a garden. Most of the time, weeds are hardly noticeable. When weeds become numerous and uncontrollable they often take over the garden, strangling, and obscuring from view the healthy plants. It is hardly surprising that a person can see only the weeds and often is blinded to the plants and flowers. However, if there are few weeds, and the weeds are under control, although still present, a person can focus on the plants and flowers. In fact, it will be the flowers, not the weeds that he often first notices. In all patients, but in particularly patients who are dealing with multiple and complex problems and in which deficits are pronounced, it may be all the more important for nurses to look for strengths and focus on them to restore the person to health and promote his recovery. Thus, nursing's approach to care is threefold: (a) support that which is working by reinforcing and making stronger existing strengths; (b) prevent further deterioration or weakening; and (c) contain, control, and manage deficits by working with the person's and family's strengths.

Nurses should remember that strengths are the person's "light"—those gifts that provide a window into the human spirit and define her humanity. Strengths are key to health because they are the building blocks of creating wholeness. Strengths become the fuel that enables a person to take charge, find solutions to her problems, deal with hardships, overcome vulnerabilities, and find meaning in life. In short, they are central to the healing process. Recall that healing is about restoring wholeness or finding a new wholeness. Working with strengths facilitates this process.

Nurses are always dealing with people strengths regardless of whether they label the quality or person's behavior as such. When a nurse teaches a person a new skill, she is developing a person's strength. When she decides, after assessing the situation, that the person is ready to discuss a sensitive matter or change treatment, she is capitalizing on

> Nurses are always dealing with people strengths whether or not they label the quality or person's behavior as such.

and mobilizing the person's openness (a strength) and willingness to try new treatment (two strengths: flexibility and motivation). When nurses become aware of strengths, they can work with them in a more intentional and purposeful way.

SOURCES OF STRENGTHS

A nurse needs to look for patient/client/family/community strengths to decide which capabilities are needed to deal with a particular problem or concern. He then decides which strengths are available and can be mobilized and which strengths need to be developed. Nurses need to consider three sources of strengths: (a) existing strengths and resources, (b) potential strengths, and (c) deficits that can be turned into strengths

Existing strengths are those capabilities and resources that are an integral part of the person and his environment. These strengths are readily available and easily mobilized to meet the person's needs and to help him cope with both small and large challenges. Although these strengths may be affected by changing circumstances, they are well developed and an integral part of the person; in fact, they define the person. We often talk of people in terms of their qualities—warm, caring, compassionate—or in terms of their weaknesses: closed, inflexible, judgmental. Nurses need to know how to recognize these strengths and how to help the person capitalize on them for maximum effect.

Consider Nurse Cheryl Armistead and her understanding of strengths. Cheryl works as a community nurse, and she looks for certain qualities when she is nursing families who are dealing with complex health needs. For Cheryl, hope and confidence are two essential strengths that she looks for.

Recall Mrs. Bhutto in Chapter 4 who had fled her native country and whose infant was suffering from failure to thrive as a result of a brain injury, Cheryl described the importance of hope and confidence: *"The journey with this family was very long. The child kept requiring more complex interventions to deal with her physical problems, and*

Mrs. Bhutto, through all the ups and downs, learned the skills she had to learn, including how to manage equipment. She faced the many surgeries that her daughter required with dignity. Despite all that was happening to her, she maintained an aura—this air of hope and confidence. Inner confidence is something that I always look for, because if somebody appears confident in front me, that speaks to a certain capacity. If they are confident, then they are going to move forward and they are going to learn new skills."

Potentials are the second type of strengths. Recall from Chapter 4 that the word *potential* refers to something that is possible, as opposed to something that is already developed. Potentials are precursors to strengths in that they do not as yet function as a strength but can be developed into a strength (Feeley & Gottlieb, 2000). At the appropriate time, and under the right circumstances and conditions, potentials can become strengths. Potentials often come in the form of a capacity. It may be said of a person that she has the *capacity* to be a leader or the *capacity* to learn. This means that the person possesses those raw materials that, when worked with, can be turned into a strength. Nurses need to learn how to recognize potentials and, once they have recognized them, know how to develop them into strengths.

The third category of strengths include *deficits that can be turned into strengths*. The challenge for nursing is to ask whether a weakness or deficit can become a strength and, if the answer is "yes," to ask how this can be done. Recall from Chapter 4 that a characteristic of a strength is that it is defined by its context or environment. In one circumstance a behavior can be a deficit, but when the context or circumstance changes or the environment is altered, the same behavior often is a strength. For example, Maggie, age ninety, has been living alone since her husband's death ten years ago. She prides herself on her independence and self-sufficiency. Three years ago, she noticed that her eyesight had deteriorated (i.e., a change in circumstance), and she was subsequently diagnosed with macular degeneration. In addition, her arthritic knees made it increasingly more difficult to walk and shop for herself. Her children, who live out of town, believe Maggie should no longer be living on her own; however, she refuses assistance (a deficit or weakness) because she likes to think of herself as independent. She believes she is managing fine even though all indicators point to the fact that she is not. She insists on living on her own (stubbornness) and in so doing puts herself at risk for falls, malnutrition, and so forth. Her stubbornness, at times her strength, has now become her liability. Changing Maggie's mindset and then her environment can revert this quality back to a strength.

CREATING ENVIRONMENTS FOR STRENGTHS-BASED CARE

An essential aspect of working with strengths is for nurses to be aware of the environments they create. Recall from Chapter 3 that the person and environment are integral (Value 6: The Person and Environment Are Integral). Nurses are an integral part of their patients/clients' environment. The nurse can create and modify a patient's environment by altering the physical environment and interacting with the patient/client/family in health-promoting ways.

SBC is based on a trusting relationship between the person and nurse. Both partners need to bring their own strengths to the relationship. For example, the nurse must be able to create the conditions that foster collaborative partnership

(Value 8: Collaborative Partnership) by sharing power and being open, nonjudgmental, and accepting (Gottlieb et al., 2006). They must also know how to create conditions that preserve patients' dignity and respect their right to self-determination (Value 5: Self-Determination). They must also know how to create conditions that select for health behaviors and promote healing (Value 1: Health and Healing). Because every experience involves learning, nurses have to create environments that are conducive to learning (Value 7: Learning, Readiness, and Timing). The primary ways nurses create such environments is by the way they interact with the person, the decisions they make, and the actions they take. (For a fuller discussion of the values that guide SBC, see Chapter 3, and for a fuller discussion of essential strengths that nurses need to have to practice SBC, see Chapter 5.)

Environments range from toxic, such as when the person and family's health and lives are put at risk, to benign, such as when nurses meet the person's basic safety requirements and adhere to the rules of medicine and nursing to "do no harm" to environments that are health promoting and facilitate healing. Health-promoting and healing environments are supportive, safe, and facilitative. SBC requires that the nurse create such environments.

Creating Supportive, Safe Environments

SBC requires that the nurse create a supportive, safe environment for patients so that they will feel empowered and well enough to take control over decisions affecting their medical care and lifestyle. Supportive environments select for those qualities that bring out the best in a person. They maximize people's potential and capitalize on their strengths. People feel secure in environments that accept them for whom they are and in which they are able to explore issues that are of concern to them. This happens when patients and families:

> Supportive environments maximize the person's potential and capitalize on their strengths. People feel secure in environments that accept them for whom they are and where they are able to explore issues that are of concern to them.

- Trust the nurse
- Can count on the nurse to be available in time of need and stress
- Are confident in the nurse's competency, that is, they know that the nurse has the knowledge and skills to meet their needs, keep them safe, protect them from harm, and promptly detect when something is amiss
- Believe the nurse knows them as a person—for their individuality and uniqueness and does not objectify or reduce them to a symptom or a diagnosis
- Know the nurse is engaged; is not distant, detached and/or disengaged
- Feel that the nurse is authentically present and listens attentively
- Know that the nurse will advocate for them, represent their interest, and will be their voice in the way they want to be heard

In negative, nonsupportive, and uncaring environments people become defensive. An uncaring environment is one in which the nurse shows no genuine interest in the person. Uncaring acts include ignoring the person's needs, being disrespectful, and discounting their opinions. Often, nurses who engage in such behaviors lack the requisite knowledge and skills to assess and carry out their professional responsibilities (Eliasson, Kainz, & von Post, 2008). In these environments, patients tend to be hostile, on edge, and at times violent. Patients feel vulnerable, threatened, under attack, and unsafe. In response, patients and families may become hypervigilant, relying on family and friends to watch over them or to provide basic care. These patients trust nobody in the system to protect and safeguard them and often fear for their own safety. The patient's and family's energy is directed toward self-preservation, protection, and even survival rather than toward health and healing.

Creating a Facilitative Environment

At the heart of the person-centered model of care is valuing a person's ability to be involved in making choices that are in accordance with his values and goals. Working with a person's strengths requires that the nurse create an environment that is growth promoting by supporting the person as he strives to make the most of his potentials and develop a repertoire of coping skills to manage difficulties and problems. The nurse's role is to facilitate and not to take over, criticize, blame, or tell the person what to do or how to do it (Hubble & Miller, 2004). Facilitative environments give the person time and space to explore issues. Such environments work best when the person's strengths are recognized. It is this recognition of feeling of being supported that frees the person to explore new avenues and work with the nurse to recognize opportunities, explore possibilities, and find solutions to his problems (McAllister, 2003).

Consider the work of Nurse Sonia Castiglione with Mrs. Desjardins, a mother of four. Mrs. Desjardins was overwhelmed by the demands of her family. In addition to her role of wife and mother, she was home-schooling Sammy, her middle child. Sammy had been diagnosed with attention-deficit disorder. This family had tried many treatments to deal with Sammy's unpredictable outbursts. Mrs. Desjardins was having difficulty coping with the many stressors in her life and had given up on the health care team. Somehow Sonia, after keeping in touch with Mrs. Desjardins regularly, was able to form a relationship with her and hear this mother's needs, where other health team members had not.

Sonia explained: *"I don't think Mrs. Desjardins has a problem saying what she means. I think it is more on how we as health care professionals pick up on what she is saying. I give her the space and time to say what she needs to say. I've seen how other health care professionals interact with her. They didn't give her the time to express herself. They would interrupt and finish her sentence and then discuss that part of it. I could see that wasn't what she wanted to hear or needed to hear or what she was really asking. . . . . . What's the point if you don't listen and then try to clarify what they are telling you? Mrs. Desjardins expresses herself well—she's very intelligent. It's a matter of hearing and acting on that."*

Sonia knew how to create a facilitative environment through being fully present, using attentive listening, and appreciating Mrs. Desjardins as a person with great strengths.

Creating Goodness-of-Fit Environments

Recall from Chapter 3 that goodness of fit is the "match" between a person's needs, temperament, and behavior style and the demands of the environment. When the demands of the environment do not overly exceed the person's capabilities, capacities, and competencies, then there is a good fit. Conversely, when the demands from the environment exceed the person's capabilities, these situations add stress and burden. These are poor healing environments, because patients and families fail to repair and grow. Such environments may even cause the patient and family harm because of the stress and anxiety they create and the additional demands and burdens they impose. It is important for nurses to understand their patients, what they and their families are going through, and what they need in a given situation and at a given point in time. This requires knowledge of the person, the situation, and some understanding as to why the person is responding in the way that he is.

> Goodness of fit refers to the goodness of the "match" between the person's needs, temperament, and behavioral style, and the demands of the environment and its capacity to respond accordingly. Patients recover and thrive in environments in which there is a good fit.

Nurse Virginia Lee explained the importance of appreciating the person's readiness, the demands and needs of the situation, and the timing of SBC interventions accordingly (Chapter 3): *"I think people have the capacity to use their strengths and resources when they're ready for it. It's a question of determining when they're ready. I can think of when I try to approach patients before surgery when they are experiencing high, high anxiety and high levels of uncertainty. During a highly anxious time, their readiness is not there. They need to cope in a different way—by denial, withdrawing, and distraction. Even if I knew that they could rely on a coping strategy that was built on their strengths, such as helping them to understand and process what's going to happen and what's happening to them, this is not a good time because they're not ready to work on these areas."*

Virginia understands the importance of creating an environment where there is a goodness of fit for the person and family to benefit from SBC. This can entail assessing a patient's readiness to meet his needs and thus knowing when to act and when to hold back. It involves tailoring the environment to what the patient needs and wants.

Now spend time observing different interactions on the units in which you are working to determine the nature and quality of the environment. To guide you in your observations, complete the Reflect and Connect exercise found in Exhibit 10.1.

APPROACHES FOR WORKING WITH STRENGTHS

PART 1: Approaches for Working with Existing Strengths

Listed below are some of the basic techniques nurses can use to work with an individual or family's existing strengths (ESs).

EXHIBIT 10.1

Reflect and connect *How healthy is your work environment?*

Reflect and Connect Instructions:

1. Select two interactions to observe between the following: a patient and family member, a nurse and patient, a nurse and student nurse, teacher and student nurse, nurse and fellow nurse, nurse and physician.
2. Take two to five minutes to make the observation.
3. Describe the interaction in as much detail as possible. Note the context of what is happening and the content of the interaction by observing what each person said and how the other person responded. Notice the verbal and non-verbal behavior of each person (e.g., whether eye contact is maintained), physical posturing (e.g., direct vs. nondirect), facial expression (e.g., smiling, sad, neutral), emotional tone (e.g., happy, depressed), general climate (e.g., positive–negative, relaxed–tense).

Interactions (e.g., nurse–patient, teacher–student nurse)	Describe the context (e.g., teaching a procedure, visiting, rounds) What is the major focus?	What the person actually said or did (i.e., verbal and nonverbal)	How the other person responded	Tone of the interaction (e.g., positive, facilitative, critical, demeaning)

4. Analyze your observation and categorize what type of environment has been created, that is, healthy, benign, and toxic. Also rate whether the environment felt safe, supportive, and/or facilitative or unsafe, nonsupportive, and/or obstructive. What do you base your rating on? Use the evidence from your observations to support your conclusions.

With experience, through experimentation and trial and error, nurses will add to their list of strengths to look for in a given situation. They will also recognize what strengths that are required to foster healing and the indicators to use to evaluate the effectiveness of a strength.

Being able to work with strengths requires knowledge of characteristics of how a quality becomes a strength (see Chapter 4). It is this knowledge that is the basis of the specific techniques summarized in Table 10.1.

ES 1: Make a list or inventory of existing strengths

The nurse may begin by developing a list of the person and family's strengths and resources following the initial assessment and then adding to the list after each encounter. The nurse can also modify the list when a strength is depleted and needs to be

TABLE 10.1

Techniques for working with existing strengths (ES) and the characteristics of strengths

Specific Techniques	Characteristics of Strengths: Basis for Technique
ES1: Inventorying existing strengths	Strengths are personal constructions. (9) Strengths are developing entities (1) Strengths can be depleted and replenished (7)
ES2: Ask the person about their own strengths and resources	Strengths are related to goals. (4) Strengths are transferable. (8) Strengths are personal constructions. (9)
ES3: Share observations of strengths with the person	Strengths can be learned. (2)
ES4: Teach the person how to discover their strengths	Strengths can be learned. (2) Strengths are related to goals. (4) Strengths are defined by the context and circumstance. (5)
ES5: Avoid diagnostic labels to describe the person	Strengths are personal constructions. (9)
ES6: Give commendation and praise	Strengths are developing entities. (1) Strengths can be learned. (2) Strengths coexist with weaknesses and vulnerabilities. (3)
ES7: Focus on finding solutions rather than on dwelling on the problem	Strengths coexist with weaknesses and vulnerabilities. (3) Strengths are related to goals. (4)
ES8: Find opportunities to convey hope	Strengths are defined by the context and circumstance. (5) Strengths are multidimensional. (6)

Note. Numbers in parentheses correspond to the characteristics of strengths described in Chapter 4.

replenished. The nurse should include biological, psychological, and social strengths as well as inner strengths and external resources. Depending on the level of concern, the nurse can consider listing personal strengths, family strengths, community strengths, or social system strengths. The inventory of strengths can be drawn up with the person and family and added to and modified during or after each encounter, and over time (see Table 10.2).

ES 2: Ask patients about their own strengths and resources

In Chapter 9, in Phase 1 of the Spiraling Process, namely, *Exploring and Getting to Know*, the nurse identifies a person's strengths through observation and asking questions. When the person describes what she has been experiencing, the nurse gains insights into her strengths.

It is important that people's perceptions, meanings, and explanations that govern their responses and their reactions to their illness and its treatments be understood in terms of how their families and social and cultural milieux have affected their created reality (Kleinman, Eisenberg, & Good, 2006). It is the person's reality that affects how he has come to experience and live with the disease and how he eventually responds and copes with it. It is by viewing the person's experience through his own lens that the nurse has an opportunity to learn more about the person's assets, capacities, competencies, and skills, that is, his strengths. Many qualities may not have been labeled as a strength;

TABLE 10.2

Inventory of strengths

Area	Examples of Strengths
Personal	Open Confident Excellent mother—devoted, caring Strong sense of self-awareness Good decisionmaker Good support system Good problem-solver Strong immunological system Good powers of recuperation
Family	Supportive relationships Open communication Strong belief system
Community	Access to health services Availability of fresh food Clean water and air Helpful neighbors
Social System	Medicaid/Medicare

however, if these qualities have helped the person contain, manage, or even overcome the problem, then they can be considered that person's strengths. Similarly, when the nurse completes a genogram and ecomap with the person and their family as described in Chapter 9, she learns about the person's social network and his perceived availability of support. These can be important resources on which the person and family have called in the past, and could call on in the future, to mitigate stress and promote well-being.

The nurse can ask the person directly, "What are your strengths?" Another way to uncover strengths is to ask questions such as the following:

- What do you enjoy doing?
- What comes easy to you? What are you good at?
- What is working for you right now? What do you like about yourself? About your life?

Often, people enjoy doing things that come naturally, without expending too much energy. These capabilities, skills, and competencies comprise their strengths.

Another approach to discovering strengths is to find out more about the person's way of coping with problems. The nurse may ask the person:

- Why do you think you responded in the way that you did while others in your situation responded differently?
- What helped you get through X? (a particular crisis, treatment, etc.)
- What keeps you going?
- What has enabled you to survive? (in catastrophic situations or in cases of chronic problems)
- Who has helped you to get through your treatments?

EXHIBIT 10.2

Personal experience *Jimmy and Eleanor*: A love story of existing strengths*

Jimmy was diagnosed with leukemia when he was just eighteen and underwent a course of radiation and chemotherapy. At age sixty, he was the only survivor among forty teenagers diagnosed at the same time. Despite having several relapses over the next thirty years, he had married, was the father of two, ran a successful business, and was a respected leader in his community. When Jimmy was asked "What made you survive while the 40 others did not?" Jimmy replied "My family had money and I was able to get the best medical treatment." The nurse added, "None of the others were married to Eleanor (his wife)" Although Jimmy and Eleanor had a loving marriage, and Jimmy knew how critical Eleanor was to his survival, he had not really thought of Eleanor in this way. Jimmy nodded—"[Eleanor] has always been upbeat and optimistic, even during my relapses and repeated hospitalizations. She has kept my spirits up in my darkest times. She has been my best strength, the best medicine!"

*This is a true story but the names have been changed for anonymity.

In answering these questions the person may be hearing himself for the first time. If the nurse has worked with the person over a period of time and knows his situation, he may offer an alternative explanation to bring a taken-for-granted behavior or resource to the person's awareness, as illustrated in Jimmy and Eleanor's story, told in Exhibit 10.2.

When the nurse asks directly about strengths, the person has to verbalize what she thinks are her strengths. The act of putting one's strengths into words helps bring a vague idea to a higher level of awareness and into the realm of the person's consciousness. The advantage of identifying and labeling a quality as a strength is that it then can be accessed more readily and used with greater intention in a new situation. It becomes an integral part of a person's identity: "I used to think I couldn't do anything well; now, I realize I am highly competent," or "I used to think I was weak. After that incident, I now realize that I am really a strong person." From here on in, if Jimmy is ever asked this question again, he will undoubtedly begin his answer with Eleanor—his greatest strength.

Asking people to verbalize their strengths also helps them link specific qualities with specific goals. They may gain new insights into what it takes to make something happen, thus putting themselves in a better place to capitalize on and mobilize that strength in the future.

ES 3: Share observations of strengths with the person

In the course of nursing, the nurse needs to share her observations of a patient's strengths and point out to the patient the contribution of those strengths to health and healing. Sharing observations of biological, psychological, and social strengths are important, for several reasons.

First, this information is critical if the nurse is to work with and support the person's innate healing mechanisms. Think of a situation in which the nurse notices that the person tires at 3:00 p.m. and requires a thirty-minute nap. She knows that sleep is a natural reparative process. Working with this strength, the nurse may put a "do not disturb" sign on the person's door at that time of day. Often, nurses do not share observations or the reasons behind their action. However, if this nurse explains to the patient that feeling tired or dozing off is nature's restorative process (a strength) and the body's way of self-regulating and conserving energy the person (other strengths), then the patient can use this information to help better self-regulate and thereby promote her own self-healing. She may plan regular naps in the future.

Second, when the nurse tells a person about his strengths, the nurse communicates genuine concern for and liking of the person. Showing concern and liking of one person is important in creating a connection and building trust.

Third, the nurse may also share observations of a person's strengths with that person to motivate her. Most people like to be told what's special about them, what they do well, and what's working. It makes them feel good and want to do better.

TIPS FOR SHARING OBSERVATIONS: When nurses share their observations about a person's strengths with that person, the message will be more effective if the nurse

- Is **specific** about the strength and **provides concrete examples**
- **Names and describes** what he has observed and **explains** why he considers a particular quality to be a strength
- **Uses the person's own words** when giving feedback so that the person can more easily relate to what he is saying
- **Links** the person's **qualities** to **improvements** or positive changes in responses, regardless of how subtle or small the change has been
- **Explains what impressed** him about the person's way of handling a situation

A person may be unaware of his strengths until the nurse has shared her observations with him. Nurse Lidia De Simone shares her observations with patients and why she believes sharing observations is important: *"It's important to find things a patient did well. For instance, when transferring a person from the bed to the chair, as a nurse, you may look for how well they conserve their energy. You may share this observation with them: 'You conserved your energy, you didn't move too quickly. You can do the same thing when walking to the door, conserve your energy, don't move too fast'... I feel it is very important for the person to feel good about themselves because if a person feels badly about themselves they won't be able to achieve their goals. They have to feel that they are good enough to even try."*

Some families may already be aware of their strengths, whereas others may not. For patients and families who are aware of their strengths, what the nurse shares with them about what she has observed may further reinforce what they already know about themselves. It's always nice to hear an outsider's perspective. The person may think "She really understands me," or "She really gets me!"

Let's return to Cheryl Armistead and her nursing of Mrs. Bhutto. As Cheryl described, *"This woman was trying to figure out Western society and the health care system. She was trying to have confidence in it, but she herself could clearly see that beyond anything that anyone was telling her this problem (with her baby) existed. So to me her strength is the knowing, but it's also finding out. She asked the right questions. She found a way to seek alternative resources within the system that to me was another important strength. I repeated back to her, 'You knew, you thought, you acted.' "*

Cheryl recognized Mrs. Bhutto's special qualities and shared them with her. Over a period of time, Mrs. Bhutto came to trust Cheryl and they were able to forge a very special bond.

ES 4: Teach people how to discover their own strengths

An important technique to help people identify their strengths is to teach them how to observe themselves. To learn how to observe, a person needs to step back, detach himself from the situation, and assume the role of observer. Too often, the person is so engrossed in his own problems that he fails to notice the things that are working.

The nurse needs to ask the person to describe what is happening during an event, to record what she is feeling, the actions she took, and how she felt afterward. For example, the nurse can say, "Describe what happened when you fell and broke your leg. What were your initial thoughts and feelings? What happened next? How did you calm yourself down? What things did you do well to manage the situation?" Alternatively the nurse could say, "Think of how ill you were. What functions have you recovered? What does this tell you about your body and your ability to heal?"

The nurse can also help a person become a more astute observer by *recording* his thoughts, feelings, and actions following a stressful event. When the person completes such a recording, the nurse should take the time to review it with him. The nurse can help the person better understand and discover their strengths by asking him what he was trying to achieve and what he expected from the situation. This technique is useful when the nurse uses it to help the person link his feelings to actions and his actions to goals. Recall that a strength is goal related. This exercise will help the person to uncover existing strengths.

Consider baby Rachel, who was being breastfed. At 6 months she refused to be fed with a bottle, even one containing breast milk. She shunned all nipples, including the bottle and pacifier and wanted only her mother's breasts. Her mother, Susan, was planning to return to work and needed Rachel to drink from a bottle. As the time to return to work approached, Susan became increasingly more anxious. What would happen to Rachel if during the eight hours she was away at work Rachel wouldn't take the bottle? She worried Rachel would cry incessantly for her. Taking Rachel to work was not an option; infants were not permitted in her workplace. The nurse asked Susan to step back and observe Rachel while the nurse fed her a bottle. The mother and nurse noted that Rachel indeed rejected the bottle's nipple. But what did baby Rachel do well? Rachel could hold the bottle nipple in her mouth but would not latch onto the bottle's nipple. She would not create the needed suction. Rachel, however, had an excellent swallowing reflex (strength). She also had excellent head and neck control (strength). She was sitting (strength). She was in the ninety-eighth percentile for weight (strength). What was the solution while the mother was gone? Susan in recognizing Rachel's strengths, came up with an alternative solution. She could teach Rachel to drink from a sippy cup. This would bypass the rubber nipple of the bottle that was too different from her own breast nipple. Susan asked the babysitter to feed

Rachel wrapped in her t-shirt so that baby Rachel could enjoy her mother's smell. Also, the nurse suggested that Susan could start Rachel on solids and nurse her before going to work and immediately upon her return. Both Rachel and Susan survived. Rachel never did take a bottle. She did learn to drink from a cup and took enough fluids to sustain her during her mother's absence. When Susan came home, Rachel greeted her with warmth. Rachel would nurse but spent some of the time at the breast, lovingly staring at her mother, throwing her looks of "I love you" and "I am so happy to have you home" between bursts of sucking.

ES 5: Avoid using diagnostic label to describe the person

Some nurses, when they talk to other people about their patients, refer to patients by their diagnosis: "the diabetic lady in Room 402," the "borderline personality," the "difficult family." Nurses need to know that labeling a person only serves to dehumanize and depersonalize another human being. People will assume their diagnosis, and their personhood will become nonexistent. Such a practice shifts the nurse's focus from seeing the person and how he is experiencing his health challenges to seeing only a problem, a diagnosis, a response to treatment and that which is missing or not working (Shebib, 2007).

The other problem with labels is that health care providers develop feelings of helplessness, in particular when the diagnosis is difficult to treat. Most health care professionals believe that if they can't fix the problem, they have little to offer their patients. Consider the family whom Lucia Fabijan was counseling. Lucia had been working with the Diego family, who had recently immigrated to Canada with their two teenage daughters, Maria and Connie. Lucia was working with the entire family to sort out parenting issues and to help them parent more effectively. The eldest daughter, Maria, shared in the parenting duties, looking after the younger Connie while her parents were at work. Lucia described the Diegos as an open, warm, caring, and loving family. Maria suffered from depression and was being seen by her own individual therapist, who had labeled her as "resistant."

As Lucia related, *"The individual therapist who was working with Maria was pulling his hair out because he was what not getting very far with her. He diagnosed Maria as 'resistant,' but I think Maria was scared in many ways—scared of making too many changes. Because if Maria made the changes and really grew up, what would her parents do without her? This was my sense of what was going on . . . So my job was to try strengthen the parents so that Maria could then move away from the parenting role and do what she needed to do because she was a young lady who needed to explore."*

By not assigning a label to Maria's behavior—in this case, "resistant"—Lucia could see the issues more clearly and capitalize on this family's strengths. Lucia commented on the positive qualities in the family and explained why she avoids labels: *"I don't like the word resistant. I could see how [Maria's] therapist could call her challenging. However, I would see Maria's humor. And I would also see her challenge her father, gently, eyes down, not quite sure how to do it, but nevertheless challenge him. To me it was a turtle putting their head up and trying it out, not too sure about how to do that. I thought it was quite enchanting that Maria knew what she had to do and was trying to do it. And it was easier for me to see that, commend it and reinforce it in my nursing of this family. If you label a person's behavior as awful, it becomes an awful behavior. However, if you challenge the label, you can really create it into strength rather than something that pisses everyone off, excuse the expression."*

Lucia was able to see strengths. She interpreted many of Maria's behaviors in positive terms. This process of interpreting helped Lucia develop a special feeling for Maria that she communicated to her when she commended what she saw as positives or strengths.

ES 6: Give commendation and praise

All people need praise and positive reinforcement to feel good about themselves. Commending a person and family for what they are doing well in the midst of crises and challenges often helps counterbalance the feelings of hopelessness, helplessness, failure, or blame that often accompany problems (Walsh, 2006). When a patient and family are in the "eye of the storm" there is a tendency to paint everything in a negative way. People often say that they cannot see anything good in themselves, in others, or in their situation. In such situations they often fail to recognize their own strengths and resources. When nurses point out their strengths, this may help patients realize that they do have strengths despite what they are going through or have been through.

Commenting on what the person and family are doing well also reinforces the message that they have something to be proud of. This may engender and boost their confidence, which in turn can result in adopting a can-do attitude, which is the foundation of self-efficacy, one of the most important strengths to have (Bandura, 1997). Giving commendation is an important technique nurses can use to help other people feel more empowered. When a strength is pointed out and the strength is linked to his behavior and his behavior to the goal, the person is more likely to use the strength with intention. Moreover, when the person is told what he is doing and how important this is to his progress in getting better, that person is more likely to try harder or to try something again.

Let's return to Lucia Fabijan, who uses commendation regularly in her work with families: *"I commend [someone] every time I see something good. I say something like, "It's really good what you said right there. That's really good; do you know why?" And then I'll just bring it out and reinforce it."* Lucia went on to describe why she uses commendation.

"It brings in some light to the family in terms of you've got all this going for you. I may also say 'Let me show you some of the things that you could use that you are doing so that you could in fact make more use of what you already have.' So I shine the light on a particular interaction, a particular behavior, a particular value or belief that would help them sort out some of their other problem areas."

Notable here is that Lucia goes beyond just commending: She asks the family to consider the reasons why this is an important strength. She also uses commendation to "shine light" on a strength and bring it to the forefront so that the person is more aware of its importance. Once the person is aware of the strength, it increases the possibility that the person will be able to use this strength to deal with another problem or another concern on other occasions.

For a commendation to be effective, it has to be **authentic**. Nurses must be sincere in their praise, and they must be truthful. If they are not, patients will pick up on the lack of sincerity. The nurse will be perceived as disingenuous—in other words, phony—and this will undermine any existing trust. As Nurse Lidia De Simone reflected, *"One* *of the things that I think is really important is to tell the truth. I wouldn't say a person is strong unless I really thought that they were strong. This is extremely important. I believe that people deserve that you be genuine and truthful in your interactions with you."*

Commendations also have to be **given at the appropriate time**. If the nurse commends a person when the person is preoccupied with something else, she may not hear the commendation or may not understand what and why the nurse is talking about.

ES 7: Focus on finding solutions rather than on dwelling on problems

In working with patients, clients, and families, nurses should shift the focus from dwelling on problems to looking for solutions. In doing this, both the nurse and patient need to examine realistic ways of dealing with an issue or challenge. It forces them each to examine what exists and to make the most of what the person currently has going for him. The person may suddenly see what he does well and understand how to use his strengths to deal with his problems. In this way, the nurse and patient begin to recognize and value his existing strengths and are in a better position to mobilize and capitalize on them both now and later. A solution-focused orientation is consistent with SBC in that it assumes the uniqueness of each person; works with each person's individuality; focuses on the processes of collaborative inquiry; assumes the person is competent, resilient, and resourceful; and motivates the person by building on their strengths (McAllister, 2003).

ES 8: Find opportunities to convey hope

Hope plays an integral and significant role in a patient's recovery. People who have hope are more likely to mobilize energy to cope with physical, mental, and emotional insults. When people have hope they are more likely to set goals for themselves and try to figure out ways to meet them. Thus, hope is associated with better physical health, psychological adjustment, and enhanced quality of life (Snyder et al., 2002).

Many scholars have written that hope is essential to life. Without hope, people feel immobilized and despondent, and they have a tendency to give up. In short, health and healing are compromised when hope wanes or is lost. People who are hopeful have the ability to establish clear goals for themselves and are able to think of workable ways to achieve those goals. When people feel hopeful they also discover and draw on their other inner strengths, such as courage, perseverance, and humor. These strengths often help patients and families deal with their challenges and find new meaning in their lives.

Hope is an important strength to nourish. It is particularly important when a person receives bad news, feels vulnerable, or when others around her have lost hope. A nurse listens for hope by listening for people's goals, the way they talk about their future, and the meaning and purpose they find in living. Health care professionals play an important role in helping people find hope as well as to create and sustain hope. They can help to instill hope by asking such questions as the following (Larsen, Edey, & LeMay, 2007):

- What most threatens your hope?
- What would a hopeful person do in your same situation?
- What would help you to become more hopeful?

There are many techniques that nurses have found useful in finding and creating hope. Among them is that hope is fostered by working with a person's strengths. For example, nurses communicate hope when they point out what is working (i.e., focusing on the person's strengths); when they point out what progress the person has made no matter how small the gains may seem; when they help the person set goals; and when they provide information and answer questions in a compassionate, honest, and respectful manner (Chu-Hui-Lin-Chi, 2007; Koopmeiners et al., 1997).

PART 2: Approaches for Developing Strengths

There are three approaches to developing new strengths:

1. Turn potentials into strengths
2. Turn a deficit or weakness into a strength
3. Minimize or contain a weakness to allow a strength to shine forth

These approaches and their specific techniques are summarized in Table 10.3.

Approach 1: Turning potentials into strengths

As discussed earlier, potentials are underdeveloped, ill-defined, or underutilized qualities that, in the right circumstance and under the right environmental conditions, can develop into a strength or become a resource. Humans are equipped with inborn or innate mechanisms of adaptation required for their survival. These innate mechanisms are potentials that can be developed into strengths. Potentials involve biological systems (e.g., immune, nervous, hormonal), psychological capacities (e.g., mental, emotional, cognitive, social) and social systems (e.g., social networks, ecological environments). Qualities such as plasticity, flexibility, and adaptability are potentials that can be turned into strengths. Consider what happens when heart vessels become blocked because of a buildup of plaque. If this happens over a period of time, the heart has an inborn

---

TABLE 10.3

Summary of approaches and techniques for developing strengths

Approach 1: Techniques to Develop Potentials into Strengths (DPS)
DPS 1: Provide knowledge about the strength.
DPS 2: Create opportunities to practice a new skill: Practice–rehearse–practice.
DPS 3: Raise the person's awareness of the potential strength.
DPS 4: Capitalize on an existing strength and modify it for a different situation.

Approach 2: Techniques for Turning Deficits into Strengths (TDS)
TDS 1: Treat the deficit as a strength.
TDS 2: Ask questions to stimulate new ways thinking.
TDS 3: Reframe the behavior.
TDS 4: Create a "goodness-of-fit" environment.

Approach 3: Techniques to Minimize a Deficit and Maximize Strengths (MDMS)
MDMS 1: Help the person take control.
MDMS 2: Strengthen mind–body connection through regulating arousal states (self-regulation).
MDMS 3: Point out strengths to counterbalance weknesseses.

mechanism to create detours or secondary routes that bypass the blockage, that is, the creation of a collateral circulation. This mechanism of detouring is present ensure that the heart muscle continues to have an adequate blood supply. This is an example of a potential that develops into a strength to ensure the person's survival.

Developing potentials into strengths is a two-step process. The first step is to identify the potential and, once it has been identified, to develop it into a usable strength.

Step 1: Identifying Potential Strengths. Before the nurse and person can develop a potential into a functional strength they have to identify the qualities that can be developed into strengths. Discovering such qualities occurs during all phases of the Spiraling Process. Potential strengths are found in a person's response to challenges. Literally thousands of books have been written about people who have discovered strengths they didn't know they possessed until they were confronted by an unexpected, unplanned negative event. It also can happen with an expected, planned event, such as becoming a parent, when a person discovers strengths they weren't aware existed. Every person within his own lifetime will face difficulties, disappointments, and hardships that will tax him and test his personhood and his will to survive. In the process of meeting these challenges, the person will discover qualities he did not know he had. These are potentials, the seeds of strengths that reside in every human being. Think of the late Christopher Reeve, the actor who played Superman, whose spinal cord was severed in a horse riding accident that left him a quadriplegic. He inspired millions with his remarkable courage, strength of character, sense of humor, and tenacity. He went beyond his own personal tragedy to change attitudes toward disabled individuals worldwide. With the loving devotion of his late wife, Dana, family, and countless friends, he raised awareness as well as millions of dollars for research into spinal cord injuries. Thus, an event will often call forth potentials, and in the right environment, under the right conditions, and with the right influences, potentials can blossom into strengths.

Discovering potential strengths also applies to identifying potential resources. The person may be pleasantly surprised to discover new sources of support. It is during times of crisis, when people are tested, that some will disappoint while others will surprise by their ability to give support, help, and inspire hope and courage.

There are many ways to identify potential strengths. Some of these approaches were described in Chapter 9 during the discussion of all four phases of the Spiraling Process. Three additional techniques are described here and prefaced by *IPS* (identifying potential strengths).

IPS 1: Use genogram and ecomap

Some of the techniques that are used for assessing strengths, such as the use of a genogram and ecomap, as described in Chapter 9, can also be used to identify potential resources. A nurse can use a genogram and ecomap to identify untapped potential resources by asking the person to think about each relationship anew and consider them in a new light by asking such questions as

- Some people can't help in one way but they are willing to help in other ways. Have you considered asking that person whether they would help and, if they would, what could they see themselves doing?
- Have you ever considered where people in your community get X? (name the help)

IPS 2: Observe how the person rallies from illness, injuries, treatments, and other insults

Another technique to identify potential strengths is to observe *how* the person deals with setbacks and illness and the speed with which she rallies and recovers, both physically and emotionally. The speed with which a person rallies speaks volumes about her capacity to contain, overcome, or compensate for weaknesses. The nurse also notes any signs of deterioration and those factors associated with these changes.

Nurses should ask themselves such questions as "How quickly does the person rally, and what is responsible for the rallying?" It is in noticing these "little" things that the person may discover or uncover things and areas that are working. Consider Shannon, who was prone to bladder infections. The first time she developed a urinary tract infection (UTI), she spiked a high fever and was very lethargic, and it took her ten days to fully recover. Shannon recovered much faster from her next UTI. Her immunological system had "learned" to respond but, more important, Shannon began to recognize the early signs of a UTI and began drinking cranberry juice (which changes the pH of the bladder) and large amounts of water. Shannon rallied much faster after her first UTI because she had learned how to support her immunological system. Alternatively, consider Sheila, who gets easily stressed and overwhelmed by change. The first time she had to change jobs she had several anxiety attacks, could not sleep at night, and became depressed. It took her several months to adjust to the new job. The next time she had to change jobs, she still felt stressed, but she was able to contain her anxiety from overwhelming her. Sheila had noticed the things that enabled her to cope. She learned that she could control her anxiety by meditating and doing yoga. Sheila had learned how to better self-regulate to control her arousal levels, that is, anxiety. When she noticed herself becoming anxious, she would take a short break—either go to the bathroom and have a little cry or leave the office and take a brief walk. She had observed, noticed, and learned from past events what helped. With her latest job change, Sheila's adjustment lasted weeks, not months.

IPS 3: Ask the person to monitor his thoughts, feelings, and responses

In addition to asking questions about what the person does best, the nurse may encourage the person to monitor his own thoughts, feelings, and behaviors over a specific period of time. Diaries or journals are effective tools to help the nurse and the person identify potentials by providing insights into how a person's feelings and thoughts contribute to his actions.

The nurse may show the person how to keep a diary or journal, which can range from an unstructured format, in which the person records random thoughts, ideas, feelings, to a structured one that follows a specific format and requires answers to specific questions. In reviewing the person's journal, the nurse may ask her to reflect on what she has learned about herself. The nurse can also ask her to think about what surprised her the most, what was most unexpected, what had been expected, and the like. The nurse may also ask the person what attitudes and skills she would like to develop further.

Nurse Amy Nyland described her reasons for giving twenty-four-year-old Rozanne a diary. Rozanne had been admitted to hospital in a asthmatic crisis. She had not been taking her medication. Rather than get angry with her, Amy wanted to understand Rozanne: *"I wasn't interested in why she wasn't [taking her medication] because I felt that she knew that too. She started to talk a bit more about her family and it turns out that she had had some very sad things happen to her during the last eighteen months and she felt that it had been a big transition period for her in a lot of ways. Things in her personal life were just really in flux, things that she didn't have that much control over. And I think that taking or not taking her medication was something that she could control."*

After listening to Rozanne, Amy bought her a notebook to help her get in touch with her goals and recognize her strengths: *"I got her a little notebook that I thought she might like because I felt that she could take hold of her life. She had been ill for awhile and I wanted to give her something that was aesthetically nice but also something that she could write ideas down in. It wasn't the writing so much that I was thinking about. I was thinking about goals. I got the impression that she hadn't been encouraged to have goals beyond the medical management kind of goals. And I felt that maybe if there were things that she was aiming for in the rest of her life it might give her reason to dig into the medical management side of it and bring that illness down to size. It's a part of her life, but it's not everything."*

Amy went on to explain how she introduced the notebook: *"The next day, I introduced the idea of the notebook as something that I wasn't sure if it would be helpful, but I told her that for me sometimes if I write down my goals, my ideas in small steps, that helps me to make them concrete. Sometimes you don't see how far you've come."*

Amy used a journal to help Rozanne get in touch with her goals (having a goal is a strength).

Step 2: Converting Potentials into Strengths. Once a potential has been identified, it still needs to be developed into a strength. The following techniques can be used to accomplish this purpose and are thus named *DPS techniques* (Developing Potential Strengths). They are summarized in Table 10.3.

DPS 1: Provide knowledge about the strength

Almost all strengths have a knowledge component as well as a practice skill component. Patients and families can learn more about their strengths through experience. Once a person is aware of a potential he has, he may want to learn more about it and how it can become a strength. Learning can come from many sources. The nurse can suggest books, DVDs, web-sites-- anything that is a source of information. The nurse can also refer the patient to individuals who have experienced a similar challenge.

In everyday practice, nurses are confronted with patients' and family member's potentials. When a family member shows an interest in learning to care for a loved one or a desire to help, these are potentials that can be turned into strengths. Consider Nurse Astride Bazile who was caring for Mr. Duman, diagnosed with advanced lung cancer, whose wife, Elwin, wanted to provide more of his care. Part of developing Mrs. Duman's strengths was for Astride to teach her what to look for.

As Astride explained, *"She was a very bright woman. I started coaching her. I noticed and then said to her, 'I understand that you want to do what's best for your husband, you want to do this.' And I taught her the things to look for so that she would have the tools and the knowledge to take care of her husband."*

DPS 2: Create opportunities to practice a new skill: Practice–rehearse–practice

The best way to develop a skill is to use it until it becomes a part of the person's repertoire. Any new competency, from the simple to the complex, needs to be used, refined, and honed through practice, practice, and more practice. Think of Sally, who has just become a mother. She may be a warm, loving, sensitive woman with an interest in and love for children (i.e., potential to be a good mother); however, in learning to become a mother she needs to use these potential qualities to actually mother her new infant. She needs to acquire information and skills in parenting. Mothers need general knowledge coupled with specific knowledge. General knowledge concerns information about pregnancy, parenting, child development, and the like. Specific knowledge concerns knowledge about *this* specific pregnancy, *this* child, *this* child's development, and *this* parent-child relationship. Thus, the mother needs to learn about her own baby and the many tasks involved in caring for a baby. She needs to observe how to provide for her infant's many needs, then practice using these new skills until they become incorporated into her way of thinking and doing. Alternatively, think of Allison, who is interested in assuming greater responsibility for her own health. She wants to be able to detect early signs of breast cancer. To this end, she needs to learn how to do breast self-examinations. First she needs to know about the anatomy and physiology of a breast, and then she needs to be taught the skill of how to conduct a breast self-examination. The nurse may demonstrate this technique first on a mannequin or by showing Allison a DVD about breast examination. The nurse may then coach and supervise Allison as she practices on a mannequin and then on herself. It is only through regular monthly self-examinations that Allison will become familiar with her own breasts and will be in a better position to detect early any abnormalities, irregularities, or subtle changes.

To turn a potential into a strength requires that the nurse and person:

- **Monitor** and **modify** the behavior
- **Elicit feedback** from others
- **Coach** the person in the proper use of the skill
- **Rehearse** the skill
- **Practice**, modify, practice, modify, practice, practice, practice

DPS 3: Raise the person's awareness of the potential strength

Once a potential has been developed into a strength and is used on a regular basis to deal with different situations, it now needs to become integrated into the person's identity and way of responding (Hodges & Clifton, 2004). Any potential quality first needs to be *labeled a strength* for the person to recognize it as such. The nurse may help the person in this process by actually labeling a specific behavior a strength and then by linking the quality and calling it a "strength." In this way, the asset or quality takes on a new meaning and is then perceived by the person to be one of his strengths.

When the strength becomes part of a person's way of being and how she sees herself, then the person is more likely to use it. It no longer is a potential but an actual strength to be called forth and used when needed.

DPS 4: Capitalize on an existing strength and modify it for use in a different situation

Recall that a characteristic of a strength is that it can be transferred from one situation to another and is defined by its context (see Chapter 4). In other words, a person calls forth the same strength to be used in different situations. Take, for example, compassion. This strength, which one needs to deal with people in a wide variety of situations. But what happens when a strength that functions well in one situation is less effective in another?

Consider the clinical situation told by Nurse Christina Rosmus about Mrs. Cleary, a high-powered executive whose fourteen-year-old son had been seriously injured in a skiing accident. Mrs. Cleary went into "executive managerial" mode to deal with the crisis, but her style was less effective in the health care system than it had been in the boardroom. Christina reported: *"Mrs. Cleary was giving herself permission to do things that normally other people wouldn't do in the health care system and that was interfering with her son's care."* Christina continued that *"Everybody on the team thought that she's managing her son like she manages her business."* The challenge for Christina was how best to capitalize on Mrs. Cleary's competency but in ways that were more appropriate to the hospital system: *"This way of behaving was ingrained in her. It would be better to work with it rather than to say: 'Oh I'm sorry to say that at work this might be okay, but please don't take this approach home with you.'"*

To capitalize on an existing strength is to recognize it as a potential that can be turned into a strength by modifying it so that it better fits the situation. The challenge for Christina was to help Mrs. Cleary understand why her take-charge attitude (normally a strength) was not working for her with this particular health care team.

Christina described the strategy she used to capitalize on Mrs. Cleary's potential. She used Mrs. Cleary's own experience to help her understand the problem. She said to Mrs. Cleary: *"You're in the finance business. If I came to you and I said, 'I've got a million dollars that I want to invest, and I want you to give me your best advice about what I can do with this money.' With your knowledge and experience, you might say to me, 'Well, I think it would be good to invest here.' And then if I said to you 'I read about this really good fund and I really want to put my money there. And you think that's not the best place to put it because of the risk values. But I keep insisting, what would you think?' Mrs. Cleary replied: 'There's a good chance you're going to kiss that money goodbye, or that this isn't going to work for you and then you'll be upset.'"*

Then Christina helped Mrs. Cleary make the connection between this situation and what she was doing: *"Now, put yourself in the situation here in the hospital. You're in the position of saying 'Okay, I want to invest in my son.' And everyone says: 'Great; we want to help you do that.' It is important to have your view and be part of the decision. But at the same time, we don't want you going in a direction that is going to create difficulties for your son and impede him from getting better."*

In the course of their discussion, Christina acknowledged that Mrs. Cleary wanted the best for her son (a strength). In selecting an example that used Mrs. Cleary's own language and one to which she could relate, Christina helped Mrs. Cleary gain insight into her own behavior and why it was causing the staff difficulty. The problem was not that Mrs. Cleary lacked the strength but rather how she was using that strength—in this instance, inappropriately. This was having a negative effect on some of the staff, which in turn negatively influenced the way they related to Mrs. Cleary. However, one staff member was able to look beyond Mrs. Cleary's behavior and see what Mrs. Cleary was trying to do. That staff member was Nurse Christina Rosmus, who practiced SBC.

Approach 2: Turning a deficit into a strength

A second set of approaches to developing strengths is to turn deficits or weaknesses into strengths. Doing this requires knowledge of the deficit as well as knowledge of the strength. It is by understanding the deficit and why it exists that a nurse can then use this information to turn the deficit into a strength. The techniques, prefaced with TDS (Turning Deficits into Strengths) are described in the following paragraphs and summarized in Table 9.3.

TDS 1: Treat the deficit as a strength

If the nurse is to turn a deficit into a strength, he needs to work with the person's perceptions. He may begin by listening to the person describe what she considers to be a deficit or weakness. The nurse may find a strength within the deficit. As Nurse Lidia De Simone explained, *"I listen for weaknesses and problems as a way to discover strengths."* Mr. Bellini, a sixty-year-old factory worker, came to Lidia for help to quit smoking. He was illiterate, never having learned how to read or write yet, as Lidia related, he had figured out how to travel. Lidia used this deficit to his advantage: *"Here was this man who was illiterate and he was trying to quit smoking. He had managed to survive as an illiterate person, and it was that information about him that played a big role in helping him to quit smoking."*

Lidia went on to explain: *"He managed to work all his life at a factory, and yet he couldn't read or write. He had managed to get around the city, not only the city he lived in but other cities as well. He traveled a good deal. Just the fact that he could talk about this (deficit) was fantastic. It was really something. He felt confident and strong about himself. He had this attitude 'Look at what I have done. I can manage to take this on (i.e., stop smoking).' And I capitalized on this sense of pride—his strength. He did manage to stop smoking."*

Lidia helped Mr. Bellini use his openness, self-confidence, ability to conquer fears to overcome adversity. She also used his fierce sense of pride to help him to control his addiction to cigarettes.

TDS 2: Ask questions to stimulate new ways thinking

Nurses need to look for ways to help patients think about their situation from a new perspective. This is the work of Phase 2 of the Spiraling Process, Zeroing In. It is during this phase that patients may consider new ways of meeting their challenges, dealing with their concerns, and managing their illness. One approach that nurses use to achieve this is by asking the person and family questions to have them consider their situation differently. One of the most effective and straightforward type of question is to simply ask: "What would have to change in your life to make this possible?" (Zander & Zander, 2000). The nurse could also ask:

- What is the worst thing that could happen if you tried X?
- What is the worse thing that could happen if you didn't try Y?

TDS 3: Reframe the behavior

Reframing is a commonly used technique to modify or shift the way a person perceives and interprets a situation by having her consider alternative ways of looking at it (Pesut, 1991; Shebib, 2007). Reframing helps individuals broaden their perspective and see the situation or their way of behaving through a new lens, in a new light. It is an effective strategy to help the person refocus and turn negatives into positives. A nurse can reframe a behavior by looking at the behavior in a new context or linking it to the person's goal. Anita, an eighty-five-year-old woman recounted, almost eighty years after the fact, how her mother used to let her walk to school by herself at age six but did not let Anita's other siblings do so. She retells the story to illustrate that her mother never loved her; she loved her other siblings more. This memory still evokes pain. Anita's pain is palpable.

Anita interpreted her mother's action as neglectful and nonprotective. The nurse reframed the situation for Anita: *"Perhaps the reason why your mother allowed you go to school by yourself is because she had so much confidence in you. She knew you knew the way to school. She also knew that you were a sensible and capable little girl. Unlike your other siblings, she didn't have to worry about you."*

This new interpretation resonated with Anita. She then recounted that her mother often told her how she never had to worry about her like she did her other children. She believed Anita was a capable, competent little girl. The nurse used reframing to help Anita entertain alternative explanations to see her mother in a new light.

The following are guidelines to enhance the effectiveness of reframing as a technique for changing deficits into strengths:

- *The reframed interpretation* has **to be plausible, resonate, and be meaningful** for the person to consider the new interpretation. The nurse needs to understand the person before putting forth an alternative explanation; otherwise, the person may reject the alternative interpretation out of hand. The nurse's goal is to plant a "seed" that there are other ways of seeing the negativity in the situation.
- *The reframed interpretation* should **not negate or discount** what the person believes to be true; instead, it should **be stated in tentative terms**: "Another way of looking at this might be . . . ." Is it possible that this symptom can be due to . . . . rather than . . . .?" The person will be less likely to reject the new interpretation out of hand if couched in these terms.
- *The reframed interpretation* has to be introduced in the clinical conversation at the right time. **Timing is critical**. It's important to listen to people. As Nurse Christina Rosmus cautioned, *"It is important to be careful that when someone is trying to tell you the glass is empty that you don't come and say too early 'but it's also half-full,' because then you minimize what they're trying to tell you."*
- *The reframed interpretation* should adopt **positive language**. The nurse needs to search for the "silver lining in the cloud." She may engage the person in this process by asking "Are there any positives here?" "What have you learned from this difficult experience?" "What helped you get through? Were you able to discover strengths in weakness?"
- *The reframed interpretation* **must be sincere**. If the nurse does not believe what she is telling the person, then the reframed interpretation will sound insincere, not be taken seriously, and perhaps dismissed and ignored. The nurse thus runs the risk of losing credibility.
- *The reframed interpretation* needs time to process. The person must be **given time to reflect** on the alternative explanation. The nurse may say, "You don't have to agree with what I have just said, just give it some thought. We can discuss this at a later date." And at a later date, the nurse might ask, "What are your thoughts on this other way of seeing your the situation? Do you have any new understanding of why the situation or symptom is happening?"

TDS 4: Create a "goodness-of-fit" environment

Recall from Chapter 4 that context often determines whether a behavior or quality functions as a strength or a deficit. In one situation a quality may be a strength, and in another it may function as a deficit. Often, the person does not recognize when and how to use that quality to his best advantage. The role of the nurse is to help the person understand the quality and when to use it appropriately.

Recall that goodness of fit is when there is a fit between the person and the demands of the environment (see Chapter 3). A person is able to create a good fit by modifying her ways of behaving so that are better suited to the demands of the environment. For example, people whisper when they are in a library or when visiting a sick person in hospital but may yell or shout at a baseball game or at a convention.

A person may also create a good fit by selecting environments that better suit him. A person who is not very social or does not like being around sick people should not select a career in the helping professions.

Turning a deficit into a strength requires that the person has some self-awareness, understands the nature of different environments, and knows environments in which he will not fit. The nurse's role may be to help people select environments that better suits his talents, temperament, and needs.

Nurse Christina Rosmus told the story of a very large, very angry woman, Mrs. Saunders, who used both her size and her anger to bully and intimidate the health care team. Christina saw the person behind this obese, angry façade—a loving mother who wanted the best care for her son, who was being seen by the pain management team for intractable pain of unknown origin. During their first encounter, Christina saw something that the other care team members had not seen. During that first meeting, Mrs. Saunders tried to intimidate Christina. Christina stood her ground and showed her that she could not and would not be intimidated: *"I let her blow off steam. I opened the valve and allowed her to ventilate. I created a safe space for her."* Christina saw that the person whom the health care team had labeled as "difficult," "impossible," and "uncooperative" was a mother committed to fighting for her son to receive the best care for him. She saw a woman frustrated and unable to deal with the health care system and with the health care providers whom she considered enemies, not as allies: *"I saw a fighter in this mother who did not know how to properly fight. It was my job to partner with her and help her learn how to fight effectively."* Christina described a long process of working with Mrs. Saunders to help her learn how to communicate in a different way to get what she wanted for her son. *"At first I really didn't say much about her confrontational and angry style. I just listened and asked her to describe her interaction with the health care team. I would ask her 'Well, how did you feel about what happened? Do you think that you were successful in getting what you wanted? And how could you have done it differently?'"*

Christina's goal was to help Mrs. Saunders see how her way of behaving affected others and why she was unsuccessful in getting what she wanted from them. Christina described a slow change in Mrs. Saunders's behavior. *"Over time she started to realize that certain things she was doing were putting people's backs up. We started practicing, kind of role playing different ways of responding—if she tried it this way or said something different in a different way, what might be the response from the other health care team members? And I also asked how she was interpreting their attitude to her or what she thought they understood about her. And there were times when she would say: 'I hadn't thought about it that way' or 'I hadn't seen it quite like that.'"*

Christina used a variety of approaches with Mrs. Saunders, including listening to her and asking her questions to gain insight into her own behavior to help her see how her behavior was having just the opposite effect from the one she wanted.

Thus, it is important for nurses to recognize a quality as a strength and help the person know how to use this quality more effectively.

The nurse can identify a weakness by asking such questions as:

- "I notice that you are very persistent (or any other quality). When has persistence worked well for you? When has it worked against you?"
- "How do you feel about yourself when you behave in this manner? How do others react to you?"

Approach 3: Minimize deficits to maximize strengths

The third approach to developing strengths is to minimize or contain a weakness to allow a strength to shine forth. Recall that one characteristic of strengths is that they often coexist with weaknesses.

Many factors can interfere with a person's ability to cope and to function at optimal capacity, such as high levels of stress; excessive pain; uncontrollable emotions, such as anxiety and fear; inadequate diet; lack of exercise; unchecked infection, and the like. Nursing activities are often directed at mitigating, treating, or controlling the deficit to allow for maximum functioning of the person's innate repair mechanisms. The following are examples of commonly used techniques to reduce deficits and maximize strengths in the service of promoting health and creating the conditions for healing. These are prefaced by *MDMS* (Minimize a Deficit to Maximize Strengths) and are

TABLE 10.4

Examples of how to minimize deficits and maximize strengths

Ways to Minimize Deficits	Techniques
1. Reduce stress	Active listening Presence Availability Meditation Comfort measures (e.g., backrubs) Medication Family support
2. Symptom management to promote coping (e.g., pain management)	Medication, acupuncture, TENS (Trancutaneous Electrical Nerve Stimulation) Relaxation exercise: imagery Reflective journaling
3. Support body's repair and restorative processes (e.g., wound healing)	Dressing changes Cleanliness, hand washing Comfort measures to promote rest and sleep Good nutrition

illustrated in Table 10.4. In addition to these approaches there are three additional techniques, which are summarized in Table 10.3.

MDMS 1: Help the person assume some control

Helping the person assume some control is a frequently used technique in which the nurse uses an existing strength to overcome, minimize, or neutralize a deficit. It requires that the nurse find the strength and then help the person use it to deal with his problem.

Nurse Gillian Taylor used this approach to help her patient, Suzanne, overcome her fear of injections. Gillian knew that Suzanne was a synchronized swimmer: "*I asked Suzanne 'How long do you hold your breath when you're under water?' Suzanne replied "Oh, about a minute and a half or something crazy." Gillian continued: "[I said,] 'Well, this little thing (referring to the immunization) I'm going to give you takes about six seconds.' Suzanne started laughing, and I said to her, 'It seems to me you're able to do something for a whole bunch of seconds and I'm assuming the last part of holding your breath under must take incredible courage.' And she said: 'Yeah we come out of the water and we even have to be smiling. Because you can't come out going 'blah,' you have to come out smiling' And I said, 'You don't have to smile at all while I do this. Not before, during, or after. If you can just hold still.'*"

Gillian was able to help Suzanne get in touch with strengths that she used in another situation and mobilize them and transfer them to deal with Suzanne's fear of needles. Gillian summarized her approach and how it works: "*I let children feel that I see their positives [i.e., strengths]. And then I use that to help them come up with a better way of handling something that they find difficult.*"

MDMS 2: Strengthen the mind–body connection through regulating arousal states (self-regulation)

The body and mind are an integrated whole (see Chapter 3, Value 3: Holism and embodiment). There are many approaches to promoting wholeness, including attending to lifestyle practices that replenish energy through good nutrition and proper exercise (Keegan, 1995); teaching body listening skills, and encouraging the person to practice yoga, meditation, biofeedback, hypnosis, and other such mind–body therapies (see Exhibit 10.3).

One of the most promising approaches is to help the person learn how to self-regulate. Self-regulation involves modulating one's arousal state. Most individuals function best when their state of arousal is neither too high nor too low. If the person is too stressed or overly anxious (i.e., in a high arousal state), she will be immobilized and unable to function and cannot learn. This is known as the *Yerkes–Dodson law of arousal*, and it was originally developed by psychologists Robert M. Yerkes and John Dillingham Dodson in 1908. Their law explains that a person's performance or ability to function increases with physiological or mental arousal, but only up to a point. When a person's levels of arousal becomes too high, when she experiences too much stress or feels too anxious, then her ability to function decreases. Similarly, when a person's level of arousal is too low, when she is asleep or in a very depressed state, her ability to function also decreases. The process is often illustrated graphically as a curvilinear, inverted *U*-shaped curve that depicts increasing and decreasing levels of arousal (see Figure 10.1).

Consider a person who is frightened or feels threatened. The sympathetic nervous system is activated and the person goes into a high state of alert. In this scenario,

EXHIBIT 10.3

Empirical study *Biofeedback therapy and the possible role of mind–body therapy in controlling high blood pressure*

The Problem

Can mind–body techniques be used to create biofeedback control of the body's physiological systems such as blood pressure (BP)?

The Issues

A randomized controlled study was designed to examine whether a four-week BP biofeedback program could reduce BP and BP reactivity to stress in participants with mild hypertension.

The Study

Two groups were created as part of the study. Participants in the active bio-feedback group ($n = 20$) were trained in four weekly laboratory sessions to self-regulate their BP with continuous BP feedback signals, whereas participants in the sham biofeedback group ($n = 18$) were told to manipulate their BP without feedback signals. BP, skin temperature, skin conductance, BP reactivity to stress, body weight, and anxiety were assessed before training and repeated at the eighth week after the training.

The Findings

The decreases in systolic BP (SBP; (12.6 ± 8.8 vs. 4.1 ± 5.7) and mean arterial BP (8.2 ± 6.9 vs. 3.3 ± 4.9) from baseline at week 12 follow-up were significantly greater in the active biofeedback group compared with the sham biofeedback group ($ps = .001$ and $.017$, respectively). Results showed that biofeedback training effectively lowered SBP and mean arterial BP ($ps = .013$ and $.026$, respectively). The pre–post differences in skin conductance and SBP reactivity were statistically significant for the biofeedback group ($ps = .005$ and $.01$, respectively), but not for the control group. For the sample as a whole and for the biofeedback group, the state anxiety score and body weight remained unchanged.

The Bottom Line

BP biofeedback exerts a specific treatment effect in reducing BP in individuals with mild hypertension, possibly by reducing their reactivity to stress through their mind–body connection.

Source: Adapted from Tsai, Chang, Chang, Lee, and Wang (2007).

all available energy is directed toward survival and warding off threats, leaving little energy available for other areas of bodily functioning. If this state of high alert continues for a prolonged period of time without any respite, exhaustion will set in. The patient may become exhausted even when he appears not to be doing anything. This is due to the body's defense mechanisms eventually running out of adenosine triphosphate (ATP; the body's energy molecule). It is a similar situation to what

FIGURE 10.1

The Yerkes–Dodson law of arousal

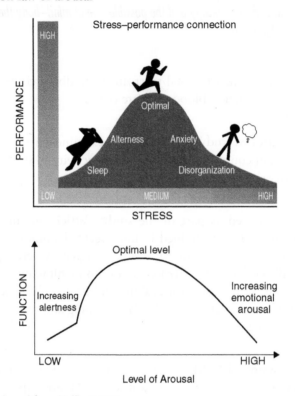

Source: Lower graph adapted from Hebb, (1966).

happens when athletes overexert themselves, their muscles run out of ATP, and they collapse from exhaustion.

At the opposite end of the spectrum, if a person is unmotivated, tired, and depressed, then messages are sent for the person to shut down—at all levels, but to varying degrees. The mind knows, and the body knows, because the person is whole and embodied. The person will be in a lowered state of arousal and therefore will have difficulty coping with and warding off challenges to her health. For the person's strengths to be fully utilized, the nurse needs to ensure that the person is in her optimal arousal zone.

Each person has his own arousal curve that is determined by personal characteristics (e.g., age, temperament, sex), the wiring of his physiological system competence (e.g., immunological, and hormonal), family factors (e.g., family history, culture, immigration status, level of support, finances), and situational factors (e.g., access to health services and information). Some individuals are better able to regulate their arousal states than are others. It is important for nurses to help their patients understand their own arousal states and how to recognize signs of energy depletion and how to replenish energy reserves.

Nurse Gillian Taylor also described how she helps children cope by asking parents how much their child can tolerate. She often tells the parents what the team is planning to do. She usually begins an appointment as follows: *"We have a couple of things we need to do today. There's a blood test, a chest X-ray, and seeing the doctor …' In some cases you can then say to the parent: 'Knowing your child as you do, what should we start with?' Some parents will understand the significance of my question right away and they'll say: 'Let's not mention the blood test quite yet. Let's do the other stuff first and when it's time to do that [the blood test] I'll prepare her and we'll do it then.'"*

By asking parents what their child is able to cope with, Gillian is in effect assessing the child's arousal curve and planning care to maximize the child's coping strengths. If Gillian did not collaborate with the parents and began with the blood test, the child might have become distraught and been unable to cope with the other medical activities.

In nurses' traditional role of attending to the body through the provision of comfort measures (e.g., changing bed linens, backrubs, bed baths) are the many ways they help patients self-regulate. These measures often help patients reduce their arousal levels and get into a zone that is conducive to rest and relaxation. When people are relaxed and able to sleep, cells and tissues repair, the mind rests, the body restores itself, and healing and growth take place.

MDMS 3: Pointing out strengths to counterbalance weaknesses

Remember that strengths can be used to counterbalance weaknesses. Nurses often observe patients engaging in unhealthy behaviors, and they may want to increase patients' awareness of these behaviors by sharing their observations. The challenge is how to do so without sounding critical or blaming the patient. The nurse needs to find a way to use a person's strengths to counterbalance unhealthy behaviors. However, for a message to be effective the person needs to listen to the message the nurse is conveying. People will listen if they feel supported and feel that the message is being communicated in a spirit of caring and compassion. Focusing on a person's strengths, what he is doing well, or pointing out why he is doing what he is doing, may help the person hear the message even if it is negative. Nurse Lidia De Simone illustrated how she always looks to counterbalance a negative message by also pointing out positives.

"If you're going to reflect on something that is negative, then don't reflect it in a way that is going to upset the person. One time I was caring for Mrs. Tremblay, who scolded her daughter, Yvonne, a lot. In a matter-of-fact way I said, 'When you become focused on Yvonne you scold her a lot. I can tell that you are very concerned about your daughter's nutrition, and obviously she is doing really well with that.' If I have to say something negative, I will also say 'I couldn't help but notice that you scolded her.' I try to balance a negative remark with a positive one; for example, 'Your house is very clean, or your daughter is so spirited and alert today.' I make a conscious effort to look for the good [strengths] in the person and not to forget to share this information with her."

Key Summary Points

- Working with strengths requires that the nurse develop a broad repertoire of approaches and techniques.
- These approaches need to be congruent with the nurse's values (see Chapter 3) and derive from knowledge of the characteristics of strengths (see Chapter 4).

- SBC requires that the nurse create facilitative, supportive, and safe environments that maximize the goodness of fit between the person and the environment to allow for health and healing.
- In caring for patients and helping them deal with their problems or concerns, nurses work with existing strengths and help to develop new ones.
- There are specific approaches to working with existing strengths.
- In helping a person to develop his unique strengths, nurses can turn potentials into strengths, turn a deficit or weakness into a strength, and minimize or contain a weakness to allow a strength to shine through by using a wide range of techniques. These approaches derive from knowledge from the biological, social, medical, and nursing sciences.

References

Abdellah, F. G. (1960). *Patient-centered approaches to nursing.* New York, NY: MacMillan Publishers.

Adam, E. (1991). *To be a nurse* (2nd ed.). Toronto, Canada: W.B. Saunders.

Aiken, L. H., Clarke, S. P., Sloane, D. M., Lake, E. T., & Cheney, T. (2008). Effects of hospital care environment on patient mortality and nurse outcomes. *The Journal of Nursing Administration, 38*(5), 223–229.

Aiken, L. H., Clarke, S. P., Sloane, D. M., Sochalski, J. A., & Silber, J. H. (2002). Hospital nurse staffing and patient mortality, nurse burnout, and job dissatisfaction. *JAMA, 288*(16), 1987–1993.

Aiken, L. H., Clarke, S. P., Sloane, D. M., Sochalski, J. A., Busse, R., Clarke, H.,...Shamian, J. (2001). Nurses' reports on hospital care in five countries. *Health Affairs, 20*(4), 43–56.

Aldwin, C. M. (2007). *Stress, coping, and development: An integrative perspective* (2nd ed.) New York, NY: Guilford Press.

Allen, D. (1998). Record-keeping and routine nursing practice: The view from the wards. *Journal of Advanced Nursing, 27,* 1223–1230.

Allen, M. (1977). Comparative theories of the expanded role in nursing and its implications for nursing practice: A working paper. *Nursing Papers, 9*(2), 38–45.

Allen, M. (1981). The health dimension in nursing practice: Notes on nursing in primary health care. *Journal of Advanced Nursing, 6*(2), 153–154.

American Nurses Association. (2010). *ANA's principles of nursing documentation: Guidance for registered nurses.* Silver Spring, MD: American Nurses Association.

Anderson, J. R., Reder, L. M., & Simon, H. A. (1996). Situated learning and education. *Educational Researcher, 25*(4), 5–11.

Aranda, S., & Brown, R. (2006). Nurses must be clever to care. In S. Nelson & S. Gordon (Eds.), *The complexities of care: Nursing reconsidered* (pp. 122–142). Ithica, NY: Cornell University Press.

Arctander, S. (1961). *Arctander's perfumed and flavor materials of natural origin.* Carol Stream, IL: Allured Books.

Arnett, J. J., & Tanner, J. L. (2009). Toward a cultural-developmental stage theory of the life course. In K. McCartney & R. A. Weinberg (Eds.), *Experience and development: A festschrift in honor of Sandra Wood Scarr* (pp. 17–38). New York, NY: APS Psychology Press.

Arnold, E. C., & Boggs K. U. (2006). *Interpersonal relationships: Professional communication skills for nurses.* (5th ed.). Philadelphia, PA: Saunders.

Atkins, S., & Murphy, K. (1993). Reflection: A review of the literature. *Journal of Advanced Nursing, 18*(8), 1188–1192.

Atkinson, S., Macnaughton, J., Saunders, C., & Evans, M. (2010). Cool intimacies of care for contemporary clinical practice. *The Lancet, 376*(9754), 1732–1733.

Audy, J. R. (1971). Measurement and diagnosis of health. In P. Shepard & D. McKinley (Eds.), *Environmental essays on the planet as a home* (pp. 140–157). Boston, MA: Houghton Mifflin.

Baker, G. R., Norton, P. G., Flintoft, V., Blais, R., Brown, A., Cox, J.,...Tamblyn, R. (2004). The Canadian adverse events study: The incidence of adverse events among hospital patients in Canada. *Canadian Medical Association Journal, 170*, 1678–1683.

Balcetus, E., & Dunning, D. (2006). See what you want to see: Motivational influences on visual perceptions. *Journal of Personality and Social Psychology, 91*(4), 612–625.

Bandura, A. (1997). *Self-efficacy: The exercise of control.* New York, NY: W.H. Freeman.

Barnard, A. (2009). Vision, technology, and the environment of care. In R. C. Locsin & M. J. Purnell (Eds.), *A contemporary nursing process: The (un)bearable weight of knowing in nursing* (pp. 357–376). New York, NY: Springer Publishing Company.

Barnard, K. E., Sumner, G., & Spietz, A. (1990). *Keys to caregiving.* University of Washington, School of Nursing: NCAST.

Barnes, E. (1961). *People in hospital.* London, UK: MacMillan.

Barry, C. D., & Gordon, S. C. (2009). Coming to know the community: Going to the mountain. In R. C. Locsin & M. J. Purnell (Eds.), *A contemporary nursing process: The (unbearable) weight of knowing in nursing* (pp. 431–444). New York, NY: Springer Publishing.

Batson, C. D., Ahmad, N., Lishner, D. A., & Tsang, J. (2002). Empathy and altruism. In C. R. Snyder, & S. J. Lopez (Eds.), *Handbook of positive psychology* (pp. 485–498). New York, NY: Oxford University Press.

Beauchemin, K. M., & Hays, P. (1996). Sunny hospital rooms expedite recovery from severe and refractory depressions. *Journal of Affective Disorders, 40*(1–2), 49–51.

Benner, P. (1984). *From novice to expert: Excellence and power in clinical nursing.* Menlo Park, CA: Addison-Wesley Publishing.

Benner, P. (1991). The role of experience, narrative, and community in skilled ethical comportment. *Advances in Nursing Science, 14*(2), 1–21.

Benner, P. (2003). Enhancing patient advocacy and social ethics. *American Journal of Critical Care, 12*(4), 374–375.

Benner, P. (2011). Formation in professional education: An examination of the relationship between theories of meaning and theories of self. *The Journal of Medicine and Philosophy, 36*, 1–12.

Benner, P., & Gordon, S. (1996). Caring practice. In S. Gordon, P. Benner, & N. Noddings (Eds.), *Caregiving: Readings in knowledge, practice, ethics, and politics* (pp. 40–55). Philadelphia, PA: University of Pennsylvannia Press.

Benner, P., Hooper-Kyriakidis, P., & Stannard, D. (2011). *Clinical wisdom and interventions in acute and critical care: A thinking-in-action approach* (2nd ed.). New York, NY: Springer Publishing Company.

Benner, P., Sutphen, M., Leonard, V., & Day, L. (2010). *Educating nurses: A call for radical transformation.* San Francisco, CA: Jossey-Bass.

Benner, P., Tanner, C. A., & Chesla, C. A. (1996). *Expertise in nursing practice: Caring, clinical judgment and ethics.* New York, NY: Springer Publishing Company.

Benner, P., & Wrubel, J. (1989). *The primacy of caring: Stress and coping in health and illness.* Menlo Park, CA: Addison-Wesley Publishing Company.

Benoleil, J. Q. (1987). Response to: Toward a holistic inquiry in nursing: A proposal for synthesis of patterns and methods. *Scholarly Inquiry for Nursing Practice: An International Journal, 1*(2), 147–152.

Berger, J. (1972). *The way of seeing*. London, UK: BBC and Penguin.

Berk, L. E. (2010). *Development through the lifespan* (5th ed.). Boston, MA: Allyn & Bacon.

Berkman, B., & D'Ambruoso, S. (2006). *Handbook of social work in health and aging*. New York, NY: Oxford University Press.

Bjork, R. A. (2011). On the symbiosis of remembering, forgetting, and learning. In A. S. Benjamin (Ed.), *Successful remembering and successful forgetting: A festschrift in honor of Robert A. Bjork* (pp. 1–22). New York, NY: Psychology Press (Taylor & Francis Group).

Bland, A. J., Topping, A., & Wood, B. (2011). A concept analysis of simulation as a learning strategy in the education of undergraduate nursing students. *Nursing Education Today, 31*, 664–670.

Blows, W. T. (2001). *The biological basis for nursing: Clinical Observations*. New York, NY: Routledge.

Bluvol, A., & Ford-Gilboe, M. (2004). Hope, health work and quality of life in families of stroke survivors. *Journal of Advanced Nursing, 48*(4), 322–332.

Borton, T. (1970). *Reach, touch and teach: Student concerns and process education*. New York, NY: McGraw Hill.

Bouchard, T. J. (2009). Strong inference: A strategy for advancing psychological science. In K. McCartney & R. A. Weinberg (Eds.), *Experience and development: A festschrift in honor of Sandra Wood Scarr* (pp. 39–59). New York, NY: APS Psychology Press.

Boyle, E., Al-Akash, M., Gallagher, A. G., Traynor, O., Hill, A. D., & Neary, P. C. (2011). Optimising surgical training: Use of feedback to reduce errors during a simulated surgical procedure. *Postgraduate Medical Journal, 87*, 524–528.

Bronfenbrenner, U. (1979). *The ecology of human development: Experiments by nature and design*. Cambridge, MA: Harvard University Press.

Brooks, D. (2009, November 10). The rush to therapy. *New York Times*, pp. A35.

Brown, J. (1997). Circular questioning: An introductory guide. *Australian & New Zealand Journal of Family Therapy, 18*(2), 109–114.

Bull, M. J. (1990). Factors influencing family caregiver burden and health. *Western Journal of Nursing Research, 12*(6), 758–776.

Buresh, B., & Gordon, S. (2006). *From silence to voice: What nurses know and must communicate to the public* (2nd ed.). Ithaca, NY: ILR.

Burnell, L. (2009). Compassionate care: A concept analysis. *Home Health Care, Management, and Practice, 21*(5), 319–324.

Burroughs, J., & Hoffbrand, B. I. (1990). A critical look at nursing observations. *Postgraduate Medical Education, 66*, 370–372.

Byrne, J. P. (2007). Some ways in which neuroscientific research can be relevant to education. In D. Coch, K. W. Fisher, & G. Dawson (Eds.), *Human behavior, learning and the developing brain: A typical development* (pp. 30–49). New York, NY: Guilford Press.

Canadian Nurses Asssociation. (2005). *Rehabilitation nursing certification*. Ottawa, Canada: Canadian Nurses Association.

Caplan, T. (2008). *Needs ABC: Acquisition and behavior change: A model for group work and other psychotherapies*. London, UK: Whiting and Birch.

Carnevale, F. A. (1995). Nursing and the body. *Canadian Journal of Nursing Research, 27*(4), 89–93.

Carpenter, J. (1995). Doctors and nurses: Stereotypes and stereotype change in interprofessional education. *Journal of Interprofessional Care, 9*(2), 151–161.

Carver, C. S., & Scheier, M. F. (2002). Optimism. In S. J. Snyder & C. R. Lopez (Eds.), *Handbook of positive psychology* (pp. 231–243). New York, NY: Oxford Press.

Casamayou, M. H. (2001). *The politics of breast cancer.* Washington, DC: Georgetown University Press.

Casey, B. J., Tottenham, N., Liston, C., & Durston, S. (2005). Imaging the developing brain: What have we learned from cognitive development? *Trends in Cognitive Science, 9,* 104–110.

Cassell, E. J. (2002). Compassion. In C. R. Snyder & S. J. Lopez (Eds.), *Handbook of positive psychology* (pp. 434–445). New York, NY: Oxford University Press.

Chamberlin, J. (1997). A working definition of empowerment. *Psychiatric Rehabilitation Journal, 20*(4), 43–46.

Charon, R. (2001). Narrative medicine: A model for empathy, reflection, profession, and trust. *JAMA, 286*(15), 1897–1902.

Chechik, G., Meilijson, I., & Ruppin, E. (1999). Neuronal regulation: A mechanism for synaptic pruning during brain maturation. *Neural Computation, 11*(8), 2061–2080.

Cheevakasemsook, A., Chapman, Y., Francis, K., & Davies, C. (2006). The study of nursing documentation complexities. *International Journal of Nursing Practice, 12*(6), 366–374.

Chen, H. (2001). Parents' attitudes and expectations regarding science education: Comparisons among Chinese, Chinese-American, and American families. *Adolescence, 36*(142), 305–313.

Chen, P. W. (2009, February 1). When doctors and nurses can't do the right thing. *New York Times.* Retrieved from www.nytimes.com/2009/02/06/health/05chen.html

Chess, S., & Thomas, A. (1996). *Temperament: Theory and practice.* New York, NY: Brunner/ Mazel Publishers.

Chklovskii, D. B., Mel, B. W., & Svoboda, K. (2004). Cortical rewiring and information storage. *Nature, 431,* 782–788.

Chu-Hui-Lin-Chi, G. (2007). The role of hope in patients with cancer. *Oncology Nursing Forum, 34*(2), 415–424.

Clarke, S. P., & Aiken, L. H. (2003). Failure to rescue: Needless deaths are prime examples of the need for more nurses at the bedside. *American Journal of Nursing, 103*(1), 42–47.

Clifton, D. O., & Harter, J. K. (2003). Strengths investment. In K. S. Cameron, J. E. Dutton, & R. E. Quinn (Eds.), *Positive organizational scholarship: Foundation of a new discipline* (pp. 111–121). San Francisco, CA: Berett-Koehler.

Cmiel, C. A., Karr, D. M., Gasser, D. M., Oliphant, L. M., & Neveau, A. J. (2004). Noise control: A nursing team's approach to sleep promotion. *American Journal of Nursing, 104*(2), 40–48.

Cody, W. K. (1994). Nursing theory-guided practice: What it is and what it is not. *Nursing Science Quarterly, 7*(4), 144–145.

Cody, W. K. (2006). Values based practice and evidence based practice: Pursuing fundamental questions in nursing philosophy and theory. In W. K. Cody (Ed.), *Philosophical and theoretical perspectives for advanced nursing practice.* (4th ed., pp. 5–12). Sudbury, MA: Jones and Bartlett Publishers.

Collins, J. W. (2007). The neuroscience of learning. *Journal Neuroscience Nursing, 39*(5), 305–310.

College and Association of Registered Nurses of Alberta. (2006). *CARNA-documentation guidelines for documentation.* Edmonton, AB: CARNA.

College of Nurses of Ontario (CNO-OIIO). (2008). *The standard of care: Documentation revised.* Ontario, Canada: CNO.

College of Registered Nurses of British Columbia. (2009). *CRNBC-Nursing documentation* (practice support, publication no. 334). Vancouver, BC: CRNBC.

College of Registered Nurses of Nova Scotia. (2005). *CRNNS-documentation guidelines for registered nurses.* Halifax, NS: CRNNS.

Cowling, W. R. (2000). Healing as appreciating wholeness. *Advances in Nursing Science, 22*(3), 16–32.

Coyle, D. (2009). *The talent code: Greatness isn't born. It's grown. Here's how.* New York, NY: Bantam Books.

Cozolino, L. (2006). *The neuroscience of human relationships: Attachment and the developing social brain.* New York, NY: W.W. Norton and Company.

D'Antonio, P., & Fairman, J. (2004). Organizing practice: Nursing, the medical model, and two case studies in historical time. *Canadian Bulletin of Medical History, 21*(2), 411–429.

D'Antonio, P., & Lewenson, S. (2010). *Nursing interventions through time: History as evidence.* New York, NY: Springer Publishing Company.

Dahnke, M. D., & Dreher, H. M. (2011). *Philosophy of science for nursing practice: Concepts and applications.* New York, NY: Springer Publishing Company.

Dalton, C., & Gottlieb, L. N. (2003). The concept of readiness to change. *Journal of Advanced Nursing, 42*(2), 108–117.

Davidson, R. J., Kabat-Zinn, J., Schumacher, J., Rosenkranz, M., Muller, D., Santorelli, S. F.,... Sheridan, J. F. (2003). Alterations in brain and immune function produced by mindfulness meditation. *Psychosomatic Medicine, 65*(4), 564–570.

Davys, D., & Jones, V. (2007). Peer observation: A tool for continuing professional development. *International Journal of Therapy and Rehabilitation, 14*(11), 489–493.

De Quincey, C. (2005). *Radical knowing: Understanding consciousness through relationships.* Rochester, VT: Park Street Press.

de Raeve, L. (2002). Trust and trustworthiness in nurse-patient relationships. *Nursing Philosophy, 3*(2), 152–162.

de Vries, K. (2004). Humility and its practice in nursing. *Nursing Ethics, 11*(6), 577–586.

Deater-Deckard, K. (2009). Parenting the genotype. In K. McCartney & R. A. Weinberg (Eds.), *Experience and development: A festschrift in honor of Sandra Wood Scarr* (pp. 141–161). New York, NY: APS Psychology Press.

Deci, E. L., & Ryan, R. M. (1985). *Intrinsic motivation and self-determination in human behavior.* New York, NY: Plenum.

Demarais, A., & White, V. (2005). *First impressions: What you don't know about how others see you.* New York, NY: Bantam Books.

Devlin, A. M., Cross, J. H., Harkness, W., Chong, W. K., Harding, B., Vargha-Khadem, F., & Neville, B. G. R. (2003). Clinical outcomes of hemispherectomy for epilepsy in childhood and adolescence. *Brain, 126*, 556–566.

Dickert, N. W., & Kass, N. E. (2009). Understanding respect: Learning from patients. *Journal of Medical Ethics, 35*(7), 419–423.

Doidge, N. (2007). *The brain that changes itself: Stories of personal triumph from the frontiers of brain science.* Toronto, Canada: Penguin.

Donahue, M. P. (2011). *Nursing the finest art: An illustrated history* (3rd ed.). New York, NY: Mosby-Elsevier.

Doona, M. E., Chase, S. K., & Haggerty, L. A. (1999). Nursing presence: As real as a Milky Way Bar. *Journal of Holistic Nursing, 17*(1), 54–70.

Dossey, B. M. (1995). Nurse as healer. In B. M. Dossey, L. Keegan, C. E. Guzetta, & L. G. Kolkmeir (Eds.), *Holistic nursing: A handbook for practice* (pp. 61–83). Gaithersberg, MD: Aspen Publisher.

Dossey, B. M., Selnaders, L. C., & Beck, D. M. (2005). Florence Nightingale today: Healing leadership and global action. Silver Spring, MD: American Nurses Association.

Dowie, J. (1993). Would decision analysis eliminate accidents? In C. Vincent, M. Ennis, & R. J. Audley (Eds.), *Medical Accidents* (pp. 116–130). Oxford, UK: Oxford University Press.

Dreyfus, H., Dreyfus, S., & Benner, P. (2009). Implications of the phenomenology of expertise in teaching and learning everyday skillful ethical comportment. In P. Benner & C. Tanner (Eds.), *Expertise in nursing practice, caring, clinical judgment, and ethics* (2nd ed., pp. 309–333). New York, NY: Springer Publishing.

Dreyfus, H. L., & Dreyfus, S. E. (1996). The relationship of theory and practice in the acquisition of skill. In P. Benner, C. A. Tanner, & C. A. Chesla. *Expertise in nursing practice: Caring, clinical judgment, & ethics.* New York, NY: Springer Publishing.

Dunn, J., & Plomin, R. (1990). *Separate lives: Why siblings are so different.* New York, NY: Basic Books.

Dunphy, L. M. (2009). With the very best of intentions: The development of the nursing process as a way of knowing. In R. C. Locsin & M. J. Purnell (Eds.), *A contemporary nursing process: The (un)bearable weight of knowing in nursing* (pp. 31–60). New York, NY: Springer Publishing.

Edgar, L. (2010). *Mastering the art of coping in good times and bad.* Vineland, Canada: Linda Edgar.

Egan, G. (2002). *The skilled helper: A problem-management and opportunity-development approach to helping.* Pacific Grove, CA: Brooks/Cole Publisher.

Egnew, T. R. (2005). The meaning of healing: Transcending suffering. *Annals of Family Medicine, 3*(2), 255–262.

Eliasson, M., Kainz, G., & von Post, I. (2008). Uncaring midwives. *Nursing Ethics, 15*(4), 500–511.

Ellefson, B., Kim, H. S., & Han, K. J. (2007). Nursing gaze framework for nursing practice: A study of acute care settings in Korea, Norway, and the USA. *Scandinavian Journal Caring, 21*(1), 98–105.

Elliot, A. J., & Dweck, C. S. (2005). Handbook of competence and motivation: Competence as the core of achievement motivation. In A. J. Elliot & C. S. Dweck (Eds.), *Handbook of competence and motivation* (pp. 3–12). New York, NY: Guilford Press.

Epp, J. (1986). *Achieving health for all: A framework for health promotion.* Ottawa, Canada: Health and Welfare Canada. Retrieved from www.hc-sc.gc.ca/hcs-sss/pubs/system-regime/1986-frame-plan-promotion/index-eng.php

Erikson, E. (1959). *Identity and the life cycle.* New York, NY: W.W. Norton.

Estabrooks, C. (1998). Will evidence-based practice make nursing perfect. *CJNR, 30*(4), 15–36.

Estabrooks, C. A., Rutakumwa, W., O'Leary, K. A., Profetto-McGrath, J., Milner, M., Levers, M. J., & Scott-Findlay. S. (2005). Sources of knowledge among practice nurses. *Qualitative Health Research, 15*(4), 460–476.

Ezer, H., Bray, C., & Gros, C. P. (1997). Families' description of the nursing intervention in a randomized control trial. In L. N. Gottlieb & H. Ezer (Eds.), *A perspective on health, family, learning, and collaborative nursing: A collection of writings on the McGill Model of Nursing* (pp. 371–376). Montreal, Canada: McGill University School of Nursing.

Fagermoen, M. S. (1997). Professional identity: Values embedded in meaningful nursing practice. *Journal of Advanced Nursing, 25*(3), 434–441.

Fawcett, J. (1984). The metaparadigm of nursing: Present status and future refinements. *Journal of Nursing Scholarship (Image), 16*(3), 77–87.

Fawcett, J. (2006). The state of nursing science: Hallmarks of the 20th and 21st centuries. In W. K. Cody (Ed.), *Philosophical and theoretical perspectives for advanced nursing practice* (4th ed., pp. 51–57). Sudbury, MA: Jones and Bartlett Publishers.

Feeley, N., & Gottlieb, L. N. (2000). Nursing approaches to working with family strengths and resources. *Journal of Family Nursing, 6*(1), 9–23.

Fenker, D., & Schutze, H. (2009). Novelty enhances memory. *Scientific American Mind, 19*(6), 47.

Ferrell, K. G. (2007). Documentation, Part 2: The best evidence of care. *American Journal of Nursing, 107*(7), 61–64.

Fine, S. B. (1991). Resilience and human adaptability: Who rises above adversity? *The American Journal of Occupational Therapy, 45*(6), 493–503.

Finfgeld-Connett, D. (2008). Qualitative comparison and synthesis of nursing presence and caring. *International Journal of Nursing Terminologies and Classifications, 19*(3), 111–119.

Finn, C. K. (2008). *Forensic nurses: Experience of receiving child abuse disclosures* (Doctoral dissertation). Denver, CO: University of Colorado Health Sciences Center.

Fontaine, D. K., Briggs, L. P., & Pope-Smith, B. (2001). Designing humanistic critical care environments. *Critical Care Nursing Quarterly, 24*(3), 21–34.

Ford-Gilboe, M. (2000). Dispelling myths and creating opportunity: A comparison of the strengths of single-parent and two-parent families. *Advances in Nursing Science, 23*(1), 41–58.

Foucault, M. (1973). *The birth of the clinic.* London, UK: Tavistock Publications.

Fraga, M. F., Ballestar, E., Paz, M. F., Ropero, F., Setien, M. L., Ballestar, D.,…Esteller, M. (2005). Epigenetic differences arisen during the lifetime of monozygotic twins. *Proceedings of the National Academy of Sciences of USA, 102,* 10604–10609.

Frank, A. W. (1998). Just listening: Narrative and deep illness. *Families, Systems, and Health, 16*(3), 197–212.

Frank, A. W. (2002). *At the will of the body: Reflections on illness.* New York, NY: Houghton Mifflin.

Frank, A. W. (2004). *The renewal of generosity: Illness, medicine, and how to live.* Chicago, IL: University of Chicago Press.

Fredrickson, B. L. (2000). Cultivating positive emotions to optimize health and well-being. *Prevention & Treatment, 3,* Article 0001a, posted March 7, 2000.

Fredrickson, B. L. (2008). Promoting positive affect. In M. Eid & R. J. Larsen (Eds.), *The science of subjective well-being* (pp. 449–468). New York, NY: Guilford Press.

Friedman, M. M., Bowden, V. R., & Jones, E. G. (2003). *Family nursing: Research, theory and practice.* Upper Saddle River, NJ: Prentice-Hall.

Gadow, S. A. (1990). Truth-telling revisited: Two approaches to the disclosure dilemma. In M. M. Leininger (Ed.), *Ethical and moral dimensions of care* (pp. 33–38). Detroit, MI: Wayne State University Press.

Gallup's annual honesty and ethics poll (November, 2008). Retrieved from www.gallup.com

Gardner, H. (1999) *Intelligence reframed. Multiple intelligences for the 21st century,* New York, NY: Basic Books.

Gates, M. G., Parr, M. B., & Hughen, J. E. (2011). Enhancing nursing knowledge using high-fidelity simulation. *Journal of Nursing Education 50*(11), 603–604. doi: 10.3928/01484834-20111116-01

Ge, S., Yang, C., Hsu, K., Ming, G., & Song, H. (2007). A critical period for enhanced synaptic plasticity in newly generated neurons of the adult brain. *Neuron, 54,* 559–566.

Germer, C. K. (2009). *The mindful path to self-compassion.* New York, NY: Guilford Press.

Gibson, C. H. (1991). A concept analysis of empowerment. *Journal of Advanced Nursing, 16*(3), 354–361.

Gladwell, M. (2008). *Outliers: The making of success.* New York, NY: Little, Brown and Company.

Goleman, D. (1995). *Emotional intelligence: Why it can matter more than IQ.* New York, NY: Bantam Dell Publication Group.

Goleman, D. (2006). *Social intelligence: The new science of human relationships.* New York, NY: Random House.

Goodnow, J. J. (2010). Culture. In M. H. Bornstein (Ed.), *Handbook of cultural developmental science* (pp. 3–19). New York, NY: Psychology Press.

Gordon, S. (1996). *Life support: Three nurses on the front lines.* Boston, MA: Little, Brown & Company.

Gordon, S., Benner, P., & Nodding, N. (1996). *Caregiving: Readings in knowledge, practice, ethics, and politics.* Philadelphia, PA: University of Pennsylvania Press.

Gordon, S., & Nelson, S. (2006). Moving beyond the virtue script in nursing. In S. Nelson & S. Gordon (Eds.), *The complexities of care: Nursing reconsidered* (pp. 13–29). Ithica, NY: Cornell University Press.

Gottlieb, L. N. (1982). Health promoters: Two contrasting styles in community nursing. In L. N. Gottlieb & H. Ezer (Ed.), *A perspective on health, family, learning, & collaborative nursing: A collection of writings on the McGill Model of Nursing* (pp. 87–100). Montreal, Canada: McGill University, School of Nursing.

Gottlieb, L. N., & Carnaghan-Sherrard, K. (2004). *Developing family mindedness within the McGill Model of Nursing: A guide to nursing the family.* First published in Japanese for an edited book on family nursing, Tokyo: Kazoku Kango. Copy available in English. Montreal, Canada: School of Nursing, McGill University.

Gottlieb, L. N., & Ezer, H. (1997). *A perspective on health, family, learning, and collaborative nursing: A collection of writings on the McGill Model of Nursing.* Montreal, Canada: McGill University School of Nursing.

Gottlieb, L. N., & Feeley, N. (1999). Nursing intervention studies: Issues related to change and timing. In M. Stewart (Ed.), *Community nursing: Promoting Canadians' health* (2nd ed.). Toronto, Canada: W.B. Saunders.

Gottlieb, L. N., & Feeley, N. with Dalton, C. (2006). *The collaborative partnership approach to care: A delicate balance.* Toronto, Canada: Elsevier-Mosby.

Gottlieb, L. N., & Gottlieb, B. (1998). Evolutionary principles can guide nursing's future development. *Journal of Advanced Nursing, 28*(5), 1099–1105.

Gottlieb, L. N., & Gottlieb, B. (2007). The developmental/health framework within the McGill model of nursing: "Laws of Nature" guiding whole person care. *Advances in Nursing Science, 30*(1), E43–E57.

Gottlieb, L. N., Lang, A., & Amsel, R. (1996). The long-term effects of grief on marital intimacy following infant death. *Omega: International journal for the study of death and dying, 33*, 1–19.

Gottlieb, L. N., & Rowat, K. (1987). The McGill model of nursing: A practice-derived model. *Advances in Nursing Science, 9*(4), 51–61.

Greenwood, J. (1998). The role of reflection in single and double loop learning. *Journal of Advanced Nursing, 27*, 1048–1053.

Gros, C., Jarvis, S., Mulvogue, T., & Renaud, J. (August 26, 2011). Nursing patients at risk for suicide: Adolescents' perceptions of "helpful" interventions. Presented at *Reseau de Quebecoise Recherche Sur Le Suicide*, Montreal, Canada.

Grossman, M. (2011). Whole person care and complementary and alternative therapies. In T.A. Hutchison (Ed.), *Whole person care: A new paradigm for the 21st century* (pp. 133–147). New York, NY: Springer.

Hagerty, B. M., & Patusky, K. L. (2003). Reconceptualizing the nurse-patient relationship. *Journal of Nursing Scholarship, 35*(2), 145–150.

Hallett, C. (2007). Editorial: A 'gallop' through history: Nursing in social context. *Journal of Clinical Nursing, 16*(3), 429–430.

Hames, C. C., & Joseph, D. H. (1980). *Basic concepts of helping: A holistic approach*. New York, NY: Appleton-Century Croft.

Harmer, B. (1922). *Textbook of the principles and practice of nursing*. New York, NY: MacMillan.

Harris, J. (1998). *The nurture assumption*. New York, NY: Free Press.

Harris, J. R. (2006). *No two alike: Human nature and human individuality*. New York, NY: W.W. Norton & Company.

Health Canada. (1997). *Supporting self-care*. Ottawa, Canada: Health and Welfare Canada.

Hebb, D. O. (1966). *A textbook of psychology* (2nd ed.). Philadelphia, PA: W.B. Saunders Company.

Helman, C. (2007). *Culture, health, and illness: An introduction of health professionals* (5th ed.). London, UK: Hodder Arnold.

Henderson, J. (2011). The physical exam and society's regard for physicians: A history. *The Health Culture*. Retrieved from www.thehealthculture.com/2011/01/the-physical-exam-and-societys-regard-for-physicians-a-history

Hendricks, C. S., Hendricks, S. J., Webb, S. J., Bonner-Davis, J., & Spencer-Morgan, B. (2005). Fostering self-efficacy as an ethical mandate in health promotion practice and research. *Online Journal of Health Ethics, 2*(1).

Hill, A. (1997). The promotion of a healing environment for the preterm infant: A utilization model. In P. B. Kritek (Ed.), *Reflections on healing: A central nursing construct* (pp. 287–293). New York, NY: WLW Press.

Hodges, T. D., & Clifton, D. O. (2004). Strengths-based development in practice. In P. A. Linley & S. Joseph (Eds.), *Positive psychology in practice* (pp. 256–268). Hoboken, NJ: John Wiley & Sons.

Howell, J. D. (2001). A history of caring in medicine. In L. F. Cluff & R. H. Binstock (Eds.), *The lost art of caring: A challenge to health professionals, families, communities, and society* (pp. 77–104). Baltimore, MD: Johns Hopkins University Press.

Hubble, M. A., & Miller, S. D. (2004). The client: Psychotherapy's missing link for promoting a positive psychology. In P. A. Linley & S. Joseph (Eds.), *Positive psychology in practice* (pp. 335–353). Hoboken, NJ: John Wiley & Sons.

Hutchison, T. A. (2011). *Whole person care: A new paradigm for the 21st century*. New York, NY: Springer.

Ignatieff, M. (2000). *The rights revolution*. Toronto, Canada: House of Anansi Press.

Insel, T. (2011, February 10). How does memory work? The plot thickens. *Director's Blog of National Institute of Mental Health*. Retrieved from www.nimh.nih.gov/about/director/2011/how-does-memory-work-the-plot-thickens.shtml

Kramer, G., Melco-Meyer, F., & Turner, M. L. (2008). Cultivating mindfulness in relationship: Insight dialogue and the interpersonal mindfulness program. In S. F. Hick & T. Bein (Eds.), *Mindfulness and the therapeutic relationship*. New York, NY: Guilford Press.

IOM. (2010). *The future of nursing: Leading change, advancing health*. Washington, DC: Institute of Medicine.

Ironside, P. M. (2003). New pedagogies for teaching thinking: The lived experiences of students and teachers in enacting the narrative pedagogy. *Journal of Nursing Education, 42*(11), 509–516.

Ironside, P. M. (2006). Reforming nursing education using narrative pedagogy: Learning and practicing interpretive thinking. *Journal of Advanced Nursing, 55*, 478–486.

Jacelon, C. S. (1997). The trait and process of resiliency. *Journal of Advanced Nursing, 25*(1), 123–129.

Jacobs, P., & Rapport, J. (2004). *The economics of health and medical care* (5th ed.) Boston, MA: Jones & Bartlett Publishers.

Jansson, A., Petersson, K., & Uden, G. (2001). Nurses' first encounters with parents of new-born children public health nurses' views of a good meeting. *Journal of Clinical Nursing, 10*(1), 140–151.

Jasper, M. (2003). *Beginning reflective practice*. Cheltenham, UK: Nelson Thornes Ltd.

Jha, A. K., Orav, E. J., Zheng, J., & Epstein, A. M. (2008). Patients' perception of hospital care in the United States. *The New England Journal of Medicine, 359*(18), 1921–1931.

Johansen-Berg, H. (2006). Structural plasticity: Rewiring the brain. *Current Biology, 17*, R141–R144.

Johnson, J. L. (1994). A dialectical examination of nursing art. *Advances in Nursing Science, 17*(1), 1–14.

Johnston, C. C., Stevens, B., Pinelli, J., Gibbons, S., Fillion, F., Jack, A., . . . Veilleux, A. (2003). Kangaroo care is effective in diminishing pain response in preterm neonates. *Archives of Pediatric Adolescent Medicine, 157*(11), 1084–1088.

Kabat-Zinn, J. (1994). *Wherever you go, there you are: Mindfulness meditation in everyday life*. New York, NY: Hyperion.

Kabat-Zinn, J. (2007). *Mindfulness with Jon Kabat-Zinn*. Retrieved October 25, 2009, from www.youtube.com/watch?v=3nwwKbM_vJc

Kachorek, L. V., Exline, J. J., Campbell, W. K., Baumeister, R. F., Joiner, T. E., & Krueger, J. I. (2004). Humility and modesty. In C. Peterson & M. E. P. Seligman (Eds.), *Character strengths and virtues: A handbook and classification* (pp. 461–475). New York, NY: Oxford University Press.

Kagan, J. (1989). Temperamental contributions to social behavior. *American Psychologist, 44*(4), 668–674.

Kagan, J., Reznick, J. S., & Gibbons, J. (1989). Inhibited and uninhibited types of children. *Child Development, 60*(4), 838–845.

Kalinovsky, A., Boukhtouche, F., Blazeski, R., Bornmann, C., Suzuki, N., Mason, C. A., & Scheiffele, P. (2011). Development of axon-target specificity of ponto-cerebellar afferents. *PLoS Biol, 9*, e1001013.

Kashdan, T. B. (2004). Curiosity. In C. Peterson & M. E. P. Seligman (Eds.), *Character strengths and virtues: A handbook and classification* (pp. 125–141). New York, NY: Oxford University Press.

Kawachi, I., & Berkman, L. F. (2003). *Neighborhoods and health*. New York, NY: Oxford University Press.

Keegan, L. (1995). Nutrition, exercise, and movement. In B. M. Dossey, L. Keegan, C. E. Guzzetta, & L. G. Kolkmeier (Eds.), *Holistic nursing: A handbook for practice* (pp. 257–288). Gaithersberg, MD: Aspen Publishers.

Keeling, A. W. (2010). Treating influenza 1918 and 2010: Recycled interventions. In P. D'Antonio & S. Lewenson (Eds.), *Nursing interventions through time: History as evidence* (pp. 31–41). New York, NY: Springer Publishing.

Keighley, T. (2006). From sickness to health. In S. Nelson & S. Gordon (Eds.), *The complexities of care: Nursing reconsidered* (pp. 88–103). Ithaca, NY: ILR Press.

Kickbusch, I. (1989). Self-care in health promotion. *Social Science and Medicine, 29*(2), 125–130.

Kim, H. S. (2010). *The nature of theoretical thinking in nursing* (3rd ed.). New York, NY: Springer Publishing.

King, L. A. (2008). Interventions for enhancing subjective well-being: Can we make people happier and should we? In M. Eid & R. J. Larsen (Eds.), *The science of subjective well-being* (pp. 431–448). New York, NY: Guilford Press.

Kisilevsky, B. S., Hains, S. M., Brown, C. A., Lee, C. T., Cowperthwaite, B., Stutzman, S. S.,...Wang, Z. (2009). Fetal sensitivity to properties of maternal speech and language. *Infant Behavior Development, 32*(1), 59–71.

Klausner, E. J., Snyder, C. R., & Cheavens, J. (2000). A hoped-based group treatment for depressed older adult outpatients. In G. M. Williamson, D. R. Shaffer, & P. A. Parmelee (Eds.), *Physical illness and depression in older adults: A handbook of theory, research, and practice* (pp. 295–310). New York, NY: Kluwer Academic/Plenum Publishers.

Kleinman, A., Eisenberg, L., & Good, B. (2006). Culture, illness, and care: Clinical lessons from anthropologic and cross-cultural research. *FOCUS: The Journal of Lifelong Learning in Psychiatry, 4*(1), 140–149.

Koerner, J. (2011). *Healing presence: The essence of nursing* (2nd ed.). New York, NY: Springer Publishing.

Kohn, L. T., Corrigan, J. M., & Donaldson, M. S. (2000). *To err is human: Building a safer health care system.* Washington, DC: Institute of Medicine, The National Academy Press.

Koopmeiners, L., Post-White, J., Gutknecht, S., Ceronsky, C., Nickelson, K., Drew, D.,...Kreitzer, M. (1997). How healthcare professionals contribute to hope in patients with cancer. *Oncology Nursing Forum, 24*(9), 1507–1513.

Kritek, P. B. (1997). Healing: A central nursing construct-reflections on meaning. In P. B. Kritek (Ed.), *Reflections on healing: A central nursing construct.* New York, NY: WLW Press.

Lakoff, G., & Johnson, M. (1980). *Metaphors we live by.* Chicago, IL: The University of Chicago Press.

Larsen, D., Edey, W., & LeMay, L. (2007). Understanding the role of hope in counselling: Exploring the intentional uses of hope. *Counselling Psychology Quarterly, 20*(4), 401–416.

Lawlor, L. C. (2003). Gazing anew: The shift from a clinical gaze to an ethnographic lens. *American Journal of Occupational Therapy, 57*(1), 29–39

Leddy, S. K. (2006). *Health promotion: Mobilizing strengths to enhance health, wellness, and wellbeing.* Philadelphia, PA: F.A. Davis.

Lee, S. H., Juang, Y. Y., Su, Y. J., Lee, H. L., Lin, Y. H., & Chao, C. C. (2005). Facing SARS: Psychological impacts on SARS team nurses and psychiatric services in a Taiwan general hospital. *General Hospital Psychiatry, 27*(5), 352–358.

Leiberman, M. D. (2000). Intuition: A social cognitive neuroscience approach. *Psychological Bulletin, 126*(1), 109–137.

Levine, M. E. (1973). *Introduction to clinical nursing.* Philadelphia, PA: F.A. Davis.

Levinson, D. (1987). *A guide to the clinical interview.* Philadelphia, PA: Saunders.

Levinson, W. R., Gorawara-Bhat, R., Dueck, R., Egener, B., Kao, A., Kerr, C.,...Kemp-White, M. (1999). Resolving disagreements in the patient-physician relationship: Tools for improving communication in managed care. *JAMA, 282*(15), 1477–1483.

Levitan, D. J. (2008). *The world in six songs: How the musical brain created human relations.* Toronto, Canada: Penguin Press.

Lewis, D. A., & Lieberman, J. A. (2000). Catching up on schizophrenia natural history and neurobiology *Neuron, 28*, 325–334.

Lewis, K., & Burd-Sharps, S. (2010). *The measure of America 2010–2011: Mapping risks and resilience.* New York, NY: New York University Press.

Lieberman, M. D. (2000). Intuition: A social cognitive neuroscience. *Psychological Bulletin, 126*(1), 109–137.

Liehr, P. R. & Smith, M. J. (2008). Story theory. In M. J. Smith & P. R. Liehr (Eds.), *Middle range theory for nursing* (2nd ed., pp. 205–224). New York, NY: Springer Publishing.

Lightman, L. R, Windle, R. J., Wood, S. A., Kershaw, Y. M., Shanks, N., & Ingram, C. D. (2001). Peri-partum plasticity within the hypothalamus-pituitary-adrenal axis. *Progress in Brain Research, 133*, 111–129.

Lloyd, L. F., & Dunn, L. R. (2007). Mind-body-spirit medicine: Interventions and resources. *Journal of the American Academy of Physicians Assistants, 20*(10), 31–35.

Locsin, R. C., & Purnell, M. J. (2009). *A contemporary nursing process: The (un) bearable weight of knowing in nursing.* New York, NY: Springer Publishing Company.

Lofman, P., Pietila, A., & Haggman-Laitila, A. (2007). Self-evaluation and peer review– an example of action research in promoting self-determination of patients with rheumatoid arthritis. *Journal of Clinical Nursing, 16*(2), 84–94.

Lopez, S. J., O'Bryne, K. K., & Peterson, S. (2003). Profiling courage. In S. J. Lopez & C. R. Snyder (Eds.), *Positive psychology assessment: A handbook of models and measures* (pp. 185–197). Washington, DC: American Psychological Association.

Luker, K. A, Austin, L., Caress, A, & Hallett, C. E. (2000). The importance of 'knowing the patient': community nurses' construction of quality in providing palliative care. *Journal of Advanced Nursing, 31*(4), 775–782.

Lynaugh, J. E., & Fagin, C. M. (1988). Nursing comes of age. *Image: Nursing Scholarship, 20*(4), 184–190.

Maddux, J. E. (2002a). Stopping the "madness": Positive psychology and the deconstruction of the illness ideology and the DSM. In C. R. Snyder & S. J. Lopez (Eds.), *Handbook of positive psychology* (pp. 13–25). New York, NY: Oxford University Press.

Maddux, J. E. (2002b). Self-efficacy: The power believing you can. In C. R. Snyder & S. J. Lopez (Eds.), *Handbook of positive psychology* (pp. 277–287). New York, NY: Oxford University Press.

Markel, H. (2008, January 1). When hospitals kept children from parents. *New York Times.* Retrieved from http://www.nytimes.com/2008/01/01/health/01visi.html

Marlier, L., & Schaal, B. (2005). Human newborns prefer human milk: Conspecific milk odor is attractive without postnatal exposure. *Child Development, 76*, 155–168.

Masten, A. S., & Coatsworth, J. D. (1998). The development of competence in favorable and unfavorable environments: Lessons from research on successful children. *American Psychologist, 53*(2), 205–220.

Masten, A. S., & Reed, M. (2002). Resilience in development. In C. R. Snyder & S. J. Lopez (Eds.), *Handbook of positive psychology* (pp. 74–88). New York, NY: Oxford University Press.

Masten, A. S., & Wright, M. O. (2010). Resilience over the lifespan: Developmental perspectives on resistance, recovery, and transformation. In J. W. Reich, A. J. Zautra, & J. S. Hall (Eds.), *Handbook of adult resilience* (pp. 211–237). New York, NY: Guilford Press.

Mattingly, C. (1998). *Healing dramas and clinical plots: The narrative structure of experience.* Cambridge, UK: Cambridge University Press.

Mayeroff, M. (1971). *On caring.* New York, NY: Harper-Row.

McAllister, M. (2003). Doing practice differently: Solution-focused nursing. *Journal of Advanced Nursing, 41*(6), 528–535.

McCaffery, R. (2009). Clinical knowing in advanced practice. In R. C. Locsin & M. J. Purnell (Eds.), *A contemporary nursing process: The (un) bearable weight of knowing in nursing* (pp. 329–365). New York, NY: Springer Publishing Company.

McCormack, B. (2003). Researching nursing practice: Does person-centeredness matter? *Nursing Philosophy, 4*(3), 179–188.

McDaniel, M. A., & Butler, A. C. (2011). A contextual framework for understanding when difficulties are desirable. In A. S. Benjamin (Ed.), *Successful remembering and successful forgetting: A festschrift in honor of Robert A. Bjork* (pp. 175–198). New York, NY: Psychology Press (Taylor and Francis Group).

MacDonald, L. (Ed.) (2008). *Florence Nightingale's suggestions for thought: collected works of Florence Nightingale, Volume 11.* Waterloo, Ontario: Wilfrid Laurier University Press.

McElligott, D. (2010). Healing: The journey from concept to nursing practice. *Journal of Holistic Nursing, 28*(4), 251–259.

McGinnis, J. M., Williams-Russo, P., & Knickman, J. R. (2002). The case for more active policy attention to health promotion. *Health Affairs, 21*(2), 78–93.

McGlynn, E. A., Asch, S. M., Adams, J., Keesey, J., Hicks, J., DeCristofaro, A., & Kerr, E. A. (2003). The quality of health care delivered to adults in the United States. *The New England Journal of Medicine, 348*(26), 2635–2645.

McKivergin, M., & Daubenmire, J. (1994). The healing process of presence. *Journal of Holistic Nursing, 12*(1), 64–81.

McLachlan, J. A. (2001). Environmental signaling: What embryos and evolution teach us about endocrine disrupting chemicals. *Endocrine Review, 22*(3), 319–341.

McNay Art Museum (2011, January 20,). *McNay Art Museum helps medical students improve observation skills.* Retrieved from www.mcnayart.org/index.php? option=com_content&view =article&id= 208%3Amcnay-art-museum-helps-ut-medical-students-improve-observation-skills&Itemid=188

McQueen, A. (2000). Nurse-patient relationships and partnership in hospital care. *Journal of Clinical Nursing, 9*, 723–731.

Meleis, A. (1997). *Theoretical nursing: Development and progress* (3rd ed.) Philadelphia, PA: Lippincott.

Meleis, A. I., Sawyer, L. M., Im, E. O, Hilfinger, M. D. K., & Schumacher, K. (2000). Experiencing transitions: An emerging middle range theory. *Advances in Nursing Science, 23*(1), 12–28.

Melzack, R. (2005). The McGill Pain Questionnaire: From description to measurement. *Anesthesiology, 103*(1), 199–202.

Metcalfe, J. (2011). Desirable difficulties and studying in the region of proximal learning. In A. S. Benjamin (Ed.), *Successful remembering and successful forgetting: A festschrift in honor of Robert A. Bjork* (pp. 259–276). New York, NY: Psychology Press (Taylor and Francis Group).

Miller, S., Wackman, D., Nunnally, E., & Miller, P. (1998). *Connecting with self and others.* Evergreen, CO: Interpersonal Communications Programs.

Miller, W. R., & Rollnick, S. (2002). *Motivational interviewing: Preparing people for change* (2nd ed.) New York, NY: Guilford Press

Minicucci, D. S., Schmitt, M. H., Dombeck, M. T., & Williams, G. C. (2003). Actualizing Gadow's moral framework for nursing through research. *Nursing Philosophy, 4*(2), 92–103.

Mintzberg, H. (2009). *Managing.* San Francisco, CA: Berrett-Koehler publications.

Monarch, K. (2007). Documentation, part I: Principles of self-protection. *American Journal of Nursing, 107*(7), 58–60.

Moore, P., Berman, K., Knight, M., & Devine, J. (1995). Constant observation: Implications for nursing practice. *Journal of Psychosocial Nursing Mental Health Service, 33*, 46–50.

Morse, J. M., & Mitcham, C. (1998). The experience of agonizing pain and the signals of disembodiment. *Journal of Psychosomatic Research, 44*(6), 667–680.

Mosby's medical dictionary (8th ed.). (2009). Toronto, Canada: Mosby/Elsevier Health Sciences.

Mount, B. (1993). Whole person care: Beyond psychosocial and physical needs. *The American Journal of Hospice and Palliative Care, 10*(1), 28–37.

Mount, B. M., Boston, P. H., & Cohen, S. R. (2007). Healing connections: On moving from suffering to a sense of well-being. *Journal of Pain and Symptom Management, 33*(4), 372–388.

Munhall, P. L. (2009). Unknowing: Towards the understanding of the multiple realities and manifold perceptions. In R. C. Locsin & M. J. Purnell. *A contemporary nursing process: The (unbearable) weight of knowing in nursing* (pp. 153–174). New York, NY: Springer Publishing.

Muraven, M., & Baumeister, R. F. (2000). Self-regulation and depletion of limited resources: Does self-control resemble a muscle? *Psychological Bulletin, 126*(2), 247–259.

Murphy, F., Taylor, G., & Townsend, J. (1997). Assessing and promoting families' readiness for change and growth. In L. N. Gottlieb & H. Ezer (Eds.), *A perspective on health, family, learning and collaborative nursing: A collection of writing on the McGill model of nursing* (pp. 365–370). Montreal, Canada: McGill University School of Nursing.

Murray, J. P., Wenger, A. F. Z, Downes, E. A., & Terrazas, S. B. (2011). *Educating professionals in low-resource countries: A global approach.* New York, NY: Springer Publishing Company.

National Institute of Health. (1998). *Cognitive rehabilitation.* Source: NIH Pub. No. 98–4315, Brain injury resource center. Seattle, WA. Retrieved from www.headinjury.com

Neff, K. (2003). Self-compassion: An alternative conceptualization of a healthy attitude toward oneself. *Self and Identity, 2*(2), 85–101.

Nelson, C. A. (2001). The development and neural bases of face recognition. *Infant and Child Development, 10*, 3–18.

Nelson, S., & Gordon, S. (2006). *The complexities of care: Nursing reconsidered.* Ithaca, NY: ILR Press.

Neufield, A., & Harrison, M. (2010). *Nursing family caregiving: Social Support and non-support.* New York, NY: Springer Publishing Company.

Newman, M. A. (2008). *Transforming presence: The difference that nursing makes.* Philadelphia, PA: F.A. Davis Company.

Nightingale, F. (1860). *Notes on nursing: What it is and what it is not.* London, UK: Harrison.

Nightingale, N. (n.d.). FinestQuotes.com. Retrieved on July 22, 2011, from www.finestquotes.com/author_quotes-author-Florence Nightingale page-0.htm

Nodding, N. (1996). The caring professional. In S. Gordon, P. Benner, & N. Nodding (Eds.), *Caregiving: Readings in knowledge, practice, ethics, and politics* (pp. 160–171). Philadelphia, PA: University of Pennsylvania Press.

Nordgren, S., & Fridlund, B. (2001). Patients' perceptions of self-determination as expressed in the context of care. *Journal of Advanced Nursing, 35*(1), 117–125.

Novak, J. D., & Canas, A. J. (2008). The theory underlying the use of concept maps and how to construct and use them. *Technical Report, IHMC CmapTools*, 1ñ36. Retrieved from www.ihmc.us

O'Regan, J. K., & Noe, A. (2001). What it is like to see: A sensorimotor theory of perceptual experience. *Synthese, 129*(1), 79–103.

Ohlen, J., & Segesten, K. (1998). The professional identity of the nurse: Concept analysis and development. *Journal of Advanced Nursing, 28*(4), 720–727.

Ohman, A. (2008). Fear and anxiety: Evolutionary, cognitive, and clinical perspectives. In M. Lewis & J. M. Haviland-Jones (Eds.), *Handbook of emotions* (2nd ed., pp. 573–593). New York, NY: Guilford Press.

Olds, D. L., Eckenrode, J., Henderson, C. R., Kitzman, H., Powers, J., Cole, R., . . . Luckey, D. (1997). Long-term effects of home visitation on maternal life course and child abuse and neglect. *JAMA, 278*(8), 637–643.

Orlando, I. J. (1961). *The dynamic nurse-patient relationship: Function, process and principles.* New York, NY: G.P. Putnam Sons.

Parse, R. R. (1999). Nursing science: The transformation of practice. *Journal of Advanced Nursing, 30*(6), 1383–1387.

Pearce, R. (2003). *Profiles and portfolios of evidence.* Cheltenham, UK: Nelson Thornes Ltd.

Peden-McAlpine, C., & Clark, N. (2002). Early recognition of client status changes: The importance of time. *Dimensions of Critical Care Nursing, 21*(4), 144–151.

Pellico, L. H., Friedlaender, L., & Fennie, K. P. (2009). Looking is not seeing: Using art to improve observational skills. *Journal of Nursing Education, 48*(11), 648–653.

Penfield, W. (1975). *The mystery of the mind: A critical study of consciousness and the human brain.* Princeton, NJ: Princeton University Press.

Peplau, H. (1952). *Interpersonal relations in nursing: A conceptual frame of reference for psychodynamic nursing.* New York, NY: Putnam.

Pesut, D. J. (1991). The art, science and techniques of reframing in psychiatric mental health nursing. *Issues in Mental Health Nursing, 12*(1), 9–18.

Peterson, C., & Seligman, M. E. P. (2004). *Character strengths and virtues: A handbook and classification.* New York, NY: Oxford University Press and Washington, DC: American Psychological Association.

Peterson, C., & Seligman, M. E. P. (2004a). Introduction: Strengths of courage. In C. Peterson & M. E. P. Seligman (Eds.), *Character strengths and virtues: A handbook and classification* (pp. 199–212). New York, NY: Oxford University Press.

Peterson, C., & Seligman, M. E. P. (2004b). Open-mindedness. In C. Peterson & M. E. P. Seligman (Eds.), *Character strengths and virtues: A handbook and classification* (pp. 143–159). New York, NY: Oxford University Press.

Pittet, D., Simon, A., Hugonnet, S., Pessoa-Silva, C. L., Sauvan, V., & Perneger, T. V. (2004). Hand hygiene among physicians: Performance, beliefs, and perceptions. *Annals of Internal Medicine, 141*(1), 1–8.

Pless, I. B., Feeley, N., Gottlieb, L. N., Rowat, K., Dougherty, G., & Willard, B. (1994). A randomized trial of a nursing intervention to promote the adjustment of children with chronic physical disorders. *Pediatrics, 94*(1), 70–75.

Plomin, R. (2009). The nature of nurture. In K. McCartney & R. A. Weinberg (Eds.), *Experience and development: A festschrift in honor of Sandra Wood Scarr* (pp. 61–80). New York, NY: APS Psychology Press.

Polifroni, E. C. (2011). Philosophy of science: An introduction. In J. B. Butts & K. L. Rich (Eds.), *Philosophies and theories for advanced nursing practice* (pp. 1–18). Sudbury, MA: Jones and Bartlett.

Post, S. G., & McCullough, M. E. (2004). Kindness: Generosity, nurturance, care, compassion, altruistic love (niceness). In C. Peterson & M. E. P. Seligman (Eds.), *Character strengths and virtues: A handbook and classification* (pp. 325–335). New York, NY: Oxford University Press.

Powell. D. S., Batsche, C. J., Ferro, J., Fox, L., & Dunlap, G. (1997). A strength-based approach in support of multi-risk families: Principles and issues. *Topics in Early Childhood Education, 17,* 1–26.

Pritchard, M. T., Ostberg, J. R., Evans, S. S., Burd, R., Kraybill, W., Bull, J. M., & Repasky, E. A. (2004). Protocols for simulating the thermal component of fever: preclinical and clinical experience. *Methods, 32*(1), 54–62.

Rachlis, M. (2004). *Prescription for excellence: How innovation is saving Canada's health care system.* Toronto, Canada: Harper collins.

Rafferty, A. M. (1996). *Politics of nursing knowledge.* London, UK: Routledge Publishers.

Rafferty, A. M., & Wall, R. (2010). An icon and iconoclast for today. (pp. 130–141). In S. Nelson & A. M. Rafferty. *Notes on Nightingale: An influence and legacy of a nursing icon*. Ithica, NY: ILR Press.

Random house dictionary (2010). New York, NY: Random House.

Rashotte, J., & Carnevale, F. A. (2004). Medical and nursing clinical decision-making: A comparative epistemological analysis. *Nursing Philosophy, 5*(2), 160–174.

Rashotte, J., King, J., Thomas, M., & Cragg, B. (2011). The moral experience of nurses' decision-making concerning prn anti-seizure medication administration to children receiving palliative care. *Canadian Journal of Nursing Research (CJNR), 43*(3), 58–77.

Reed, P. A. (2009). Inspired knowing in nursing: Walking on moonbeams. In R. C. Locsin & M. J. Purnell (Eds.), *A contemporary nursing process: The (Un) bearable weight of knowing in nursing* (pp. 61–71). New York, NY: Springer Publishing Company.

Reed, P. G. (1997). Nursing: The ontology of the discipline. *Nursing Science Quarterly, 10,* 76–79.

Registered Nurses of Ontario, (2010). RNAO-

Reverby, S. M. (1987). *Ordered to care: The dilemma of American nursing, 1850–1945*. Cambridge, UK: The Cambridge University Press.

Richardson, G. E. (2002). The metatheory of resilience and resiliency. *Journal of Clinical Psychology, 58*(3), 307–321.

Robinson, C. A., & Wright, L. M. (1995). Family nursing interventions: What families say makes a difference. *Journal of Family Nursing, 1*(3), 327–345.

Rogers, C. (1992). The necessary and sufficient conditions of therapeutic personality change. *Journal of Consulting and Clinical Psychology, 60*(6), 827–832.

Rogers, M. E. (1970). *An introduction to the theoretical basis of nursing*. Philadelphia, PA: F.A. Davis Company.

Rolfe, G., Freshwater, D., & Jasper, M. (2001). *Critical reflection for nursing and the helping professions: A user's guide*. Basingstoke, UK: Palgrave Macmillan Publishers Limited.

Rollnick, S., Miller, W. R., & Butler, C. C. (2007). *Interviewing in health care: Helping patients change behavior*. New York, NY: Guilford Press.

Rothbart, M. K. (2011). *Becoming who we are: Temperament and personality in development*. New York, NY: Guilford Press.

Rubak, S., Sandbaek, A., Lauritzen, T., & Christensen, B. (2005). Motivational interviewing: A systematic review and meta-analysis. *The British Journal of General Practice, 55*(513), 305–312.

Russell, G., & Ng, A. (2009). Taking time to watch: Observation and learning in family practice. *Canadian Family Physician, 55*(9), 948–950.

Ryan, R. M., & Deci, E. L. (2006). Self-regulation and the problem of human autonomy: Does psychology need choice, self-determination, and will? *Journal of Personality, 74*(6), 1557–1586.

Sabin, L. (2010). Sweating, purging, and a passion for care: The Yellow Fever nurse in the deep south in the early nineteenth century. In P. D'Antonio & S. B. Lewenson, (Eds.), *Nursing interventions through time: History as evidence* (pp. 3–16). New York, NY: Springer Publishing Company.

Sacks, J. (2004). *Celebrating life: Finding happiness in unexpected places*. London, UK: Continuum.

Sakalys, J. A. (2006). Bringing bodies back in: Embodiment and caring science. *International Journal for Human Caring, 10*(3), 17–21.

Saleebey D. (1996). The strengths perspective in social work practice: Extensions and cautions. *Social Work, 41*(3), 296–305.

Saleebey, D. (2008). *The srengths perspective in social work practice* (4th ed.). Boston, MA: Pearson/Allyn & Bacon.

Sandelowski, M. (2000). The physician's eyes: American nursing and the diagnostic revolution in medicine. *Nursing History Review, 8,* 3–38.

Scarr, S., & McCartney, K. (1983). How people make their own environments: A theory of genotype environment effects. *Child Development, 54*(2), 424–435.

Scherbring, M. (2002). Effect of caregiver perception of preparedness on burden in an oncology population. *Oncology Nursing Forum, 29*(6), E70–E76.

Schon, D. A. (1983). *The reflective practitioner: How professionals think in action.* New York, NY: Basic Books.

Schumacher, K. L., & Meleis, A. I. (1994). Transitions: A central concept in nursing. *Image, Journal of Nursing Scholarship, 26*(2), 119–126.

Schuman, M. (2002). The passion to know: A developmental perspective. In C. R. Snyder & S. J. Lopez (Eds.), *Handbook of positive psychology* (pp. 313–326). New York, NY: Oxford University Press.

Seligman, M. E. P. (2006). *Learned optimism: How to change your mind and your life.* New York, NY: Vantage (Random House).

Sense. (n.d.). *In Dictionary.com Unabridged.* Retrieved May 25, 2011, from HYPERLINK "http://www.dictionary.reference.com/browse/sense" www.dictionary.reference.com/browse/sense

Senge, P. M. (2006). *The fifth discipline: The art and practice of the learning organization.* New York, NY: Random House (Currency Publication).

Shapiro, J. (2002). (Re)Examining the clinical gaze through the prism of literature. *Families, Systems & Health, 20*(2), 161–170.

See (n.d.). In *Merriam-Webster's on-line dictionary.* Retrieved from www.merriam-webster.com/dictionary/see

Shapiro, S. L., Carlson, L. E., Astin, J. A., & Freedman, B. (2006). Mechanisms of mindfulness. *Journal of Clinical Psychology, 62(3),* 373–386.

Shebib, B. (2007). *Choices: Interviewing and counseling skills for Canadians* (3rd ed.). Toronto, Canada: Pearson Prentice Hall.

Sheldon, K. M., Davidson, L., & Pollard, E. (2004). Integrity: Authenticity, honesty. In C. Peterson & M. E. P. Seligman (Eds.), *Character strengths and virtues: A handbook and classification* (pp. 249–271). New York, NY: Oxford University Press.

Short, P. (1997). Picturing the body in nursing, In J. Lawler (Ed.), *The body in nursing.* South Melbourne, VIC: Churchill Livingstone.

Siegel, D. J. (1999). *The developing mind: Toward a neurobiology of interpersonal experience.* New York, NY: Guilford Press.

Siegel, D. J. (2007). *The mindful brain: Reflection and attunement in the cultivation of well-being.* New York, NY: W. W. Norton.

Siegel, D. J. (2010). *The mindful therapist: A clinician's guide to mindsight and neural integration.* New York, NY: W. W. Norton.

Silberman, M. (1996). *Active learning: 101 strategies to teach any subject.* Boston, MA: Allyn and Bacon. Retrieved from www.activetraining.com

Simmons, P. F. (2002). *Learning to fall: The blessings of an imperfect life.* New York, NY: Bantam Books.

Skodol, A. E. (2010). The resilient personality. In J. W. Reich, A. J. Zautra, & J. S. Hall (Eds.), *Handbook of adult resilience* (pp. 112–125). New York, NY: Guilford Press.

Skott, C. (2001). Caring narratives and the strategy of presence: Narrative communication in nursing practice and research. *Nursing Science Quarterly, 14*(3), 249–254.

Smith, E. J. (2006). The strength-based counseling model. *The Counseling Psychologist, 34,* 13–79.

Smith, J. A. (1981). The idea of health: A philosophical inquiry. *Advances in Nursing Science, 3*(3), 43–50.

Smith, M. C., Persson, H. K., & Lynn, C. E. (2008). President's message on the threshold of the 20th anniversary of SRS: Honoring our past and growing our future. *Visions: The Journal of Rogerian Nursing Science, 15*(1), 58–60.

Smith, T. D. (2001). The concept of nursing presence: State of the science. *Nursing Scholarly for Nursing Practice: An International Journal, 15*(4), 299–322.

Smotherman, W. P., & Robinson, S. R. (1995). Tracing developmental trajectories into the prenatal period. In J. P. Lecanuet, W. P. Fifer, N. A. Krasnegor, & W. P. Smotherman (Eds.), *Fetal Development* (pp. 15–32). Hillsdale, NJ: Erlbaum and Associates.

Snyder, C. R., & Lopez, S. J. (2002). *Handbook of positive psychology.* New York, NY: Oxford Press.

Snyder, C. R., Lopez, S. J., & Pedrotti, J. T. (2011). *Positive psychology: the scientific and practical explorations of human strengths* (2nd ed.,Chapter 12). Thousand Oaks, CA: Sage Publications.

Snyder, C. R., Rand, K. L., & Sigmon, D. R. (2002). Hope theory: A member of the positive psychology family. In C. R. Snyder & S. J. Lopez (Eds.), *Handbook of positive psychology* (pp. 257–276). New York, NY: Oxford University Press.

Solomon, M. R. (2009). *Consumer behavior: Buying, having, and being* (8th ed.). Englewood, NJ: Prentice-Hall.

Steiner, J. E., Glaser, D., Hawilo, M. E., & Berridge, D. C. (2001). Comparative expression of hedonic impact: Affective reactions to taste by human infants and other primates. *Neuroscience and Biobehavioral Review, 25*(1), 53–74.

Stewart, M., Brown, J. B., Weston, W. W., McWhinney, I. R., McWilliam, C. L., & Freeman, T. R. (2003). *Patient-centered medicine: Transforming the clinical method* (2nd ed.). Abingdon, UK: Radcliffe Medical Press Ltd.

Sullivan, M. (2003). The new subjective medicine: Taking the patient's point of view on health care and health. *Social Science and Medicine, 56*(7), 1595–1604.

Sullivan, W. M. (2005). *Work and integrity: The crisis and promise of professionalism in America.* San Francisco, CA: Jossey-Bass.

Sullivan, T. J. (1998). Consumers in health care. Part II: Expert viewpoints. In T. J. Sullivan (Ed.), *Collaboration: A health care imperative* (pp. 561–593). New York, NY: McGraw Hill.

Sumner, G., & Spietz, A. (2004). *NCAST-AVENUW Caregiver/Parent-child interaction feeding manual.* Seattle, WA: NCAST-AVENUW, University of Washington, School of Nursing.

Swanson, K. M. (1993). Nursing as informed caring for the well-being of others. *Image: Journal of nursing scholarship, 25*(4), 352–357.

Swanson, K. M., & Wojnar, D. M. (2004). Optimal healing environments in nursing. *The Journal of Alternative and Complementary Medicine, 10,* S43–S48.

Tamis-Lemonda, C. S., & McFadden, K. E. (2010). Development in different places: The United States of America. In M. H. Bornstein (Ed.), *Handbook of cultural developmental science* (pp. 299–322). New York, NY: Psychology Press (Taylor & Francis Group).

Tangney, J. P. (2002). Humility. In C. R. Snyder & S. L. Lopez (Eds.), *Handbook of positive psychology* (pp. 411–419). New York, NY: Oxford University Press.

Tartaglia, E. M., Barmert, L., Mast, F. W., Herzog, M. H. (2009). Human perceptual learning by mental imagery. *Current Biology, 19*(24), 2081–2085.

Taylor, C. (1991). *The malaise of modernity.* Concord, Canada: Anansi Press.

Taylor, C. (2004). *Modern social imaginaries*. Durham, NC: Duke University Press.

Teicher, M. H. (2002). Scars that won't heal: The neurobiology of child abuse. *Scientific American, 286*(3), 68–75.

Templeton, J. (1997). *Worldwide laws of life*. Philadelphia, PA: Templeton Foundation Press.

Tickle-Degnen, L., & Rosenthal, R. (1990). The nature of rapport and its nonverbal correlates. *Psychological Inquiry, 1*(4), 285–293.

The Times of London (April 17, 2009). *"Whistleblower" Nurse Margaret Hayward Struck Off (Nursing Registry) Over Panorama Film*. Author.

Travelbee, J. (1971). *Interpersonal aspects of nursing* (2nd ed.). Philadelphia, PA: F.A. Davis.

Troy, G. (2011, September 15). The 'blinkisher' rabbi. *Canadian Jewish News*.

Tsai, P., Chang, N., Chang, W., Lee, P., & Wang, M. (2007). Blood pressure biofeedback exerts intermediate-term effects on blood pressure and pressure reactivity in individuals with mild hypertension: a randomized controlled study. *Journal Alternative & Complementary Medicine 13*(5), 547–554.

Uchino, B. N. (2009). Understanding the links between social support and physical health. *Perspectives on Psychology Science, 4*(3), 236–255.

Uustal, D. B. (1978). Values clarification in nursing: Application to practice. *American Journal of Nursing, 78*(12), 2058–2063.

Vanier, J. (1998). *Becoming human*. Toronto, Canada: Anansi Press.

Vygotsky, L. S. (1978). *Mind and society: The development of higher mental processes*. Cambridge, MA: Harvard University Press.

Wallin, D. J. (2007). *Attachment in psychotherapy*. New York, NY: Guilford Press.

Walsh, F. (2006). *Strengthening family resilience* (2nd ed.). New York, NY: Guilford Press.

Walsh, R. A. (2008). Mindfulness and empathy. In S. F. Hick & T. Bien (Eds.), *Mindfulness and the therapeutic relationship* (pp. 72–86). New York, NY: Guilford Press.

Wanzer, M. B., Wojtaszczyk, A. M., & Kelly, J. (2009). Nurses' perceptions of physicians' communication: The relationship among communication practices, satisfaction, and collaboration. *Health Communication, 24*(8), 683–691.

Ward, N. S., & Cohen, L. G. (2004). Mechanisms underlying recovery of motor function after stroke. *Archives of Neurology, 61*(12), 1844–1848.

Watson, J. (1997). The theory of human caring: Retrospective and prospective. *Nursing Science Quarterly, 10*(1), 49–52.

Watson, M., & Ecken, L. (2003). *Learning to trust: Transforming difficult elementary classrooms through developmental discipline*. San-Francisco, CA: Jossey-Bass.

Weber, R. J. (2000). *The created self: Reinventing body, persona, and spirit*. New York, NY: W.W. Norton & Company.

Weinberg, D. B., Aranda, S., & Brown, R. (2006). When little things are big things: The importance of relationship for nurses' professional practice. In S. Nelson & S. Gordon (Eds.), *The complexities of care: Nursing reconsidered* (pp. 30–43). Ithaca NY: ILR Press.

Weiss, S. M., Malone, R. E., Merighi, J. R., & Benner, P. (2001). Economism, efficiency, and the moral ecology of good nursing. *CJNR (Canadian Journal of Nursing Research), 35*(2), 95–119.

Whitman, M. C., & Greer, C. A. (2007). Synaptic integration of adult-generated olfactory bulb granule cells: Basal axodendritic centrifugal input precedes apical dendrodendritic local circuits. *Journal of Neuroscience, 27*(37), 9951–9961.

Wiedenbach, E. (1964). *Clinical nursing: The helping art*. New York, NY: Springer Publishing Company.

Wolf, O. T. (2009). Stress and memory in humans: Twelve years of progress? *Brain Research, 1293*, 142–154.

Wolf, Z. R. (2009). Know patient's bodies: Nurses' bodywork. In R. C. Locsin & M. J. Purnell (Eds.), *A contemporary nursing process: The (un)bearable weight of knowing in nursing* (pp. 175–204). New York, NY: Springer Publishing Company.

Wolin, S. (2003). What is a strength? *Reclaiming Children and Youth, 12*(1), 18–21.

Worthington, E. L., Hight, T. L., Ripley, J. S., Perrone, K. M., Kurusu, T. A., & Jones, D. R. (1997). Strategic hope-focused relationship-enrichment counseling with individual couples. *Journal of counseling psychology, 44*(4), 381–389.

Wright, L., & Leahey, M. (2009). *Nurses and families: A guide to family assessment and intervention* (5th ed.). Philadelphia, PA: F.A. Davis.

Wright, L. M., & Bell, J. M. (2009). *Belief and illness: A model for healing.* Calgary, Al: 4th Floor Press.

Wright, L. M., & Leahey, M. (2005). *Nurses and families: A guide to family assessment.* Philadelphia, PA: F.A. Davies.

Wright, L. M., Watson, W. L., & Bell, J. M. (1996). *Beliefs: The heart of healing in families in illness.* New York, NY: Basic Books.

Wuest, J. (1994). Professionalism and evolution of nursing as a discipline: A feminist perspective. *Journal of Professional Nursing, 10*(6), 357–367.

Yu, J., & Kirk, M. (2008). Measurement of empathy in nursing research: A systematic review. *Journal of Advanced Nursing, 64,* 440–454.

Zander, R. S., & Zander, B. (2000). *The art of possibility: Transforming professional and personal life.* Boston, MA: Harvard Business School Press.

Zukav, G. (1979). *The dancing of the Wu Li masters: An overview of the new physics.* New York, NY: Morrow.

Zuzelo, P. R., Gettis, C., Hansel, A. W., & Thomas, L. (2008). Describing the influence of technologies on registered nurses' work. *Clinical Nurse Specialist, 22*(3), 132–140).

Index